HANDBOOK OF VETERINARY PREVENTIVE MEDICINE

HANDBOOK OF VETERINARY PREVENTIVE MEDICINE

Debra Russell
Teresa Pedro

Kruger Brentt
Publishers
2024

Kruger Brentt Publishers UK. LTD.
Company Number 9728962

Regd. Office: 68 St Margarets Road, Edgware, Middlesex HA8 9UU

ISBN: 978-1-78715-195-6

For information on all our publications visit our website at http://krugerbrentt.com/

PREFACE

Veterinary preventive medicine is a branch of veterinary medicine that focuses on the prevention and control of animal diseases. Preventive medicine involves the use of various measures to prevent diseases from occurring or spreading, including vaccination, biosecurity measures, and hygiene practices. This essay will discuss the importance of veterinary preventive medicine and its various aspects. Veterinary preventive medicine plays a crucial role in ensuring animal health and welfare, protecting public health, and ensuring sustainable animal production. The prevention of animal diseases reduces the need for costly treatment and minimizes the risk of zoonotic diseases, which can be transmitted from animals to humans. Preventive medicine also helps to minimize the risk of animal diseases spreading between countries, thereby supporting global trade and food security. Aspects of Veterinary Preventive Medicine: There are various aspects of veterinary preventive medicine, including vaccination, biosecurity measures, and hygiene practices.

Vaccination is one of the most effective preventive measures against infectious diseases. Vaccines help to stimulate the animal's immune system to produce antibodies against specific diseases, thereby reducing the risk of infection. Vaccination is essential for both domestic animals and livestock, and it is critical in preventing zoonotic diseases such as rabies, anthrax, and avian influenza.

Biosecurity measures refer to a range of measures aimed at preventing the introduction and spread of infectious diseases in animal populations. Biosecurity measures include quarantine, restriction of movement, and disinfection. These measures are essential in controlling infectious diseases and reducing the risk of disease spread between animals and humans. Hygiene practices involve the use of practices that promote cleanliness and good health in animal populations. Hygiene practices include regular cleaning of animal housing, proper waste management, and the use of appropriate disinfectants. These measures help to reduce the risk of infectious diseases by eliminating potential sources of infection. Veterinary preventive medicine is crucial in ensuring animal health and welfare, protecting public health, and ensuring sustainable animal production. Vaccination, biosecurity measures, and hygiene practices are some of the essential aspects of veterinary preventive medicine. By implementing these measures, veterinary professionals can prevent and control animal diseases, reduce the risk of zoonotic diseases, and support global trade and food security.

The present book explores the principles and practice of veterinary medicine and it includes diagnosis and prognosis. It addresses major animal diseases, including foreign animals. The subject matter is presented in a lucid and succinct style so that even those who do not have a prerequisite knowledge of the subject can easily understand it. The book will be ideal for practitioner's students, teachers and researchers engaged in veterinary medicine and clinical pathology.

We are grateful to all those persons as well as various books, manuals, periodicals, magazines, journals etc. that helped in the preparation of this book. In spite of the best efforts, it is possible that some errors may have occurred into the compilation and editing of the book. Further queries, constructive suggestions and criticisms for the improvement of the book are always welcomed and shall be thankfully acknowledged.

Debra Russell

Teresa Pedro

CONTENTS

CHAPTER-1

RELATED TERMINOLOGY

ANIMAL TERMINOLOGY

POULTRY	Broiler / fryer	Chicken Raised for Meat
	**Capon**	castrated male chicken or turkey
	Chick	new born chicken or turkey
	Cock or rooster	male chicken of breeding age
	Cockerel	young male chicken
	Hen	mature female chicken or turkey
	Hen poult	young female turkey
	Jake	young male turkey
	Poult	young turkey
	Pullet	immature laying hen
	Spent hen	egg-laying hen that is no longer producing eggs that are of grade A quality (approximately 2 years of age)
	Tom	male turkey of breeding age

CATTLE	Bull	Male of Breeding Age
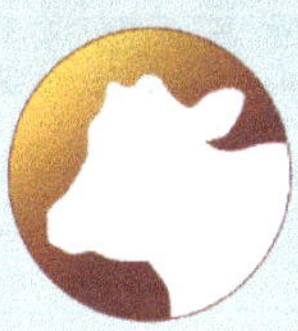	**Bullock**	young male, typically less than 20 months of age
	Calf	newborn (generally any male or female less than 1 year of age)
	Cow	mature female; a female that has produced a calf
	Dry cow	a cow that has finished one lactation and has not yet given birth and started a subsequent lactation
	Heifer	young female; a female that has not produced a calf (term may be used whether or not they're currently pregnant)
	One-calf heifer	young female that has produced only one calf and is in her first lactation

CATTLE	Bull	Male of Breeding Age
	Heiferette	a heifer that has calved once, is not lactating, and is fed for slaughter
	Springer	breeding age heifer that has not yet given birth to her first calf and is within the last 6 weeks of gestation
	Steer	castrated male
	Stocker	weaned cattle that are run on grass or are fed high roughage diets
	Yearling	male or female that is 1-2 years of age

HORSES	Colt	young male
	**Filly**	young female
	Foal	newborn
	Gelding	castrated male
	Mare	mature female
	Stallion or stud	male of breeding age

SHEEP	Ewe	mature female
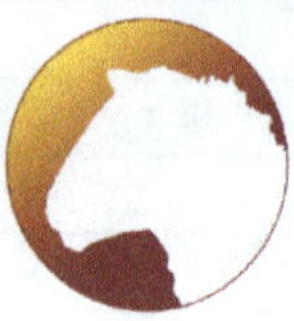	**Ewe lamb**	young female
	Lamb	newborn
	Ram	male of breeding age
	Ram lamb	young male
	Wether	castrated male

GOATS	Buck or billy	male of breeding age
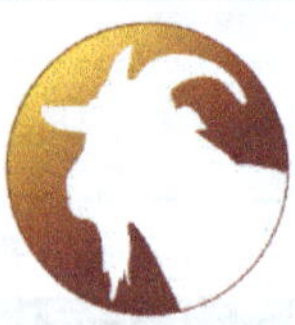	**Buck kid**	young male
	Doe	mature female
	Doe kid	young female
	Kid	newborn
	Wether	castrated male

SWINE	Barrow	castrated male
	**Boar**	male of breeding age
	Finishing Pig	pig aged from about 10 weeks to slaughter age (about 6 months of age)
	Gilt	young female; a female that has not had a litter
	Nursery pig	pig aged 21 days to 10-12 weeks
	Piglet	newborn, up to 21 days of age
	Shoat	young male
	Sow	mature female; a female that has had a litter
	Weaned pig	piglet that has been separated from the sow

DOGS	Bitch	intact female
	Dog or stud	mature male
	Puppy	newborn

CATS	Queen	intact female
	Tom	mature male
	Kitten	newborn

Production Terminology

POULTRY	Aviary house	cageless layer house with litter floor and multiple layers of perches and nests, allowing birds to freely move between all levels
	Furnished cages	large enclosed cages, holding 30-60 laying hens, that have perches and scratch pads
	Grandparent stock	first generation, highest biosecurity level poultry stock owned by breeder companies
	Litter	wood chips or seed (rice, peanut) hulls used for footing
	Multiplier stock	offspring of grandparent stock; owned by poultry companies and bred for production of growing turkeys, broilers, and layers

CATTLE	Backgrounding	growing program for feeder cattle from time calves are weaned until they are on a finishing ration in the feedlot
	Biological type	refers to size of cattle (small, medium or large), growth rate, milk production (high, medium or low), and age at puberty
	Calf crop	number or percentage of calves produced within a herd in a given year relative to the number of cows and heifers in the breeding herd
	Calving	act of giving birth
	Conditioning	treatment of cattle by vaccination and other procedures before introducing them into the feedlot
	Cow-calf operation	a management unit that maintains a breeding herd of cows and produces weaned calves for sale
	Crossbred	an animal that is the product of the crossing of two or more breeds
	Culling	removing cattle from the herd for sale or slaughter

	Dry period	rest period at the end of a lactation before a cow gives birth again
	Feeder cattle	those requiring more growth and/or fattening before slaughter
	Feedlot	beef cattle enterprise where cattle are placed in confinement, fed harvested feeds, and fattened for slaughter
	Finished cattle	cattle whose time in the feedlot is completed and are now ready for slaughter
	Freestall	loose housing system for cows indoors, in which cows can move freely in groups within a large space
	Fresh cow	cow that has given birth within the last 3 weeks
	Freshening	calving
	Lactation	period between two calvings during which the cow gives milk, usually lasting about one year. A cow that has just given birth to her second calf is in her second lactation
	Preconditioning	preparation of feeder calves for marketing and shipment, may include vaccinations, castration, training calves to eat and drink in pens
	Seedstock producer	enterprise that produces breeding animals for the commercial segment of the industry
	Serving	act of breeding
	Tiestall	confined housing system with cow tethered by their head and held in one place
HORSES	**Foaling**	act of giving birth
	**Covering**	act of breeding
SHEEP	**Lambing**	act of giving birth
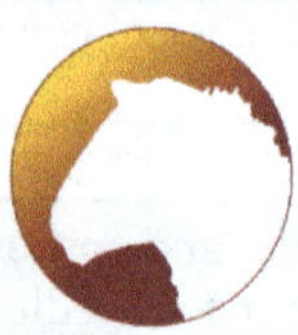	**Tupping**	act of breeding
GOATS	**Kidding**	act of giving birth
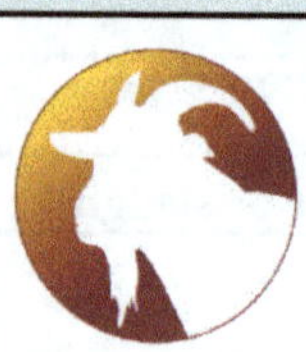	**Serving**	act of breeding

PIGS	**Farrowing**	act of giving birth
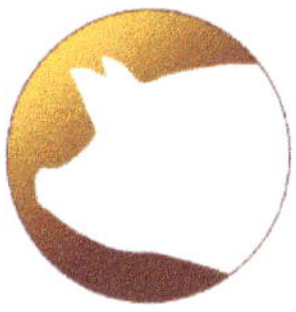	**Coupling**	act of breeding
	Farrowing rate	(# farrowing / # bred) x 100
	Non-productive days	days a given sow or gilt of breeding age is present in the herd but is not pregnant or lactating
	Not-in-pig	female diagnosed pregnant (usually by ultrasound) that does not go on to farrow = mortality of all fetuses during gestation

DOGS		
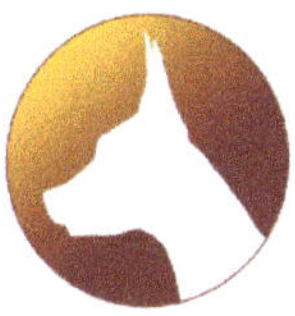	**Whelping**	act of giving birth

CATS		
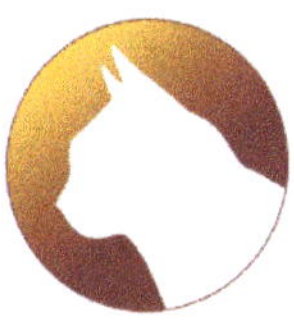	**Queening**	act of giving birth

CHAPTER-2

VACCINES AND VACCINATIONS: AN OVERVIEW

BENEFITS OF VACCINATION

The primary benefit of vaccination is the decrease in the number of animals becoming infected with and dying from infections. When many animals are vaccinated, this "herd effect" has benefit for the vaccinated animals, which are unlikely to become ill from a disease for which they have been vaccinated, and for all animals in the population, who are less likely to be exposed to the disease. This also has public health significance; rabies would be a significant threat to human health in the United States without vaccination of domestic animals.

Objectives of Vaccination

- To vaccinate the largest possible number of individuals in the population at risk
- To vaccinate each individual no more frequently than necessary
- To vaccinate only against agents to which the animal has a realistic risk of exposure and subsequent development of serious disease

VACCINATION CONFERS PROTECTIVE IMMUNITY

Vaccination is controlled exposure of an animal's immune system to something that causes disease. Vaccination is the act; immunization is the desired result. In veterinary medicine, most vaccines are developed against viruses; some protect against specific bacteria or toxins. When an animal is vaccinated, its immune system recognizes the foreign proteins and builds up a response to them. Part of that response is the creation of antibodies, proteins that bind to the pathogen and lead to its destruction (humoral immunity). Another part of that response is creation of cells within the animal's body that will destroy that pathogen (cellular immunity). Some of those cells are memory cells and are capable of generating a faster and stronger response every time the animal is re-exposed to the pathogen. This means that vaccinated animals, which have created a store of memory cells, can respond quickly to any natural exposure to the pathogen and are significantly less likely to become ill.

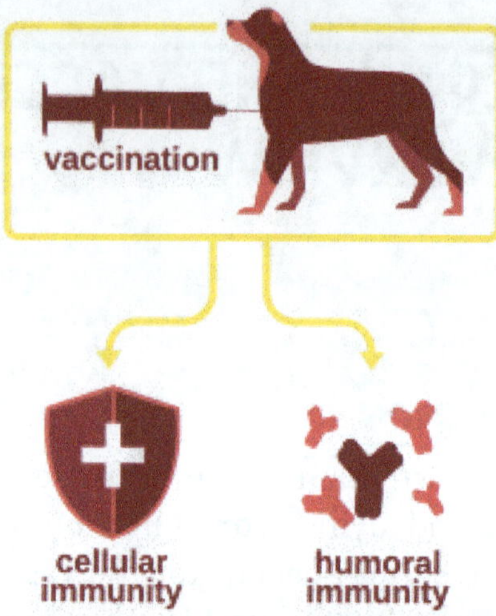

TYPES OF VACCINES

There are three types of vaccines available for use by veterinarians. Killed vaccines (also called inactivated vaccines) contain inactivated whole viruses or bacteria. Killed vaccines are more stable for handling and storage and are incapable of causing disease in the animal but require use of an adjuvant, which may be associated with vaccine reactions, and may not generate a long-lasting immune response, often requiring them to be given more frequently to be effective. The first time a killed vaccine is given, it primes the immune system but does not evoke an immune response; the animal must get a booster or be naturally exposed for an immune response to occur. Modified live virus (MLV) vaccines (also called attenuated vaccines) contain whole viruses that are not dead but are treated such that they can no longer cause disease. Because the organism in the MLV vaccine is alive and can replicate, these may occasionally cause diseases in vaccinated animals. These vaccines generally stimulate a much stronger and long-lived immune response.

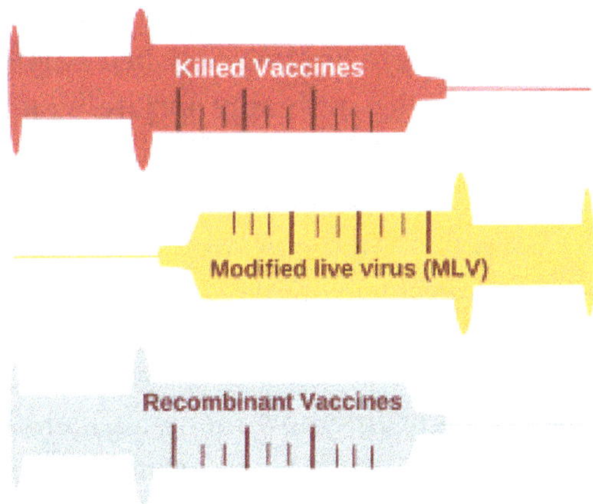

Because these may occasionally cause disease in vaccinated animals, their use must be timed carefully; for example, many MLV vaccines cannot be given to pregnant animals as they may cause abortion. Caution also must be used in giving these vaccines to immunosuppressed animals. Recombinant or subunit vaccines use portions of viruses or bacteria to generate an immune response. These cannot cause disease in vaccinated animals but do not always generate an adequate immune response. Recombinant technology is improving steadily and it is anticipated that in the future, recombinant vaccines will be the preferred type. Because an animal's response to vaccination is not dependent on "dose" of vaccine provided, the same amount of vaccine is given to all animals in a given species.

VACCINATION SERIES

The earliest age at which vaccines can be given and the need for boostering is defined by the manufacturer. Young animals that nursed from their dam within the first day of life will have antibodies from her first milk (colostrum) that were taken up across their GI tract into their general circulation (passive immunity). Those antibodies will interfere with vaccines and often we do not know when those antibody concentrations decline. Young animals also are variable in timing of function of their own immune function (active immunity). Because of this, young animals often receive a series of vaccines, with timing of boosters defined by the manufacturer. In adult animals, some vaccines are boostered when first given and others are not; directions for use on the vaccine label always should be followed.

The goal of boostering vaccines in adult animals is to create an elevation in immune response to protect against disease challenge. Timing of boosters is dependent on the type of vaccine used (killed versus MLV, for example) and on the characteristics of the organism itself. The manufacturer provides guidelines for optimal intervals for boostering of vaccine. What if the animal (young or adult) is overdue for vaccines? There are no published studies evaluating immune response in animals vaccinated with an inappropriately long boostering interval. Veterinarians must use their common sense and knowledge of immunology (or in the case of rabies, they must follow the law). Guidelines are available from the American Animal Hospital Association and American Association of Feline Practitioners to answer this concern for dogs and cats.

REGULATORY ASPECTS OF VACCINATION

There is a lot of controversy regarding how many antigens one should include at one time for vaccination against disease. Some argue that the immune system has built-in systems to be duplicative, so even if only a couple of B cells respond to a given antigen, that will trigger production of more B cells and a quick amplification of antibody concentrations. Others argue that the body can only respond to so many attacks at one time because there are a finite number of B cells and T cells available as antigens are introduced, so the animal (or person) either won't respond to some of the antigens or will do so improperly. Those who argue this latter point often make the jump that what we are doing is inducing an abnormal immune response, and autoimmune disease, where antibodies or T cells are triggered to destroy host tissue. None of this is particularly well evaluated using the scientific method. A non-medical piece to the puzzle is client compliance; if you get one chance to vaccinate that animal, is it wisest to vaccinate against all diseases of concern, recognizing that the client may not return with that animal for further vaccines if you choose to limit what you offer at a given time?

All vaccines used by veterinarians must be approved by the United States Department of Agriculture (USDA) and demonstrated to be pure, safe, potent, and effective. It is from this USDA approval process that the manufacturer determines what information will be on the vaccine label. The USDA considers a vaccine safe if it does not cause "undue local or systemic responses." After the vaccine is licensed and marketed, no continuing measurement of risk is required. An adverse reaction is defined by the USDA as "any undesirable side effect or unintended effect (including lack of desired result) associated with the administration of a licensed biological product". All adverse reactions reported by veterinarians to the manufacturer are reported to the USDA. If veterinarians do not report adverse effects, the manufacturer may not be aware they are occurring. Here is information from Dr. Richard Ford: "In veterinary medicine, there is no mandate to report a vaccine adverse reaction, whether the reaction is known to have been caused by a vaccine or merely suspected to have been. Although encouraged to do so, formal reports from the veterinarians to the USDA are seldom filed. Veterinarians who do report known or suspected reactions tend to contact the manufacturer directly. However, neither the licensing agencies nor the vaccine manufacturers are under obligation to provide a veterinarian with additional information regarding either the number of type of vaccine adverse events. Today, there are no data available to veterinarians that specifically address surveillance or documentation of vaccine adverse reactions in companion animals. Manufacturers are under no obligation to compensate the owner or the veterinarian for diagnostic or treatment services related to a known or suspected adverse event."

True effectiveness of a vaccine often is unknown. Challenge testing, in which unvaccinated and vaccinated animals are exposed to the virus and the number that become ill compared, is not always performed. Duration of immunity (the amount of time an animal is protected from disease after vaccination) is not known for all vaccines approved by the USDA.

RISK FACTORS OF VACCINATIONS

Risk factors to be considered include host factors specific to that animal, environmental factors, and agent factors specific to that vaccine. Animals that are malnourished, are ill with another disease or condition, or are stressed are unlikely to respond well to vaccination. Young animals (for example, puppies and kittens less than 16 weeks of age) may still have significant levels of antibodies from their mother, taken in when they nursed in their first day of life. These antibodies may inactivate the vaccine, rendering it useless. Environmental factors look at the population as a whole. The more animals there are in the population, the greater the likelihood any one animal will be exposed to a given virus. Those animals that are exposed to new animals, for example by introduction of a new pet, or by boarding or grooming, are at greater risk. The final thing to assess is the virus and disease itself. Rabies is an example of a virus that kills all the dogs and cats it infects and can kill exposed humans if they are not treated promptly. Any risk of vaccination is outweighed by the huge risk of death if infected with the virus.

Examples of Risk Factors of a Vaccine Regimen for Horses

- Risk of infection and disease (geography, horse age, occupation, movement patterns)
- Medical, economic, and logistic consequences of disease should it occur
- Potential for spread of infection to other horses and/or humans
- Farm size and type
- Vaccine cost, availability, and efficacy
- Risk of adverse reactions to vaccination

Factors to Consider in Disease Prevention

Diseases occur due to multiple factors. Their relationship is sometimes called the infection triangle.All three factors (environment (e.g. management practices), host, and pathogen) are important for the development or prevention of disease and all three need to be considered during disease prevention.

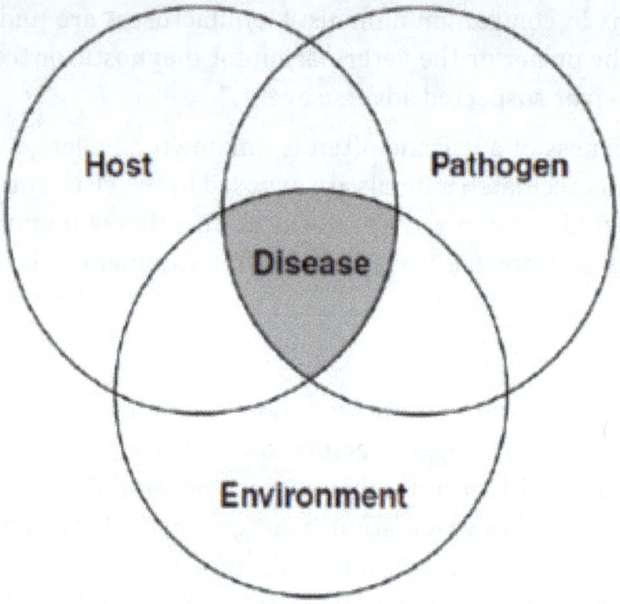

"The Epidemiological Triad", https://www.nap.edu/read/13147/chapter/1#xviii

ADVERSE EFFECTS OF VACCINATION

Adverse effects of vaccination have been attributed to preservatives in the vaccine, contaminants, the organism itself, products added to enhance the immune response (adjuvants), and to the administration of multiple vaccines at one time. In most cases, neither the cause nor the exact likelihood of an adverse effect is known.

There are two main types of vaccine reactions, systemic and local. Systemic reactions occur throughout the body, not just at the site of administration of the vaccine, and usually are non-specific. Examples include lack of appetite, fever and soreness. Allergic reactions may occur. These may be sudden, with onset immediately after vaccination and clinical signs lasting for up to two days. Signs of an allergic reaction include swelling of the face and respiratory distress. Some advocate giving less vaccine to minimize allergic reactions but since neither allergic reactions nor immunization are "dose" dependent, there is little wisdom in this practice. Autoimmune diseases are those conditions in which the immune system of an animal or person starts to destroy that individual's normal tissue. While people have hypothesized that autoimmune disease could be induced by vaccination, there is little scientific evidence of such a connection.

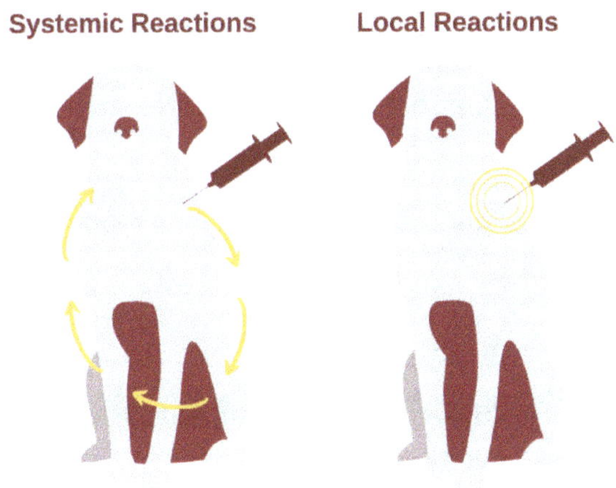

Local adverse vaccine reactions include pain at the injection site, hair loss or change in hair color at the injection site, and swellings. Swellings that develop fairly soon after the vaccination, are non-painful, and feel soft usually are benign sites of inflammation. They resolve over weeks to months. Pain may develop if the vaccine is inadvertently administered near a nerve. Some vaccines cause more pain than others when administered because of their chemical composition.

A final possible adverse effect of a vaccine is vaccine virulence, in which the vaccine causes the disease it was designed to protect against. This can only occur with modified live vaccines, which contain the whole virus. Likelihood of this occurring is very dependent on the host into which the vaccine is being injected. For example, a vaccine that is safe for adult animals may cause disease in very young animals. Some modified live vaccines can induce birth defects if given to pregnant animals. Vaccines are more likely to become virulent if used in the wrong species (for example, using an unapproved feline vaccine in ferrets) or if given by the wrong route (for example, cats that lick at the injection site may take some vaccine in by mouth, with a return to virulence when the vaccine contacts the mucous membranes of their gums).

Vaccines are designated as core or non-core (risk-based). Core vaccines are those that are recommended for administration to every animal, based on (1) universal susceptibility to disease caused by a specific infectious organism; (2) significant risk that animals in the area will become infected; (3) likelihood of significant medical consequences to the animal as a result of infection and disease; (4) availability of a vaccine that is both safe and highly effective; and (5) possible risk of zoonosis. In other words, core vaccines are those for infectious diseases for which the benefit-risk-cost relationship is clear for all animals and the decision to vaccinate is straightforward. Non-core, or *risk-based,* vaccines are recommended only when an animal's lifestyle is such that they are at increased risk of exposure to the disease. These diseases usually will resolve spontaneously or respond readily to treatment. One method of determining whether or not a vaccine should be given to a specific animal is to use some sort of scoring rubric such as that below.

Define "core" and "non-core" as related to vaccinations.

Scoring Rubric for Vaccination Needs

dvm TABLE 1

THE VACCINOMETER

Practitioners can gauge a vaccine's necessity by adding the points for a total score. A score of six to nine would not require vaccination, while a score of 10 to 13 leaves vaccination optional. A score totaling 14 or more would require inoculation.

Individualized Evaluation Criteria	Low (1)	Moderate (2)	High (3)
What is the prevalence and risk of exposure/infection in your area? (e.g. infectiousness)			
How great is the risk of severe disease once the dog is infected? (e.g. pathogenicity and virulence)			
How effective is the vaccine?			
How safe is the vaccine?			
What is the potential for zoonotic spread to human contacts?			
What is the potential for spread to other dogs?			
Total Score Minimum Score = 6 Maximum Score = 18			

6 - 9 Vaccination unnecessary
10 - 13 Vaccination optional
14 + Vaccinate

Credit: Glickman, Purdue University

"Researcher creates tool to gauge vaccine needs", http://veterinarynews.dvm360.com/researcher-creates-tool-gauge-vaccine-needs

CHAPTER-3

INDIVIDUAL ANIMALS: VACCINES & VACCINATIONS

ADVERSE EFFECTS OF VACCINATION IN DOGS AND CATS

Currently there is much controversy among small animal veterinarians and pet owners regarding how frequently vaccinations should be administered to animals. There is no vaccine that is 100% effective and no vaccine that is 100% safe. Vaccines do not induce the same degree of protection in all animals. Knowing, this, how can we decide whether or not to vaccinate a given animal? Your veterinarian does this by assessing the risk factors for your animal and by considering possible adverse effects.

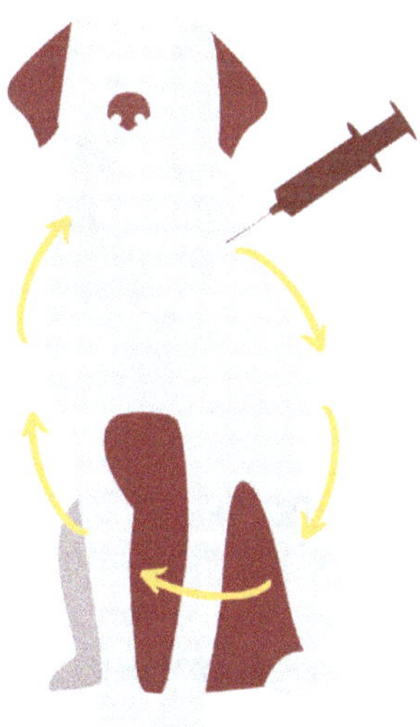

Systemic reactions occur throughout the body, not just at the site of administration of the vaccine. These can be non-specific, causing lack of appetite, fever and soreness that lasts for up to 36 hours after vaccination. This non-specific response is most likely to occur after multiple vaccines are administered and in patients greater than 1 year of age. Allergic reactions may occur. These may be sudden, with onset immediately after vaccination and clinical signs lasting for up to two days. In dogs, 51% of these reactions affect the skin, usually as swellings of the face and ears, and 40% affect the intestinal tract, causing vomiting with or without diarrhea. In cats, 66% of these reactions affect the intestinal tract, 22% affect the respiratory tract, and 12% affect the skin. No particular type of vaccine or manufacturer has been demonstrated to be more likely to cause allergic reactions in dogs and cats. Autoimmune diseases are those conditions in which the immune system of an animal or person starts to destroy that individual's normal tissue. While people have hypothesized that autoimmune disease could be induced by vaccination, there is no scientific evidence of such a connection in dogs and cats.

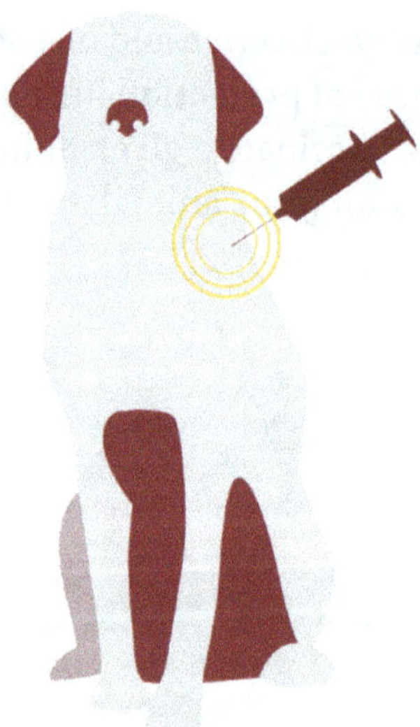

Local adverse vaccine reactions include pain at the injection site, hair loss or change in hair color at the injection site, and swellings. Swellings that develop fairly soon after the vaccination and are soft and non-painful usually are benign sites of inflammation. They resolve over weeks to months and are most commonly seen in dogs after vaccination with rabies vaccine or the distemper combination, and in cats after receiving the rabies vaccination.

Dogs with a history of adverse reactions, especially allergic reactions, may be treated with an antihistamine, a corticosteroid, or both, prior to vaccination.

This should not impact how they respond to the vaccine as a single dose of a corticosteroid is not sufficient to cause immunosuppression.

Vaccine-associated feline sarcoma is a malignant tumor that may develop following vaccination in cats. It is reported to occur in 1 in every 1000-10,000 vaccinated cats and is most frequently associated with killed rabies vaccines and vaccines against the feline leukemia virus. Tumors develop weeks to years after vaccination. These tumors are highly invasive, requiring surgical removal and possible chemotherapy. The American Association of Feline Practitioners (AAFP) recommends using non-adjuvanted rabies vaccines for cats in an attempt to decrease the risk of developing vaccine-associated sarcomas. It is unknown at this point if use of non-adjuvanted vaccines decreases the incidence of sarcomas. Because of concerns about development of sarcomas, it is recommended that vaccines not be given in the scruff of the neck, where surgical removal of tumors would be difficult. In North America, vaccines are commonly given in the distal limb, with many practices creating specific practices ("leukemia left, rabies right, rest in the front", for example, with feline leukemia and rabies vaccines given in the distal left and right rear limbs, respectively, and other vaccines given in the distal forelimbs). Another alternative, described in only one study to date, is vaccination in the tail.

Recommended Vaccination Techniques to Minimize Pain and Fear in Dogs and Cats

- Use one needle to reconstitute and draw up the reconstituted vaccine, and use a new needle to inject the animal.
- Use the smallest gauge needle possible.
- Deaden the area to be vaccinated using a topical anesthetic cream, such as lidocaine or prilocaine.
- Distract the animal by giving a tasty treat, petting or massaging the animal, catnip, or any other delightful distraction appropriate to the animal and the setting.
- Before vaccinating, dimple or pinch the skin in the area where the needle will puncture the skin.
- Deliver the vaccine slowly.

"Fear Free", https://fearfreepets.com/veterinary-professionals/

CONDITIONS FOR WHICH WE VACCINATE DOGS AND CATS

Diseases of Dogs and Cats for which Vaccines are Commonly Recommended

DISEASE	CAUSATIVE ORGANISM	CLINICAL SIGNS	CURABLE?	CONTAGIOUS?
CANINE DISTEMPER	Distemper virus	This does not cause a change in the dog's behavior or temperament. Clinical signs include coughing, sneezing, runny eyes, and neurologic changes.	No specific treatment is available.	Yes, to other dogs and to ferrets
INFECTIOUS CANINE HEPATITIS	Adenovirus	Clinical signs are of liver disease with decreased appetite, fever, vomiting, diarrhea, and edema of the cornea, and discharge from the eyes and nose.	No specific treatment is available.	Yes, to other dogs
CANINE PARVOVIRUS	Parvovirus	Clinical signs are of severe destruction of the intestinal tract with vomiting and bloody diarrhea.	No specific treatment is available.	Yes, to other dogs and wild canids (wolves)
KENNEL COUGH	**Bordetella bronchiseptica** and parainfluenza virus	Infected dogs have a chronic harsh cough.	Bacterial infection is treatable with antibiotics.	Yes, to other dogs, cats, and pocket pets
CANINE INFLUENZA	Canine influenza virus (H3N8, H3N2)	Upper and lower respiratory signs (nasal discharge and cough, respectively), lethargy	No specific treatment is available.	Yes, to other dogs.
LEPTOSPIROSIS	**Leptospira** spp	Clinical signs are those of kidney and liver disease and include fever, lack of appetite, vomiting, and increased thirst.	Yes, with antibiotics.	Yes, through contact with urine from infected animals
LYME DISEASE	**Borrelia burgdorferei**	The most common clinical signs are lameness shifting from leg to leg, and fever.	Yes, with antibiotics.	No, this disease must be transmitted by an infected tick

DISEASE	CAUSATIVE ORGANISM	CLINICAL SIGNS	CURABLE?	CONTAGIOUS?
RABIES	Rabies virus	Clinical signs are neurologic; there is a "dumb" form (paralysis) and a "furious" form (aggression, seizures).	No – this disease is invariably fatal.	Yes, to all mammals, including humans
FELINE DISTEMPER	Panleukopenia virus	This does not cause a change in the cat's behavior or temperament. Clinical signs are of severe destruction of the intestinal tract with vomiting and diarrhea.	No specific treatment is available.	Yes, to other cats
CALICIVIRUS	Calicivirus	Clinical signs are of severe respiratory disease.	No specific treatment is available.	Yes, to other cats
FELINE RHINOTRACHEITIS	Herpesvirus	Rhinotracheitis is inflammation of the nose and respiratory tract, evidenced as discharge from the eyes and nose and sneezing.	No specific treatment is available.	Yes, to other cats
FELINE LEUKEMIA	Feline leukemia virus	The immune system is suppressed so chronic infections may be seen. Associated problems are anemia and cancer.	No specific treatment is available.	Yes, to other cats

Veterinarians are required to follow the label directions for use of all vaccines

- Frequency of rabies vaccination legally is controlled by municipalities and may be linked to animal licensing
- Puppies and kittens require a series of boosters and revaccination at about 1 year after completion of the initial vaccine series to develop protection against disease
- Vaccines can be designated as "core" or "non-core"

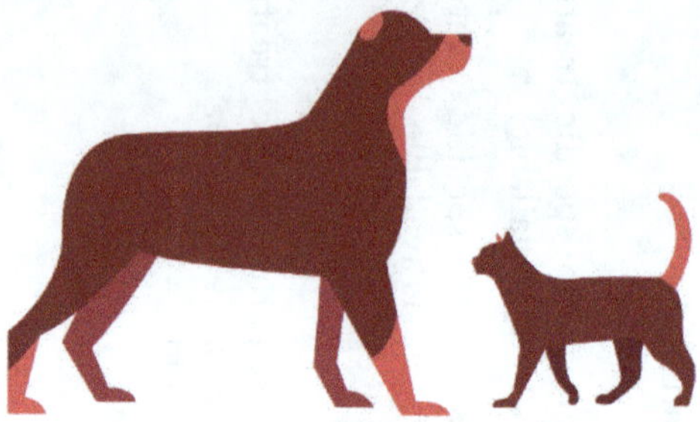

Some vaccination protocols in small animals are being questioned. The vaccine protocols that are being questioned are those for the core vaccines administered to adult dogs and cats. Some data suggest that adult animals may maintain immunity for 5-7 years after their initial vaccinations as young animals, suggesting that the annual revaccination veterinarians had recommended for years is not necessary. Certainly in human medicine, adults are not revaccinated frequently for serious disease but instead in many cases maintain lifelong protection after childhood vaccination. It has been suggested that measurement of antibody concentrations (titers) in animals could be used to determine if vaccination was indicated in a given animal; however, there is confusion regarding how best to measure antibodies in animals and we do not know what concentration of antibody actually is protective against disease. This also is an inaccurate measure of immune status of the animal as it does not account for cell-mediated immunity.

Increased antibody titers have been demonstrated to be well correlated with protection for canine distemper, canine parvovirus, canine adenovirus (hepatitis), and feline parvovirus (panleukopenia). Antibody titers, if high, can be used to support the contention that vaccination has induced immunity. However, if they are low, that does not mean that an anamnestic response cannot be generated by the animal. Examples of patients for whom antibody titer testing may be useful are young animals at the end of their core vaccine series, dogs from breeds with genetic lack of response to parvovirus vaccination (rottweilers, Doberman pinschers, pit bull terriers), dogs with a history of adverse vaccine reactions, dogs with chronic disease, and aged dogs.

Rabies is a special case on all fronts. Frequency of rabies vaccination is mandated by law and that law may not be based in science. Veterinarians do not have the authority to waive the legal requirement for rabies vaccination for dogs with a history of adverse reactions or chronic disease. All rabies vaccines are boostered one year after initial vaccination. Rabies antibody titers are a legal indicator of adequate vaccination and are not considered a legal index of immunity.

The American Animal Hospital Association (AAHA) and AAFP have developed guidelines for vaccination protocols for adult animals.

Vaccination Protocols for Adult Animals

VACCINES	DOG		CAT	
	CORE	NON-CORE	CORE	NON-CORE
CANINE DISTEMPER VIRUS	X			
CANINE PARVOVIRUS	X			
CANINE ADENOVIRUS-2 (hepatitis)	X			
RABIES	X		X	
FELINE PANLEUKOPENIA VIRUS (distemper)			X	
FELINE HERPESVIRUS-1			X	
FELINE CALICIVIRUS			X	
FELINE LEUKEMIA VIRUS			X*	
CANINE PARAINFLUENZA VIRUS (kennel cough)		X		
LEPTOSPIRA SP.		X		
BORDETELLA BRONCHISEPTICA (kennel cough)		X		
CANINE INFLUENZA VIRUS		X		
BORRELIA BURGDORFEREI (Lyme disease)		X		
CANINE CORONAVIRUS		X		
CHLAMYDIA (CHLAMYDOPHILA) FELIS				X
FELINE INFECTIOUS PERITONITIS VIRUS				X

* Considered core for cats less than 2 years of age and for cats that are outside part- or full-time and for cats that live inside but are exposed to outside cats

The University of Minnesota Veterinary Medical Center's currently recommended vaccination protocols for pediatric and adult dogs and cats are based on the reports and recommendations of the American Veterinary Medical Association (AVMA), AAHA and AAFP. Pros and cons of use of a given vaccine are discussed with the owner, who works in concert with the veterinarian to create the protocol that will be used for their animal. As more research results become available, the recommended vaccines and vaccination intervals may change.

Young animals receive a series of boosters to try to ensure immunization while waiting for maternal antibodies to wane and for the young animal to become immunocompetent. Antibody titers in the bitch can be used as a rough guide to help determine how quickly antibody titers will wane in their offspring; bitches with high titers will have higher concentrations of antibody in their colostrum so pups that receive that colostrum will have transfer of more passive transfer of antibodies and it will take longer for those maternal antibodies to clear, suggesting that those pups will not benefit from very early vaccination. Vaccines should not be given any more frequently than every two weeks, as cytokine release at the time of vaccination may interfere with new vaccines introduced too quickly.

Preventive Health Care Recommendations for Puppies

VISIT NUMBER: AGE	VACCINATIONS GIVEN	PARASITE CONTROL
Visit One: 6-8 weeks	**Distemper / Hepatitis / Parvovirus** Kennel cough	**Fecal examination** **Deworming medication** **Heartworm medication** **Flea and tick prevention** (check label for appropriate age to start a given product)
Visit Two: 9-12 weeks	**Distemper / Hepatitis / Parvovirus** **Rabies** (follow label directions – give at 12 weeks)	**Deworming medication** **Heartworm medication** **Flea and tick prevention**
Visits Three +/- Four: 14-16 weeks*	**Distemper / Hepatitis / Parvovirus** Leptospira (repeat in 2-3 wk) Lyme disease (repeat in 2-3 wk)	**Heartworm medication** **Fecal examination** **Flea and tick prevention**

The core vaccines (those recommended for all dogs) and parasite control necessary for every puppy are in bold print.

Vaccinations are boostered every 3-4 weeks until 16 weeks of age. Rabies is given once at 12 weeks of age and again 1 year later.

*= Current recommendations are for the final distemper combination booster to be given at 16 weeks of age or older.

Preventive Health Care Recommendations for Kittens

VISIT NUMBER: AGE	VACCINATIONS GIVEN	PARASITE CONTROL	TESTS
Visit One: 6-8 weeks	**Distemper / Calicivirus / Herpesvirus**	**Fecal examination** **Deworming medication** **Heartworm medication**	**Feline leukemia / Feline immuno-deficiency virus**
Visit Two: 9-12 weeks	**Distemper / Calicivirus / Herpesvirus** **Feline leukemia** **Rabies** (follow label directions – give at 12 weeks)	**Deworming medication** **Heartworm medication**	You may decide to test for feline leukemia at this visit
Visits Three +/- Four: 13-16 weeks*	**Distemper / Calicivirus / Herpesvirus** **Feline leukemia**	**Deworming medication** **Heartworm medication** Flea and tick prevention (if outdoors)	

The core vaccines (those recommended for all cats) and parasite control necessary for every kitten are in bold print.

- Vaccinations are boostered every 3-4 weeks until 16 weeks of age. Rabies is given once at 12 weeks of age and again 1 year later.
- *= Current recommendations are for the final distemper combination booster to be given at 16 weeks of age or older.

Preventive Health Care Recommendations for Adult Dogs

EXAMINATION	VACCINES	PARASITE CONTROL	TESTS
1 YEAR OF AGE			
Annual physical examination	◉ **Distemper / Hepatitis / Parvovirus**– booster at 1 year* ◉ **Rabies**– booster at 1 year* ◉ Leptospira – booster at 1 year* ◉ Lyme disease– booster at 1 year* ◉ Kennel cough– repeat in 1 year	◉ **Deworming medication** (if fecal examination positive) ◉ **Heartworm medication** ◉ **Flea and tick prevention**	**Fecal examination** **Heartworm test**
2-6 YEARS OF AGE			

Annual physical examination	◉ **Distemper / Hepatitis / Parvovirus** – booster every 3 years ◉ **Rabies** – booster every 3 years ◉ Leptospira – booster every year ◉ Lyme disease – booster every year ◉ Kennel cough – booster every year	◉ **Deworming medication** (if fecal examination positive) ◉ **Heartworm medication** ◉ **Flea and tick prevention**	**Fecal examination** **Heartworm test**
GREATER THAN 6 YEARS OF AGE			
Annual physical examination	**Distemper / Hepatitis / Parvovirus**– booster every 3 years **Rabies** – booster every 3 years Leptospira – booster every year Lyme disease – booster every year Kennel cough – booster every year	**Deworming medication** (if fecal examination positive) **Heartworm medication** **Flea and tick prevention**	**Fecal examination** **Heartworm test** **Senior screening tests**

* or at the 1 year anniversary of the last vaccine received as a puppy

- The items in bold print are recommended for every dog. Items not highlighted may or may not be recommended based on the lifestyle of your pet.
- Leptospira vaccine is recommended for all dogs in Minnesota. In general, it is recommended for breeding dogs, duck hunting dogs and farm dogs, or any dog that has routine access to sources of standing water.
- The Lyme vaccine is recommended for dogs that travel in areas where Lyme disease is known to occur commonly, including New England and the upper Midwest. In Minnesota, the area where dogs are most at risk is north of the Twin Cities. Tick prevention is strongly recommended to prevent this disease and other tick-borne illnesses.
- Kennel cough vaccine is recommended for dogs that are exposed to a large number of other dogs, such as dogs that are boarded, show dogs, breeding dogs, and dogs that are housed at "doggy day care" or visit dog parks. Some grooming facilities require this vaccine.

- Frequency of rabies vaccinations legally is mandated by local, not state or federal, law.
- Veterinarians are required to follow the label directions for use of all vaccines.

Preventive Health Care Recommendations for Adult Cats

EXAMINATION	VACCINES	PARASITE CONTROL	TESTS
1 YEAR OF AGE			
Annual physical examination	**Distemper / Calicivirus / Herpesvirus** – booster at 1 year of age* **Rabies (Purevax)** – booster at 1 year of age* **Feline leukemia** – booster at 1 year of age*	**Deworming medication (if fecal examination positive)** **Heartworm medication** Flea and tick prevention (if outdoors)	**Fecal examination** **Feline leukemia test**
2-7 YEARS OF AGE			
Annual physical examination	**Distemper / Calicivirus / Herpesvirus** – booster every 3 years **Rabies (Purevax)** – booster every 3 years Feline leukemia – booster every year	**Deworming medication** (if fecal examination positive) **Heartworm medication** Flea and tick prevention (if outdoors)	Consider annual testing for feline leukemia if your cat is at risk
GREATER THAN 7 YEARS OF AGE			
Annual physical examination	**Distemper / Calicivirus / Herpesvirus** – booster every 3 years **Rabies (Purevax)** – booster every 3 years Feline leukemia – booster every year	**Deworming medication** (if fecal examination positive) **Heartworm medication** Flea and tick prevention (if outdoors)	**Senior screening tests**

* or at the 1 year anniversary of the last vaccine received as a kitten

- The items in bold print are recommended for every cat. Outdoor or patio cats should receive all of the above vaccinations, parasite control measures, and tests.
- Frequency of rabies vaccinations legally is mandated by local, not state or federal, law.

- Veterinarians are required to follow the label directions for use of all vaccines.

VACCINATION OF HORSES

Commercial vaccines are available for only a small subset of the infectious diseases to which horses are susceptible. Despite this, vaccination plays an important role in reducing the incidence and severity of common viral and bacterial diseases. There is no such thing as a "one-size-fits-all" vaccination program that is appropriate for use in all horses!

Vaccination programs are tailored to the individual and the farm based on an assessment of:

- Risk of infection and disease (geography, horse age, occupation, movement patterns)
- Medical, economic, and logistic consequences of disease should it occur
- Potential for spread of infection to other horses and/or humans
- Farm size and type
- Vaccine cost, availability, and efficacy
- Risk of adverse reactions to vaccination

Many equine vaccines are available for purchase "over-the-counter", but horse owners rarely have the knowledge and experience to conduct this type of analysis. Horse owners/managers should therefore make decisions about optimal vaccination programs for each individual horse with the guidance of an equine veterinarian that is familiar with their farm, animals, training/performance goals, and budget. That said, within a given geographical region there is typically a set of core vaccines that are promoted for use in all horses, similar to what was described for small animals. As an example, all horses are highly susceptible to tetanus, a devastating and often fatal disease caused by the bacterium *Clostridium tetani*. This bacterial organism is widespread in the soil and environment, and readily contaminates the minor wounds and punctures that horses tend to sustain on a frequent basis. Available vaccines are very safe and effective, so are recommended for use in all horses. If you had to identify the single most important core vaccine for horses, it would be tetanus toxoid!

For the remainder of commercial vaccine products, the benefit-risk-cost relationship is less clear and can vary widely between individual horses, different farms, and different geographical regions. These products are categorized as risk-based (non-core) vaccines, which are recommended for some horses and not others. Equine veterinarians use their knowledge and experience to identify horses and farms that may benefit from specific risk-based vaccines. For example, diarrhea caused by rotavirus affects young foals only. Adult horses often carry the virus within their gastrointestinal tracts, but only young foals in the first few months of life develop disease as a result of infection. Some breeding farms suffer high rates of disease caused by this pathogen year after year, while others experience no disease whatsoever. Farms with a significant history of rotavirus enteritis are good candidates for use of the rotavirus vaccine, which is administered to pregnant mares late in gestation to stimulate high levels of anti-rotavirus antibodies in colostrum. These antibodies are consumed and absorbed by the foal in the first day of life, and help to reduce the subsequent risk of infection and disease. There is no reason for adult horses other than broodmares to be vaccinated with this product, nor do all broodmares require such vaccination.

Vaccination is only one element of an infectious disease control program. Horse owners and managers should be aware that farm management practices play just as important a role (for example, sanitation practices, good nutrition and parasite control, controlling horse traffic, quarantine of new arrivals, and quarantine of horses with known contagious disease). They should understand that vaccination does not provide a guarantee of protection at the individual animal level – it lowers the risk of infectious disease but cannot eliminate that risk entirely. Some vaccines are more effective than others, some horses respond to vaccination better than others, many vaccines require multiple doses before protective immunity is achieved, and protective immunity may not be achieved for days to weeks following vaccine administration. Owners who manage their own vaccines should be advised that improper storage, handling, and administration of vaccine products will undermine their effectiveness.

Equine Infectious Disease Control

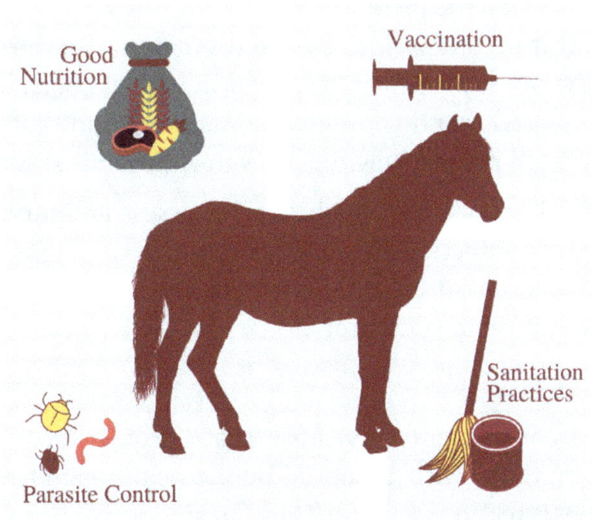

Immune protection of foals is generally achieved through vaccination of the dam in late gestation. Antibodies produced by the mare are concentrated in her colostrum, and then transferred to the foal as it suckles colostrum in the first hours of life. These antibodies provide protection for several months, after which levels gradually decline and the foal must be vaccinated to stimulate its own active immunity. For foals that received adequate amounts of colostrum from a properly vaccinated mare, first vaccines are administered at 4-6 months of age. If they are vaccinated earlier than this, maternal antibody will interfere with an effective immune response to vaccination. By contrast, foals of unvaccinated mares do not have significant concentrations of maternal antibody so vaccination should be initiated earlier. Since it is difficult to predict the precise timeframe during which maternal antibody concentrations wane, foals often receive more doses of vaccine in the initial series compared to adult horses being vaccinated for the first time. For example, a 2-dose initial series is recommended for first-time vaccination of adult horses against tetanus. By contrast, a 3-dose initial series is recommended for foals. This approach helps to ensure that all foals are adequately protected, even those in which maternal antibody may have persisted longer than usual.

The vast majority of equine vaccines are administered by intramuscular (IM) injection, and a few are administered intranasally. Adverse reactions to vaccination are common but in most cases are limited to minor transient muscle swelling and tenderness at the injection site. Occasional horses develop hives, lethargy, fever, or inappetance that may be self-limiting or may require veterinary support. A very small percentage of horses experience serious, and potentially life-threatening, systemic reactions such as anaphylaxis, purpura hemorrhagica, endotoxemia, laminitis, or infection of muscle tissue with the anaerobic bacterium *Clostridium* sp. (clostridial myonecrosis). Owners should be aware that all vaccines carry an inherent risk of adverse effects, even when the product has been stored, handled, and administered correctly. Administration of vaccines by the veterinarian rather than the owner/manager ensures that an appropriate vaccine product has been chosen; the product has been properly stored, handled, and administered; and that peracute adverse reactions can be treated promptly while the veterinarian is still on the premises.

Serum antibody titers are not widely used to assess an individual horse's level of immunity to a given infectious disease, or to guide decisions about whether or not vaccination is warranted. Insufficient data are currently available to guide meaningful interpretation of such titers.

CORE VACCINATIONS

The AVMA defines core vaccines as those that "protect from diseases that are endemic to a region, those with potential public health significance, required by law, virulent/highly infectious, and/or those posing a risk of severe disease. Core vaccines have clearly demonstrated efficacy and safety, and thus exhibit a high enough level of patient benefit and low enough level of risk to justify their use in the majority of patients." The following equine vaccines are considered to meet these criteria:

- Tetanus (tetanus toxoid)
- Western Equine Encephalitis (WEE) and Eastern Equine Encephalitis (EEE)
- West Nile Virus
- Rabies

Tetanus

This is a horrifying and often fatal disease caused by the bacterium *Clostridium tetani*. Spores of the organism are ubiquitous and reside primarily in soil, from where they gain ready access to the body through lacerations, punctures, surgical incisions, and exposed tissue such as the umbilicus of neonatal foals. Bacteria multiply within devitalized tissues at the site of injury or invasion, then produce a neurotoxin that migrates along motor nerves to the spinal cord and central nervous system (CNS). Most mammals are susceptible to this neurotoxin, including humans, but horses are exquisitely sensitive to its effects. Within the CNS, tetanus toxin inhibits the release of inhibitory neurotransmitters, resulting in loss of normal balance and control of muscular contraction. Over 10-7 days, affected horses develop progressive localized and generalized muscle contraction, rigidity, and spasms that are aggravated by stimulation and excitement. Horses often exhibit a characteristic sawhorse stance, raised tail head, prolapse of the third eyelid, and difficulties prehending and masticating feed due to excessive contraction of masticatory muscles ("lockjaw"). They suffer great pain and anxiety related to the muscle spasms and their inability to move or eat normally. Death is often the result of respiratory failure when the muscles of the larynx, intercostal muscles, and diaphragm become affected. Affected horses may be treated with a combination of tetanus antitoxin (antibodies targeting the neurotoxin), penicillin to kill the *C. tetani*, wound debridement and management to prevent further production of neurotoxin, sedatives, nutritional support, extensive nursing care, and a quiet environment. Whether or not a horse can survive depends upon how early the disease was diagnosed, the speed and severity of disease onset, and how aggressively it can be treated. The good news about tetanus is that it is easily prevented through vaccination! All available vaccines contain tetanus toxoid, a formalin-inactivated form of the tetanus neurotoxin that stimulates a strong humoral immune response following IM administration. The antibodies produced in response to vaccination bind and inactivate the neurotoxin before it can reach the CNS to wreak havoc. Many brands of tetanus toxoid are available and individual products may contain tetanus toxoid alone, or in combination with other antigens as part of a multivalent vaccine. Some products contain all of the core equine vaccines, and others also contain one or more risk-based vaccines. Initial vaccination of a previously unvaccinated adult horse consists of a 2-dose series administered by IM injection 4-6 weeks apart, after which horses are boostered with a single dose annually. Broodmares receive their annual vaccination 4-6 weeks prior to foaling to ensure that high levels of protective antibody may be transferred to the foal via colostrum. Foals then receive a 3-dose series beginning at 4-6 months of age, followed by single annual booster doses as for adults. It is common for horses to receive supplemental boosters if they need surgery or sustain a wound/puncture more than 6 months following their previous vaccination. True protection probably lasts much longer than this, but we err on the side of caution given the horse's unique susceptibility to this devastating disease.

Western & Eastern Equine Encephalitis

This neurological disease is caused by the related Western (WEE) and Eastern Equine Encephalitis (EEE) alphaviruses, which are endemic in North America. Birds and rodents are the major reservoirs of these viruses, but they may be transmitted to horses and humans by mosquitoes. Following the bite of an infected mosquito, the virus replicates and moves through the bloodstream to the brain, where it causes inflammation and neurological dysfunction. Affected horses exhibit fever, incoordination and weakness, stupor (the common name of the disease is "sleeping sickness"), head-pressing, and terminal seizures and coma. No known antiviral agents are effective in the treatment of this disease, so treatment focuses on supportive care and reduction of CNS inflammation. Fatality rates are 50% for WEE and over 90% for EEE. Horses that survive typically exhibit permanent neurological injury and deficits. The viruses are not directly transmissible from infected horses to other horses or their human handlers, even through mosquitoes, but horses serve as sentinels for increased regional risk of human and equine exposure. The good news about WEE/EEE is that it is easily prevented through vaccination! All available vaccines contain formalin-inactivated WEE and EEE viruses, and they are considered to be very safe and effective in preventing disease. Most vaccines are multivalent products containing WEE/EEE in combination with other core antigens such as tetanus toxoid and West Nile Virus, but versions containing additional antigens are also available. Initial vaccination of a previously unvaccinated adult horse consists of a 2-dose series administered by IM injection 4-6 weeks apart, after which horses are boostered with a single dose annually. Annual boosters are administered in early spring to ensure that horses are well-protected during the summer and fall vector seasons. Broodmares receive their annual vaccination 4-6 weeks prior to foaling to ensure that high levels of protective antibody may be transferred to the foal via colostrum. Foals then receive a 3-dose series beginning at 4-6 months of age, followed by single annual booster doses as for adults. In southeastern states where mosquitoes are active year-round, it is common practice to (1) use a 4-dose primary series for foals beginning at 3 months of age, and to (2) administer boosters every 6 months rather than on an annual basis to ensure that protective immunity is maintained year-round. Because horses are an important part of the surveillance network for arboviruses that also affect humans, WEE/EEE is a reportable disease in Minnesota. When you suspect or confirm this diagnosis you must notify your state veterinary regulatory authorities immediately. In Minnesota, this is the Board of Animal Health.

West Nile Virus Encephalitis

This neurological disease is caused by the West Nile Virus (WNV), a flavivirus for which birds throughout North America are the major reservoir. The virus is transmitted to horses and humans by mosquitoes. After an incubation period of 7-10 days, affected horses develop inflammation of the brain and spinal cord that results in behavior changes, tremors, facial fasciculations, hyperesthesia, weakness, incoordination, and recumbency, seizures, and coma in severe cases. Approximately 30% of cases progress to recumbency and paralysis; these cases carry a poor prognosis and usually are euthanized. No known antiviral agents are effective in the treatment of this disease, so treatment focuses on supportive care and reduction of CNS inflammation. Horses that recover often exhibit neurological deficits that may or may not resolve over the next 6-12 months. The good news about West Nile Virus is that it is easily prevented through vaccination! Four commercial vaccine products are currently available: two contain inactivated virus, one is a live canary pox recombinant vector vaccine, and one is an inactivated flavivirus chimera vaccine. Some versions contain only WNV antigen, while others are multivalent products containing supplemental core or risk-based vaccines. These vaccines are considered to be safe and effective. Specific recommendations vary by product, and the manufacturer's instructions should be followed. For most of the commercial products, initial vaccination of a previously unvaccinated adult horse consists of a 2-dose series administered by IM injection 4-6 weeks apart, after which horses are boostered with a single dose annually. Annual boosters are administered in early spring to ensure that horses are well-protected during the summer and fall vector seasons. Broodmares receive their annual vaccination 4-6 weeks prior to foaling to ensure that high levels of protective antibody may be transferred to the foal via colostrum. Foals then receive a 3-dose series beginning at 4-6 months of age, followed by single annual booster doses as for adults. In southeastern states where mosquitoes are active year-round, it is common practice to (1) use a 4-dose primary series for foals beginning at 3 months of age, and to (2) administer boosters every 6 months rather than on an annual basis to ensure that protective immunity is maintained year-round. Many veterinarians also use a 6-month booster interval for geriatric and immunocompromised horses. Because horses are an important part of the surveillance network for human disease, WNV is a reportable disease in Minnesota.

Rabies

Rabies is rare in horses, but it is given special consideration because of its public health significance and the fact that disease is almost always fatal. The rabies virus is transmitted in saliva through the bite of an infected wild or domestic animal. The most common vectors vary by geographical region, but in the United States are typically skunks, foxes, raccoons, and bats; in Minnesota, rabies usually is carried by skunks. Horses are typically bitten on the muzzle, face, or lower limbs, but bite wounds may not be visible at the time of diagnosis. Following the bite, the virus migrates along nerves to the spinal cord and brain, where is causes progressive encephalomyelitis that invariably proves fatal. The time period between the bite and onset of neurological symptoms is highly variable, and in other species can range from 1 week to 6 years! Clinical signs of equine rabies are highly variable, but most horses exhibit changes in behavior that are clearly recognized by their owners as uncharacteristic. These may include hyper-alertness, anxiety and mental distress, aggression, hyperactivity such as persistent running, persistent abnormal vocalization, or simply profound depression/somnolence. Affected horses can be extremely dangerous to their owners/handlers as a result of their altered mental status, even in the absence of overtly aggressive behavior. Animals that are not euthanized at this stage will progress to recumbency, paralysis, seizures, coma, and death. The time between first recognition of a problem and death is rarely more than 5-7 days. Definitive diagnosis of rabies requires laboratory testing on the brain. The good news about rabies is that it is easily prevented through vaccination! All commercial vaccines contain killed rabies virus, a potent antigen that triggers strong antibody responses; they are generally considered to be very safe and effective. Initial vaccination of a previously unvaccinated adult horse consists of a single dose of vaccine administered by IM injection, followed by annual booster doses to maintain protective immunity. Broodmares typically receive their annual vaccination 4-6 weeks prior to foaling to ensure that high levels of protective antibody may be transferred to the foal via colostrum, but available evidence regarding duration of immunity indicates that annual vaccination prior to breeding is also acceptable. Foals then receive a 2-dose series (4-6 weeks apart) beginning at 6 months of age, followed by single annual booster doses as for adults. At present, none of the rabies vaccines licensed for use in horses carry a 3-year label as is common for small animal products. Rabies vaccines are available over-the-counter in some states, while other states (including Minnesota) mandate that vaccines be administered by licensed veterinarians only. Because of its zoonotic potential, rabies is a reportable disease of great medical and legal concern.

RISK-BASED (NON-CORE) VACCINATIONS

Risk-based vaccines are included in the vaccination program on the basis of risk-benefit-cost analysis. Their use varies regionally, between different horse populations within a region, and even between different horses on a single farm. The use of risk-based vaccines should be guided by an equine veterinarian, as horse owners and managers rarely have the knowledge and experience needed for optimum program design. The most commonly used risk-based vaccines in North America include:

- Equine herpesvirus (EHV; rhinopneumonitis or "rhino")
- Influenza
- Strangles
- Botulism
- Potomac Horse Fever (PHF)
- Equine viral arteritis (EVA)
- Rotavirus diarrhea
- Anthrax
- Leptospirosis

EQUINE HERPESVIRUS

Equine herpesviruses 1 and 4 (EHV-1 and EHV-4) are respiratory viruses that cause typical signs of upper respiratory disease: acute fever, lethargy, inappetance, serous nasal discharge, and cough, with full recovery within 2-3 weeks. Clinical disease is most likely to occur in young horses, especially those entering training at facilities in which extensive comingling occurs. EHV-1 is also an important cause of abortion in pregnant broodmares, however, and in rare cases it invades the CNS to cause weakness, incoordination, and inability to urinate and defecate. Epidemics of the neurological form of the disease occur with some regularity, especially among horses assembled at racing or show venues. The virus is spread via direct contact with nasal secretions, aerosolized virus from coughing and sneezing, and in the case of EHV-1 from contact with aborted fetuses, fetal fluids, and the infected placenta. The viruses are ubiquitous and most horses become infected early in life and remain so; the viruses have a complex biology that features a latency state, from which reactivation, viremia, and viral shedding can occur during periods of stress. These factors make infection virtually impossible to control, and explains why outbreaks of EHV can occur in closed populations of horses. Most adult horses develop some immunity as a result of repeated exposure to the viruses; these horses rarely develop significant respiratory disease when infected but can still contribute to spread of the virus within a population. This age- and exposure-related immunity does not protect horses from abortion or neurological involvement, unfortunately. Relegation of EHV vaccines to the risk-based category is the result of this complex virus biology, the high prevalence of latent infection, the fact that most horses develop only mild respiratory disease as a consequence of active infection, and the fact that vaccines are only partially protective. The primary indications for use of EHV vaccines are:

- Prevention of EHV-1 induced abortion in pregnant mares
- Reduction of symptoms and spread of respiratory tract disease (rhinopneumonitis) in foals, weanlings, yearlings, and young performance/show horses that are at particularly high risk of exposure to EHV-1 and EHV-4

EHV-1/EHV-4 vaccines are licensed as aids in prevention of respiratory disease, while specific EHV-1 vaccines are licensed and labeled for prevention of abortion in broodmares. None of the current EHV vaccines are licensed for prevention of herpes myeloencephalitis, the CNS form of EHV-1 infection, nor have any available vaccines been shown to be effective in this regard. All except one vaccine contain formalin-inactivated EHV-1 and EHV-4 (respiratory vaccines) or EHV-1 only (abortion vaccines). Most of these are administered by IM administration only, while one product carries an option for intranasal use once an initial series of IM injections has been administered. Products licensed for prevention of abortion tend to contain larger amounts of viral antigen than those licensed for control of respiratory disease, and these products stimulate stronger immune responses. There is a single modified-live EHV-1 vaccine on the market that is licensed as an aid in preventing respiratory disease due to EHV-1. Initial vaccination of a previously unvaccinated adult horse with a killed virus respiratory vaccine consists of a 3-dose series administered by IM injection 4-6 weeks apart, after which horses are boostered every 6-12 months depending on the stringency of immune protection desired. Horses under 5 years of age, those on breeding farms and in contact with pregnant mares, and performance/show horses are often boostered every 6 months. For abortion prevention, broodmares are vaccinated at 5, 7, and 9 months of gestation using a high-antigen EHV-1 product. This regimen also ensures that colostrum contains significant anti-EHV-1 antibody. Foals then receive a 3-dose series beginning at 4-6 months of age, followed by boosters every 6 months.

Influenza

Influenza is a common viral respiratory disease of horses. As with EHV-1/EHV-4, affected horses exhibit acute fever, lethargy, inappetance, serous nasal discharge, and cough, with full recovery within 2-3 weeks. The virus is spread via direct contact with nasal secretions, and as virus is aerosolized from coughing and sneezing. As with EHV, disease is most likely to occur in young horses, especially those in training at facilities in which extensive comingling occurs (training/show barns, racetracks). The virus does not circulate constantly within a population the way herpesviruses do, but triggers disease when an infected horse is introduced into a naïve population. Vaccination and 14-day quarantine of new arrivals is therefore more effective for control of influenza than for rhinopneumonitis. Since the influenza virus tends to change its genetic and structural makeup over time, vaccines tend to contain multiple strains of virus and are updated on a regular basis to ensure that horses remain protected against viruses in current circulation. Horses under 6 years of age, show/performance horses, and horses boarded at stables with a high level of horse traffic are good candidates for vaccination against influenza. Older horses maintained in a closed herd are at comparatively low risk of infection and disease. There are 3 types of influenza vaccine on the market at present, most of which elicit at least 6 months of protective immunity:

- Many inactivated virus vaccines (IM administration, but for one product boosters may be administered intranasally). Often included in multivalent vaccines targeting EHV-1/EHV-4 or other infectious diseases
- One live canary pox recombinant vector vaccine (IM administration)
- One modified-live vaccine (intranasal administration)

Each of the vaccine types requires a different initial series. Initial vaccination of a previously unvaccinated adult horse with a killed virus vaccine consists of a 3-dose series administered by IM injection, after which horses are boostered every 6-12 months depending on the age of the horse, expected exposure level, and the stringency of immune protection desired. The canary pox recombinant vaccine requires a 2-dose initial series administered by IM injection 4-6 weeks apart, after which horses are boostered every 6-12 months. The modified-live intranasal vaccine requires only a single primary dose, followed by boosters every 6 or 12 months. Broodmares are vaccinated every 6 months, with one of those doses timed for administration 4-6 weeks prior to foaling. Foals are then vaccinated beginning at approximately 6 months of age; as for adults, the primary protocol varies between vaccines but subsequent boosters are administered every 6 months.

Strangles

Strangles is a common and highly contagious respiratory disease of horses caused by the bacterium *Streptococcus equi equi*. Young horses are most susceptible but horses of any age can be affected. The organism is transmitted by direct contact with infected nasal secretions or purulent material from ruptured lymph node abscesses, and is easily spread on equipment, tack, feed and water buckets, grooming supplies, and human hands or clothing. Horses with active disease shed the highest levels of bacteria, but clinically normal carriers can also shed bacteria and trigger disease outbreaks. Classical signs of disease include fever, copious purulent nasal discharge, lethargy, inappetance, and progressive enlargement, abscessation, and rupture of submandibular, retropharyngeal, and parotid lymph nodes, with subsequent drainage of purulent material. Most horses make a full recovery within several weeks but occasional horses develop life-threatening complications such as upper airway obstruction, pneumonia, spread of infection beyond the respiratory tract ("bastard strangles"), abdominal abscessation, and purpura hemorrhagica, a dangerous immune-mediated disorder. Unless rigorous biosecurity precautions are taken, strangles can sweep through a large percentage of horses in a barn, interrupting the training and show schedule for weeks or months. Even once affected horses have made a full recovery, they may harbor bacteria in the pharynx and guttural pouch for months afterward, serving as a potential source of infection for additional horses. Routine cases of strangles are not treated with antibiotics because they tend to slow progression and resolution of the disease. Treatment is primarily supportive with anti-inflammatory medications used to combat high fever and to encourage horses to eat and drink. Horses with life-threatening complications do receive antibiotic therapy, and horses with immune-mediated disease require concurrent immunosuppressive therapy with corticosteroids. Vaccination against strangles is recommended on premises where strangles is a persistent problem and for horses considered to be at high risk of exposure. Strangles cannot be completely controlled through vaccination, but it does reduce the incidence and severity of disease. Historical efforts to develop safe and effective strangles vaccines were ineffective due to the biology of the causative organism. Many of the vaccines that have been brought to market over the years have carried a high risk of adverse effects and elicited relatively poor levels of immune protection. At present, available vaccines are of two types: a single modified-live vaccine administered by intranasal inoculation, and subunit vaccines containing purified extracts of the *Streptococcus equi equi* M-protein virulence factor. The modified-live vaccine is considered to be more effective, but is more difficult to administer and carries a higher risk of adverse effects. Vaccination with either product can trigger development of purpura hemorrhagica. Initial vaccination of previously unvaccinated adult horses with the modified-live intranasal vaccine consists of a -2dose series administered 3 weeks apart, after which horses are boostered every 12-6 months depending on the expected level of exposure and the stringency of immune protection desired. The subunit vaccine requires a -2 or -3dose initial series administered 4-2 weeks apart, followed by boosters every 6 months. The intranasal modified-live vaccine is not approved for use in broodmares, so when needed the subunit product is administered 6-4 weeks prior to foaling. Foals then receive a -3dose series beginning at 6-4 months of age (subunit vaccine) or 9-6 months of age (intranasal vaccine), followed by boosters every 6 months if ongoing risk of exposure is anticipated. Horses that have recovered from strangles develop strong immune responses that provide protection for approximately 5 years. Subsequent vaccination should be done with caution, as vaccination in the face of existing immunity increases the risk of purpura hemorrhagica.

Botulism

This is a serious and life-threatening disease caused by a toxin produced by the bacterium *Clostridium botulinum*. Bacterial spores gain access to the body either through ingestion or wound contamination, after which the spores vegetate and toxin is produced. Alternatively, preformed botulinum toxin may be consumed when horses eat decaying or improperly preserved hay, haylage, or silage, or feed contaminated with rotting remnants of animal carcasses (a decomposing dead rabbit incorporated during round bale production, for example). Horses are exquisitely sensitive to the biological effects of botulinum toxin, which blocks acetylcholine release at the neuromuscular junction to cause profound flaccid paralysis of muscle. Clinical signs in horses include generalized weakness progressing rapidly to recumbency, tremors, inability to prehend and swallow feed (dysphagia), secondary injury related to falls, and death by respiratory paralysis. There are 8 distinct toxins produced by different subtypes of *Cl. botulinum*; types B (90% of cases) and C (10% of cases) are responsible for most cases of equine botulism. Type B botulism occurs most often in the Mid-Atlantic states and Kentucky, while Type C botulism is most common in Florida. Affected horses may be treated with a combination of antitoxin (antibodies targeting the neurotoxin), antibiotics to kill the *C. botulinum* organism, laxatives to encourage passage of any toxin within the gut, nutritional support, extensive nursing care, and mechanical respiratory ventilation for horses in respiratory failure. Prognosis for life depends upon how early the disease was diagnosed, the speed and severity of disease onset, how aggressively it can be treated, and whether the horse remains standing. Horses that survive can take weeks to recover fully. Vaccination is recommended for horses in endemic regions, or horses scheduled for transport to endemic regions. Minnesota horses are not routinely vaccinated against botulism, as the disease is rare here. By contrast, Minnesota broodmares that will be transported to Kentucky in the spring for foaling and breeding are typically vaccinated to optimize protection for the mare and her foal in that environment. Available vaccines contain inactivated Type B botulinum toxin (toxoid). There are no licensed vaccines containing Type C or any other toxin sub-type. Initial vaccination of previously unvaccinated adult horses with botulinum toxoid consists of a -3dose series administered by IM injection 4 weeks apart, after which horses receive annual boosters. Broodmares typically receive their annual vaccination 6-4 weeks prior to foaling to ensure high levels of antibody in colostrum. Foals then receive a -3dose series (4 weeks apart) beginning at 3-2 months of age, then boostered at 12 months of age, and annually thereafter. This vaccine may be administered earlier than others because maternal antibody shows little interference with vaccination.

Potomac Horse Fever

Potomac Horse Fever (PHF) is caused by *Neorickettsia risticii*, a bacterial organism that is transferred to horses when they inadvertently ingest aquatic insects near rivers, streams, ponds, or marshland. Most infections are subclinical, but some horses develop fever, diarrhea, endotoxemia, and laminitis. Severe cases may be fatal or result in euthanasia of the case due to cost of management and/or occurrence of severe laminitis. In Minnesota most cases are seen from July to September. Young foals are less susceptible to this disease than adults. Commercial killed bacterin products are available but efficacy is questionable; clients should not expect prevention of disease in endemic regions. Not only is there little scientific evidence that vaccination induces protective immunity, but vaccines contain a single strain of *Neorickettsia risticii* while natural disease has been attributed to multiple field strains. Anecdotally, veterinarians in endemic regions believe that vaccination may reduce the incidence and severity of disease. Vaccinations should be timed to precede the peak period of exposure during summer/fall months. PHF is available as both a standalone vaccine and as a combination PHF-rabies vaccine. Initial vaccination of a previously unvaccinated adult horse with the killed bacterin consists of a -2dose series administered by IM injection 4-3 weeks apart, after which the horse is boostered every 12-6 months depending on the regional level of exposure and risk of disease. Broodmares typically receive their annual vaccination 6-4 weeks prior to foaling. Foals then receive a 2-dose series (3-4 weeks apart) beginning at 5 months of age, and are then boostered at 12 months of age, and every 6-12 months thereafter.

Equine Viral Arteritis

Equine viral arteritis (EVA) is a viral disease of particular significance to the equine breeding industry. Infection is rarely life-threatening, but the virus can establish a long-term carrier state in breeding stallions and cause abortion in pregnant broodmares. The virus is transmitted in respiratory secretions and also in the semen from infected stallions. Most horses that become infected show no signs of disease, but clinical signs that do occur include fever, edema of the lower limbs and ventral abdomen, hives, serous nasal and ocular discharge, and abortion. Infection of intact males can result in a life-long carrier state within the reproductive tract, and these horses are the key reservoirs of infection within the population. A modified-live EVA vaccine is commercially available, and is considered safe and effective in stallions and non-pregnant mares. It is not widely used, but is reserved for use in specific circumstances. Reasons for vaccination include:

- To protect stallions against infection and subsequent development of a carrier state
- To immunize seronegative mares before being bred with known-positive semen
- To stop outbreaks in non-breeding populations

EVA is a reportable disease because of its significance to the breeding industry. When planning a vaccination program against EVA veterinarians should consult with state veterinary officials. Since is not possible to differentiate serological responses to vaccination from those induced by natural infection, horses being vaccinated for the first time are tested first to confirm that they are seronegative. Vaccination status may also influence the ability to export a horse in future; vaccinated horses become seropositive and this can bar them from export to certain countries. Initial vaccination of a previously unvaccinated seronegative adult horse with the modified-live EVA vaccine consists of a single dose administered by IM injection, followed by annual boosters. Broodmares are vaccinated prior to breeding, and stallions are vaccinated approximately 4 weeks prior to the breeding season.

Rotavirus Diarrhea

Rotavirus is a major cause of infectious and contagious diarrhea in young foals. Adults can become infected and shed rotavirus in manure, but do not develop clinical disease. The virus is transmitted by the fecal-oral route and destroys small intestinal villi, leading to maldigestion, malabsorption, and profuse diarrhea. The manure from affected foals contains high levels of virus that cause widespread contamination of barns and paddocks. Fatality rates are low as long as foals receive adequate supportive therapy including fluids, electrolytes, and nutritional support. Although vaccination is a useful aid in reducing the incidence and severity of rotaviral enteritis, biosecurity procedures play an even more important role. An inactivated vaccine containing Group A rotavirus is commercially available, and is used on breeding farms with a history of significant rotaviral disease. This vaccine is not administered to foals, but to pregnant broodmares in late gestation with the goal of eliciting high levels of anti-rotavirus antibody in the colostrum. The vaccine is considered to be safe and effective. Pregnant mares receive a 3-dose series of IM vaccinations at 8, 9, and 10 months of gestation. In order for colostral antibody to protect the foal, the foal must consume an adequate volume of colostrum and absorb the antibody it contains.

Anthrax

This is a rapidly fatal type of septicemia caused by the bacterium *Bacillus anthracis*. Horses and other species (including humans) become infected through ingestion, inhalation, or wound contamination by bacterial spores within the soil. Survival of spores is enhanced by alkaline soil conditions, so the disease tends to occur only in specific geographical regions, including pockets of North and South Dakota. Vaccination is warranted only for horses that are pastured in endemic regions. A single vaccine product is licensed for use in horses. It contains live non-encapsulated bacterial spores administered by subcutaneous injection. Vaccination of pregnant mares is not recommended. Initial vaccination of a previously unvaccinated adult horse consists of a 2-dose series (2-3 weeks apart) administered by subcutaneous injection, followed by annual boosters. If broodmares are vaccinated, this should be done when they are open (non-pregnant) prior to the breeding season. There is little information to guide vaccination programs in foals, and foals are more likely to experience adverse effects following vaccination compared to adult horses.

Leptospirosis

Leptospirosis is a zoonotic disease, caused by bacteria of the genus *Leptospira*. There are many different serotypes of disease and prevalence varies with geographic location. Healthy horses may carry multiple serovars and clinical disease occurs sporadically. The serovar most commonly associated with disease in horses is pomona. Infection is acquired through exposure to the organism via the mucous membranes or abraded skin. The leptospiral organisms are shed in the urine of infected horses (additionally the placenta, fetal fluids, and urine of the mare in abortion cases) and a number of wildlife hosts can shed *Leptospira spp.* in the urine as well. Clinical manifestations of disease include inflammation within the eye (uveitis), late-term abortion, and acute renal failure. There is one vaccine approved for use in horses in the United States. It is a killed vaccine and is labeled for use in healthy horses 6 months of age or older. Duration of immunity of this product has not been determined. Vaccination will prevent animals from shedding leptospiral organisms in urine. Horses 6 months of age or older should receive two initial doses, 3-4 weeks apart with annual revaccination. The product can safely be used in mares up through the second trimester of pregnancy.

CHAPTER-4

PRODUCTION ANIMALS FOR VACCINES AND VACCINATIONS

DAIRY CATTLE

Dairy and beef cattle generally always live in a herd. Management practices will therefore affect multiple animals. Likewise, from an infectious disease standpoint, it has to be kept in mind that not one, but multiple animals will be exposed to a particular pathogen. As a result, the prevention of disease on dairy farms needs to be targeted towards groups of animals and the entire herd rather than individual animals. Disease prevention is crucial to allow the economic survival of the farm and to ensure animal welfare. Specific brands of vaccines will not be discussed for beef or dairy cattle because there is tremendous variability in vaccines used. Examples of diseases for which cattle may be vaccinated include bovine viral diarrhea (BVD), infectious bovine rhinotracheitis (IBR), parainfluenza (PI3), bovine respiratory syncytial virus (BRSV), leptospirosis, *Pasteurella*, *Histophilus* (*Hemophilus*), *Campylobacter* (*Vibrio*), and clostridial diseases. Specifics of vaccines and their use will be covered in species-specific coursework later in the curriculum. An example of which vaccines are used at which life stage is included in the section on beef cattle as are descriptions of the diseases we protect against with vaccination in cattle.

Risks and Management Factors

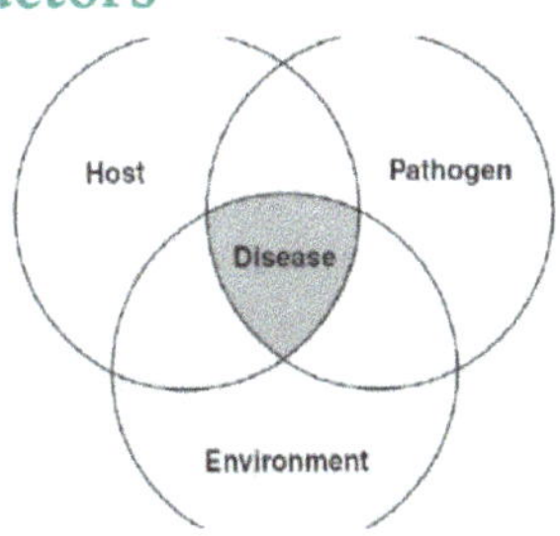

"The Epidemiological Triad", https://www.nap.edu/read/13147/chapter/1#xviii

Factors to Consider in Disease Prevention

Diseases occur due to multiple factors. Their relationship is sometimes called the infection triangle.All three factors (environment (e.g. management practices), host, and pathogen) are important for the development or prevention of disease and all three need to be considered during disease prevention.

The host has various defense mechanisms to prevent or to deal with infections. A given species or animal might not be susceptible to a certain disease. For example, *E. coli* O157:H7, a potentially fatal bacterium for humans, is a normal gut commensal for cattle. Cattle do not have the receptors for the toxins of this bacterium in their kidneys and so they cannot develop the hemolytic uremia syndrome that affects humans. Other defense mechanisms, specific and non-specific, are part of the immune system. These defense mechanisms may be impaired due to the animal's age, inadequate nutrition, and other stressors from within the animal, or may be impaired due to management practices. Stress due to heat, weaning, malnutrition, infection pressure (amount of exposure to a given pathogen), transport, and other factors will negatively impact how the immune system can react to a "pathogen attack".

Furthermore, an infectious disease can only spread through a population if the pathogen 'finds' susceptible animals to infect. Some animals might get sick, but if a population (herd) has many resistant animals, the probability of new infections can be so low that the disease 'dies out' even if not all animals are resistant to the disease. This is called "herd immunity". In human medicine this principle is used every year as we receive flu shots. The aim is to reduce the number of susceptible humans through flu vaccinations and so reduce the likelihood of new infections, particularly in children and immunocompromised people.

So for obvious reasons, the environment and management practices play a crucial role in disease prevention on farm by influencing the animal and the pathogen. Any management practices that decrease the infection pressure on animals (for example, hygiene or biosecurity) will support animals in coping with infection pressure and will reduce the likelihood that animals will even get exposed to the pathogens.

Vaccination is only part of this puzzle and cannot be used as a standalone practice to prevent disease or infection on farm. Vaccination is not a miracle intervention. It does not result in immediate immunity or resistance against diseases in all vaccinated animals. First, it takes time for the immune system of the animal to react to the vaccine and second, just because an animal is vaccinated, it does not automatically mean that the animal cannot be infected or develop the disease. However, vaccination can be used as one of many management practices to help animals cope with potential infection threats.

Vaccinating Production Animals

When thinking about vaccinating a dairy herd, you have to understand the production system and the diseases that are of importance for that particular dairy farm. You need to ask several questions:

- What management practices are already in use on this dairy farm and where could improvements possibly be made to decrease infection pressure? Examples include improving hygiene, not bringing in animals from unknown sources, and limiting foot traffic between age groups.
- Which pathogens are of concern for their impact on the health and production of animals? If an animal is unlikely to ever encounter a pathogen, it is probably not necessary (and is possibly too costly) to vaccinate against it. Do not over-vaccinate animals, and tailor the vaccine program toward each herd individually.
- Do benefits of a possible vaccination outweigh the costs of the disease or could vaccination be economically detrimental? For example, Foot-and-Mouth-Disease (FMD) has not been diagnosed in the United States since the 1920s and the detection of positive antibody titers in animals would result in serious trade restrictions. Therefore, routine vaccination against FMD is probably not economically sound.
- When is the best time to vaccinate the animals? On farms, it is always groups of animals, not individuals, that are vaccinated with a given vaccine. The timing of the vaccination has to take into account which age groups are at the highest risk for diseases, how long it takes for an animal to build up immunity, when the animals are going to be handled for any reason, and when the potential stressors occur in an animal's life. For example, when is the best time to vaccinate a dairy cow against pathogens associated with calfhood diarrhea? Calves desperately need to ingest the antibodies in the colostrum of its dam (passive immunization) to allow them to handle infections until they were able to build their own immune response. The cow needs several weeks after vaccination to develop significant antibody concentrations that can be deposited into colostrum. So, keeping biology and management practices in mind, in this example, it is best to vaccinate the dam in the weeks before calving so the dam can deliver these antibodies through the colostrum to the calf to prepare the calf's immune system for a potential exposure in the first week of life.
- Read the label of the vaccines! What is the dosage and route for vaccine administration? How long will the immunity last? Some vaccines are for heifers only and some must not be given during pregnancy.

Other vaccines (in particular those against zoonotic pathogens) are to be administered by the veterinarian only. Additionally, you have to remember that you are administering a biological drug to a food production animal. Therefore, you need to consider withdrawal times to ensure safety of meat and milk from that animal as products from that animal may enter the human food chain. Withdrawal times may be based on the organism itself or on other components of the vaccine (for example, preservatives or adjuvants).

BEEF CATTLE

The role of vaccines in a preventative health program for beef cattle is to prevent or eliminate clinical disease in an individual or a population of cattle. This is accomplished by decreasing the incidence and severity of disease through increased level of immunity as part of a preventive health program. No vaccine is 100% effective. Vaccines are part of a preventive health program that should include management procedures and handling, parasite control, and nutritional considerations that reflect an in-depth understanding of not only the beef production system but also farm-specific issues and goals.

Factors to Consider in Developing a Vaccination Strategy

When developing a vaccination strategy, several factors must be considered. Some of these factors are:

- Class of cattle (age)
    - Nursing calves, weaned calves, yearling cattle, replacement heifers, pregnant cows, open cows, breeding bulls
- Production system the cattle are in
    - Cow-Calf, Stocker/Backgrounder, Feedlot
    - Open system (purchasing and bringing in cattle) vs. Closed system
- What to vaccinate for
    - Reproductive Diseases
    - Respiratory Diseases
    - Systemic Diseases
- Goals of the producer / history
    - Future plans, direction, etc.
    - Previous challenges/approaches
- Risk tolerance of the producer
    - High vs. Low

    - Expectations
- Facility availability / husbandry skills
    - Ease of handling, stress of handling
    - Labor needed/available
    - Compliance ability

Vaccination does not equal immunization, so designing the vaccine program also requires consideration of factors affecting immune response. These factors can include:

- **Age of calf**
    - The bovine's immune system begins to develop prior to birth but does not reach maximum responsiveness until later in life.
    - In addition there is thought to be "maternal interference" where passive immunity obtained through colostrum consumption may interfere with ability for young calves to respond to some vaccines.
- **Nutritional Status**
    - Current and previous nutritional status should be considered. Cattle that have been deficient in key components (protein, energy, vitamins, and minerals) may have a decreased ability to mount an immune response.
- **Stressors**
    - Vaccines should be administered at times of low or minimized stress and, if possible, prior to expected stressors. Common stressors include environmental temperature, disease status, parasite load, transport, weaning, nutritional changes, handling, management practices (castration, dehorning, etc), and comingling.
- **Timing of vaccination**
    - The time between vaccination and challenge by infectious agents is important. If using a killed vaccine, you need adequate time for a booster dose when first administering.
    - Additional considerations such as time following parturition or prior to breeding, colostrum production, pregnancy status, and avoiding stressors are important as well.
    - Try to incorporate vaccination with other herd management procedures when possible to take full advantage of handling efficiencies; your goal is to minimize frequency of handling, which is a stressor.

Recommended Vaccination Schedules

Preventive health programs for beef cattle in the upper Midwest provide recommendations for vaccines at specific lifestages.

Calves

LIFESTAGE	RECOMMENDED VACCINE
Birth	+/- Oral Scours vaccine +/-IBR, PI3, BRSV(intranasal)
Branding (mid summer) or Prebreeding	IBR, PI3, BRSV, BVD I & II 7/8 way Clostridia (+/- tetanus) +/- **Mannheimia-Pasteurella** +/- Pinkeye (**Moraxella bovis**)
Preweaning	IBR, PI3, BRSV, BVD I & II **Mannheimia-Pasteurella** 7/8 way Clostridia (+/- tetanus) +/- **Histophilus (Hemophilus)**
Weaning	IBR, PI3, BRSV, BVD I & II +/- 7/8 way Clostridia (+/- tetanus)
At entry to feedlot (Variable; based on vaccine history and risk class)	IBR, PI3, BRSV, BVD I & II **Mannheimia-Pasteurella** 7/8 way Clostridia (+/- tetanus) +/- **Histophilus (Hemophilus)**
Revaccination (Variable; based on vaccine history and risk class)	+/-IBR, PI3, BRSV, BVD I & II +/-**Mannheimia-Pasteurella** +/-7/8 way Clostridia (+/- tetanus) booster +/- **Histophilus (Hemophilus)** booster

Beef Replacement Heifers

LIFESTAGE	RECOMMENDED VACCINES
Prebreeding 1 (8-10 months)	IBR, PI3, BRSV, BVD I & II 5 way Lepto +/- **Lepto hardjo-bovis** +/- Vibrio (**Campylobacter fetus**) **Brucellosis**
Prebreeding 2 (30 days before breeding)	IBR, PI3, BRSV, BVD I & II 5 way Lepto booster +/- **Lepto hardjo-bovis** booster +/- Vibrio (**Campylobacter fetus**) booster +/- 7/8 way Clostridia booster

LIFESTAGE	RECOMMENDED VACCINES
Precalving 1 if on a fall (pregnant cow) vaccine schedule	IBR, PI3, BRSV, BVD I & II (May use MLV if vaccinated prebreeding with MLV) 5 way Lepto +/- **Lepto hardjo-bovis** +/- Vibrio (**Campylobacter fetus**) +/-Scours vaccine
Precalving 2 (5-7 weeks precalving)	+/-Scours vaccine booster
Move to cow schedule	

Adult Cows and Bulls

LIFESTAGE	RECOMMENDED VACCINES
Fall Pregnancy Check or Prebreeding	IBR, PI3, BRSV, BVD I & II 5 way Lepto +/- **Lepto hardjo-bovis** +/- Vibrio (**Campylobacter fetus**) +/- 7/8 way Clostridia booster
Precalving (3-7 weeks precalving)	+/- Scours vaccine booster

Vaccination Risks and Methods

As in small animals, side-effects can occur with vaccination in cattle. These include soreness/swelling/knots at the injection site, fever, off-feed, and potentially anaphylaxis (allergic reactions). "Endotoxin stacking," the act of giving multiple killed bacterin vaccines (often Gram negative or Gram negative-like) vaccines together, has been associated with higher incidence of adverse reactions, failed immune response, and death.To minimize vaccine risks:

- Avoid the administration of more than two killed bacterin vaccines at the same time
- Do not shake killed bacterial vaccine such as clostridial (black-leg) products
- Never vaccinate on days where cattle are heat stressed
- Store vaccines properly
- 35-45oF, DO NOT FREEZE, and avoid sunlight
- Administer with proper care
- Only use licensed, quality vaccines

Beef Quality Assurance Vaccination Administration Guidelines

Any injection has the ability to cause a detectable lesion at slaughter. Beef Quality Assurance programs offer guidelines in proper administration of injectable products with the goal of maintaining and increasing the quality of the end product.Some general recommendations include:

- Use vaccines labeled for subcutaneous route of administration whenever possible.
- Administer all vaccines in the neck region.
- Inject in a clean site.
- Replace needles frequently or use single use needles.
- Use an appropriately sized needle for the intended injection route.
- Use good sanitation when withdrawing vaccines.
- Use properly cleaned and maintained syringes.

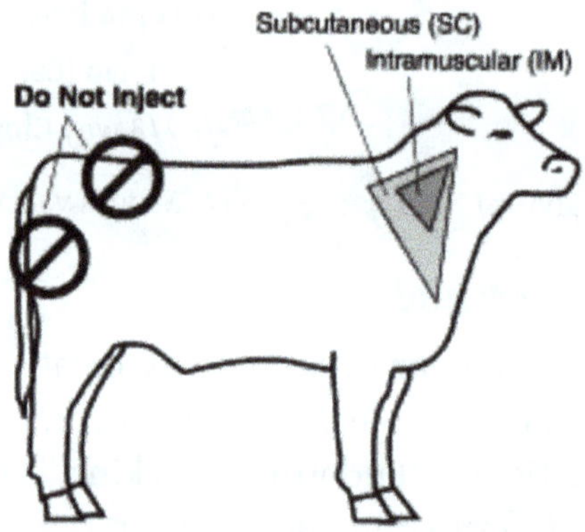

"Injection sites", https://www.ag.ndsu.edu/bqa/documents/injections

Route of Vaccine Administration in Cattle

	Subcutaneous (SC) (1/2 to 3/4 inch needle*)			Intravenous (IV) (1 1/2 inch needle*)			Intramuscular (IM) (1 to 1 1/2 inch needle*)		
Cattle Weight (lbs)	<300	300-700	>700	<300	300-700	>700	<300	300-700	>700
Gauge needle required for thin injectable viscosity (ex: saline)	18	18-16	16	18-16	16	16-14	20-18	18-16	18-16
Gauge needle required for thick injectable viscosity (ex: oxytetracycline)	18-16	18-16	16	16	16-14	16-14	18	16	16

*Select the needle to fit the cattle size (the smallest practical size without bending)
—"Recommended needle size", https://bqa.unl.edu/bqanebr-article-3

Diseases to Vaccinate Against in Beef and Dairy Cattle

Diseases in beef and dairy cattle to vaccinate against, include:

- Bovine viral diarrhea (BVD)
- Infectious bovine rhinotracheitis (IBR)
- Parainfluenza (PI3)
- Bovine respiratory disease complex
- Leptospirosis
- Campylobacter
- Clostridial diseases
- Brucellosis

Bovine Viral Diarrhea

BVD is a common cause of respiratory and reproductive issues in the herd. It is an economically important disease in many countries. The disease is caused by the bovine viral diarrhea virus, which may cause primary disease or be part of a large complex of infections. Cows infected during pregnancy may abort, give birth to a stillborn calf, or give birth to a live calf. Calves can be infected *in utero* or after birth. Calves born carrying BVD virus will never clear the infection and will shed the virus continuously into the farm environment. Signs of BVD in adults are highly variable and include fever, lethargy, loss of appetite, ocular discharge, nasal discharge, diarrhea, and decreased milk production. Infected calves may have cerebellar hypoplasia; signs of this are ataxia, tremors, a wide stance, and failure to nurse.

Infectious Bovine Rhinotracheitis

IBR is a highly contagious, infectious respiratory disease that is caused by bovine herpesvirus I. It can affect young and older cattle. IBR causes acute inflammation of the respiratory tract; clinical signs include those of respiratory disease (mucosal hyperemia, erosive mucosal lesions, nasal discharge, coughing), and also conjunctivitis, abortion, and encephalitis. After the first infection, the virus is sequestered in neurons in the brain as a latent infection. At times of stress, the virus undergoes recrudescence and can be shed from the eyes and nose. Because an infected animal never clears the virus, animals that are seropositive for bovine herpesvirus 1 cannot be shipped into countries that are free of the disease and cannot be housed in artificial insemination (AI) centers. Carrier cattle should be identified and removed from the herd.

Parainfluenza

The PI3 virus infects the upper respiratory mucosa, where it is shed in aerosols (sneezing and coughing) and by direct contact. PI3 causes only respiratory disease. In mature cattle, infection is mild. The most important consequence of PI3 infection in bovine respiratory disease is that it predisposes animals to concurrent infection with IBR or bacterial respiratory pathogens.

Bovine Respiratory Disease Complex

Bovine respiratory disease complex is caused by a variety of pathogens, including the three above. Other organisms against which cattle may be vaccinated to minimize this disease complex are bovine respiratory syncytial virus (BRSV) and bacteria including *Pasteurella multocida, Mannheimia haemolytica,* and *Histophilus* (formerly *Hemophilus) somnus*. These pathogens interact with each other to cause disease. Disease is worsened in the presence of stressors including parasites, weaning, change of feed, variation in ambient temperature and humidity, and weather. Clinical signs depend on age of the animal, organism(s) involved, and stage of the disease. Bovine respiratory disease is closely linked with fever; it is one of the most common causes of fever in cattle and fever may be the first sign of disease in affected cattle. Other signs include mental dullness, lack of appetite, rapid shallow breathing, and discharge from the nose and eyes (watery to purulent to bloody). Coughing will be mild and tentative early in the disease course and prominent ("honking") later in the disease course.

Leptospirosis

Leptospirosis is a zoonotic disease, caused by bacteria of the genus *Leptospira*. There are many different serotypes of disease and prevalence varies with geographic location. Serovars include hardjo-bovis, pomona, canicola, icterohaemmorhagiae, and grippotyphosa. Maintenance hosts, also called reservoir hosts, carry the bacteria and are a source of exposure to other susceptible animals. Maintenance hosts for leptospirosis include cattle, pigs, dogs, raccoons, skunks, and rodents. Animals can be infected by serovars maintained by their own species (host-adapted infection) or by serovars maintained by other species (non-host-adapted infection). Leptospirosis can be transmitted either directly between animals or indirectly, through the environment. Cattle are the maintenance hosts for L. hardo-bovis; disease in cattle with this serovar is less severe but can have a significant economic impact. Cattle infected with other seorvars, especially L. pomona, suffer more severe illness. Clinical signs vary with the herd's degree of resistance or immunity, the infecting serovar, and the age of the animal infected. Host-adapted infections in cattle can occur in animals of any age and mainly affect fertility and the renal system. Infected cattle may shed the organism in their urine for weeks to months. Non-host-adapted infection in cattle is typically due to L. pomona and mainly affects the hemolymphatic, urinary, and reproductive systems. Acute disease is characterized by hemolytic anemia, which causes red urine and jaundice. Reproductive effects include infertility, stillbirths, and abortion 1-3 months after infection. Lactating cows may suffer from mastitis, with decreased production and milk that is thick and yellow.

Campylobacter

Campylobacteriosis, formerly called Vibriosis, is caused by the bacterium *Campylobacter fetus* and is spread by infected bulls when they mate with susceptible cows and heifers. Once infected, a bull remains an asymptomatic carrier of the condition. Transmission is venereal; non-venereal transmission is unlikely to occur. When introduced to a herd the disease spreads rapidly because the cows and heifers have no immunity. Conception rates drop to around %40. As immunity develops, the disease rate drops but reinfection often occurs as immunity wanes about a year after the initial infection. Conception rates in chronically infected herds are usually between 65 and %75, with replacement heifers (newly introduced animals) being most severely affected. The infection can prevent implantation of a fertilized egg in the uterine lining, or more commonly, causes death of the developing embryo. When the embryo is lost, the cow goes back into heat and usually can be rebred successfully, since she has now developed immunity. Occasionally the disease results in permanent infertility.

Clostridial Diseases

Clostridial diseases strike cattle suddenly, often causing death before any clinical signs are seen. The bacteria that cause these diseases create very long-lived spores that are found everywhere in the environment and can easily be picked up by grazing cattle or enter the body through a wound. Bacteria may live in the gastrointestinal tract and spores also may be present in the tissues of healthy animals. Not all species of *Clostridium* cause disease but those that do usually are fatal. Examples include:

- *C. septicum - malignant edema*
- *C. chauvoei - blackleg*
- *C. perfringens types A, B, C, and D - enterotoxemia*
- *C. tetani - tetanus*
- *C. botulinum - botulism*

Contributing factors are necessary to allow the bacteria to multiply and cause disease. This may include injury or invasive procedures such as surgery, giving birth (parturition), or puncture wounds. Diet changes, overeating, and acidosis may permit clostridial organisms in the gut to multiply and cause disease. Clinical signs differ depending on the specific organism and may include sudden death in apparently healthy animals, lethargy or depression, high fever, anorexia, localized stiffness or muscle spasms, port wine colored urine, acute lameness and swelling in the hips and shoulders with a crackling sound when the skin is pressed (blackleg), or flaccid paralysis (botulism).

Brucellosis

Brucellosis is an infectious disease that spreads between animal species and between animals and humans. In cattle, the bacterium involved usually is *Brucella abortus*. Brucellosis is highly contagious, spreading very easily between cattle. The primary clinical sign is late-term abortion and the aborted calf, membranes, and fluids all contain large numbers of bacteria.

SMALL RUMINANTS

Vaccination Methods

Vaccines cannot replace good management practices. When vaccinating sheep and goats, make sure they are healthy animals, and that the injection site is clean and dry to prevent introducing infection with your injection. Make sure you have adequate handling facilities such as a properly constructed chute or pen. When vaccinating multiple animals using an automatic syringe, verify that the correct dose is being administered. Needles should be changed every 12-20 animals (generally every pen or chute-full) and anytime the needle is dull, burred, or bent. Some facilities will be part of specific disease-control programs (caprine arthritis encephalitis virus (CAE) or ovine progressive pneumonia (OPP)); in that instance, multi-dose syringes may be used but a new needle must be used for each animal. In general, 18 gauge 5/8" needles are used for adult animals and 20 gauge 1/2 to 5/8" needles are used for young animals. Make sure all animals are individually identified (tags, tattoos) and that there is a system for record keeping so you know which animals received which vaccines.

To vaccinate, part the wool if necessary, raise the skin to form a tent and insert the needle into the tent opening so that the needle is almost parallel with the neck. The site of injection is important if the animal you are vaccinating is to be used for food. Vaccines are given so as to minimize carcass and hide degradation due to abscess or scar formation. Vaccines should be given subcutaneously in the neck region or in the ventral aspect of the axillary space. The meat from these regions is of low value and pelt damage in these areas easily can be trimmed with minimal effect on value. Injection over the ribs is not optimal but it can be used if the animal cannot be restrained to allow you to use another location.

How to Vaccinate Sheep and Goats

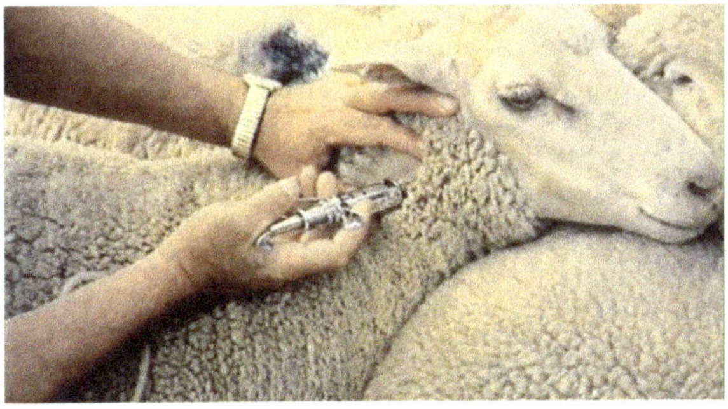

"Sheep vaccinating", https://slideplayer.com/slide/4554386/

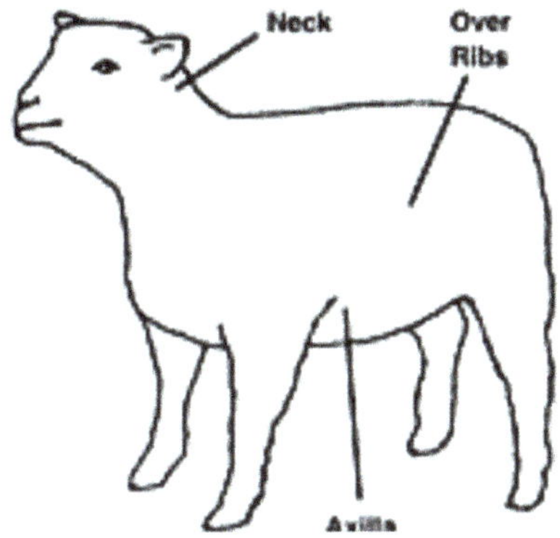

"Sheep injection sites", https://diamondhlivestockoregon.wordpress.com/tag/raisingsheep/

- Factors to Consider in Developing a Vaccination Strategy
- Which vaccines are used depends on:
- History at the individual farm
- Age of the sheep or goats
- Previous disease problems
- Open or closed flock/herd status – are animals coming and going for shows, purchases, breeding?
- Geographic region
- Soil type
- Diet and flock/herd economics
- Withdrawal time (refer to the label!)

To choose vaccines, consider:

- Real and high-likelihood risks
  - Since all ruminants are at risk for Clostridium perfringens type D, toxoid against this agent ideally should be used in all sheep flocks and goat herds
  - Show animals have considerable exposure to contagious ecthyma virus (soremouth) and caseous lymphadenitis
  - Open flocks have exposure to foot rot and abortion diseases
- All animals should be vaccinated with:

- **CD-T vaccine–** *Clostridium perfringens* is more commonly called enterotoxemia or overeating disease. Type C primarily affects lambs and kids during their first few weeks of life. Type D (pulpy kidney disease) affects lambs and kids that are usually over a month of age, particularly those that are creep-fed or finished on concentrate diets. *Clostridium tetani* is the causative agent of tetanus. CD-T toxoid is the vaccine usually used to protect healthy sheep and goats against these clostridial diseases.

- Most animals should be vaccinated against Campylobacter and Chlamydophila (abortion diseases) and contagious ecthyma (soremouth).
- Some animals should be vaccinated against contagious lymphadenitis and rabies and even more rarely, against E. coli, bluetongue virus, and Brucella ovis.
- Some people recommend use of cattle or equine vaccines in small ruminants but they are not labeled for this use and efficacy has not been well demonstrated.

Diseases in Sheep and Goats

Diseases to be vaccinated against in sheep and goats include:

- Clostridial diseases
- Abortion diseases in sheep
- Contagious ecthyma (soremouth, orf, scabby mouth or pustular dermatitis
- Caseous lymphadenitis (CLA, boils, abscesses or cheesy gland)

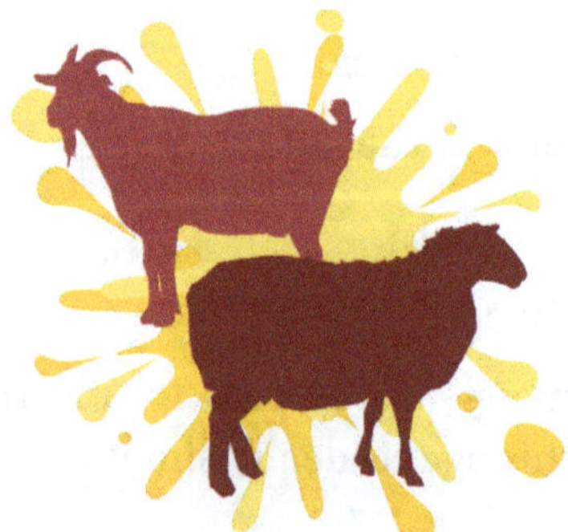

Clostridial Diseases

Clostridial organisms of various types are found in the soil, where they can survive for a very long time. Most clostridial organisms also survive naturally in the gastrointestinal tract of healthy animals. Sheep can be infected with various clostridial diseases (see diseases in cattle) but the most common are enterotoxemia types C and D and tetanus. Enterotoxemia type C (hemorrhagic enteritis or bloody scours) is caused by *Clostridium perfringens type C* and affects lambs during their first few weeks of life, causing a bloody infection of the small intestine. It is often related to indigestion and is predisposed by a sudden change in feed, for example an increase in the dam's milk supply or beginning creep feeding as lambs are being weaned. Enterotoxemia type D (overeating disease or pulpy kidney disease) is caused by *Clostridium perfringens type D* and commonly strikes the largest, fastest growing lambs in the flock. It is caused by a sudden change in the feed that causes the organism, which is already present in the lamb's gastrointestinal tract, to proliferate, causing a toxic reaction. It is most common in lambs that are on high concentrate rations but can also occur when lambs are nursing from dams that are heavy milkers. It usually affects lambs over one month of age. Sudden death may be the first sign. Other clinical manifestations include neurologic signs, seizures, and diarrhea. Tetanus is caused by *Clostridium tetani*, a soil inhabitant that is a prolific spore producer. This disease is usually related to tail docking and castration, although any wound can harbor the tetanus organism. Signs of tetanus occur from about 4 days to 3 weeks or longer after infection is established in a wound. The animal may have a stiff gait, lockjaw can develop, and the third eyelid may protrude across the eye. The animal usually will go down with all four legs held out straight and stiff and the head drawn back. Convulsions may occur.

Abortion Diseases

Ewes or does that lose their lambs early in pregnancy may not return to heat because they are seasonal breeders, and so may not be bred back that season. This is a significant loss for the producer both because of decreased lamb crop and because those dams will not lactate that season. Pregnancy also may be lost late in gestation or weak or deformed lambs may be born. For many diseases causing abortion in small ruminants, there is no vaccine in the United States (for example, Q fever, toxoplasmosis, Border disease). In the United States, the most common causes of abortion in ewes are *Chlamydia / Chlamydophila* (enzootic abortion) and *Campylobacter*. Enzootic abortion is transmitted from aborting dams to other females in the flock. Ewe lambs are the most susceptible on farms where the organism is present. Abortion usually is seen late in pregnancy or lambs may be born that die shortly after birth. Campylobacteriosis (formerly called Vibriosis) causes abortion late in pregnancy or birth of stillborn or weak lambs. Infecting organisms are *Campylobacter jejuni* and *Campylobacter fetus*. Ewes are infected orally and the incubation time from ingestion to abortion is just 2 weeks.

Contagious Ecthyma (soremouth, orf, scabby mouth, or pustular dermatitis)

Soremouth is the most common skin disease affecting sheep and goats. It is a highly contagious viral infection that also can produce painful infections in humans. The virus causes scab formation on the skin, usually around the mouth, nostrils, eyes, mammary glands, and vulva. It first appears as tiny red nodules, usually at the junctions of the lips.

Caseous Lymphadenitis (CLA, boils, abscesses, or cheesy gland)

Caseous lymphadenitis is an infectious, contagious disease that primarily infects the lymphatic system, though other organs can be affected. It is caused by *Corynebacterium pseudotuberculosis*. Infection results in abscess formation in the lymph nodes that when cut or ruptured, discharge pus containing the bacteria in the surroundings. When the infection spreads internally, affected animals slowly lose weight and eventually become emaciated.

- Vaccines for Disease in Sheep and Goats
- Specific vaccines that are available are:
- CD-T (*Clostridium perfringens types* C and D and tetanus toxoid)
- Abortion vaccines
- Contagious ecthyma (soremouth, orf)
- Caseous lymphadenitis (CLA)
- Rabies
- CD-T (***Clostridium perfringens types*** **C** and ***D*** and tetanus toxoid)

Protection against type C is needed by nursing lambs and kids on all farms, regardless of management practices. Maternal antibodies will be present in colostrum if the ewe/doe was vaccinated in the 2-4 weeks prior to parturition. This passive immunity lasts in the lamb/kid for their first 50-60 days of life. Protection against type D is needed in lambs/kids fed grain or lush forage (any high-carbohydrate diet). It is associated with production of a toxin that is acutely fatal in fast-growing lambs. Tetanus toxoid is included in this product. Ewes and does should be vaccinated 8 weeks prior to the first time they give birth, and boostered at 2-4 weeks prior to parturition. Previously vaccinated ewes and does only require the vaccination 2-4 weeks prior to parturition. Offspring from vaccinated dams are vaccinated at weaning and again 3-4 weeks later. Offspring from unvaccinated dams are vaccinated as newborns (may have systemic reaction, can be treated with epinephrine) and are boostered at 3-4 weeks of age and again at weaning. All animals, including males, should be boostered at least annually; some goats may only maintain protective antibody titers for six months after vaccination.

Abortion Vaccines

In general, do not vaccinate if there are no problems on the farm or if animals are determined to be at low risk. Risk is associated with having an open flock, with animal traffic on and off the farm, with free-roaming wildlife, feeding on the ground, or with a history of abortions in the flock. Diagnosis for abortion problems is difficult and for many diseases causing abortion in small ruminants, there is no vaccine in the United States (for example, Q fever, toxoplasmosis, Border disease).

- Chlamydia / Chlamydophila (enzootic abortion) vaccine may not be effective against all strains causing abortions and regional variations in protection may exist. The label states that the vaccine should be administered 60 days prior to breeding with a booster in 30 days.
- Campylobacter (formerly called Vibrio) vaccination induces immunity for only 4-5 months. The label states that the first dose of vaccine should be given 2 weeks prior to breeding and that it should be boostered 2-3 months later. In the face of an "abortion storm," where many abortions are occurring in the flock due to this organism, revaccination of all animals may reduce losses.

Contagious Ecthyma (Soremouth, orf)

This is a live virus vaccine that will introduce a mild infection. This vaccine should only be used if this disease is present in the flock. The vaccine is given percutaneously; an area of skin in a wool-less region (inside the thigh or ear, or under the tail) is scarified in the form of an X deeply enough to cause inflammation but not so deeply as to cause bleeding. The vaccine is brushed on. The vaccinated area will scab over and does contain live virus that will be infective even after falling off the sheep. Vaccination under the tail is preferred to that inside the thigh, as vaccination on the medial thigh region may cause irritation and scabbing over the mammary glands and teats. This is a zoonotic disease so people should wear gloves and exercise caution when handling the vaccine or sheep, or picking up scabs. On farms that have a problem with this disorder, each new lamb and kid crop should be vaccinated. Lambs moving into feedlots should be vaccinated at least 14 days before shipment. Do not use this vaccine on farms that do not already have this disorder.

Caseous Lymphadenitis (CLA)

This may be a stand-alone vaccine or combined with CD-T vaccine. Vaccination decreases severity of disease but does not prevent disease. The vaccine should not be used in flocks or herds unless they have been exposed or contain affected individuals.

Rabies

This is a killed vaccine. Several products are available for sheep. No products are specifically labeled for goats but there is a recommendation in some situations that publicly displayed goats will be vaccinated. For example, goats take to a show that will be housed in a pen probably will not be vaccinated for rabies, while goats at a petting zoo that are purposefully brought to that site to interact with people will be vaccinated for rabies. Animals are vaccinated when greater than 3 months of age and then annually.

SWINE

Vaccination is a common preventive medicine practice on commercial swine farms. Vaccination protocols for swine typically focus upon preventing diseases of the reproductive, respiratory, and gastrointestinal tracts, and preventing multi-systemic disease. Vaccines may be applied to the reproductive herd (sows and boars), replacement females (gilts), or growing pigs, depending on when the disease challenge is expected.

Forms of Vaccination Production

- Commercial (manufactured and sold by pharmaceutical companies)
- Autogenous (typically manufactured by a licensed laboratory from organisms isolated from the farm of concern)
- On Farm – Typically includes other, less controlled, methods that stimulate immunity such as oral feeding of infectious organisms ('biofeedback') or inoculation with serum from viremic animals (serum inoculation)

Routes of administration for swine vaccines typically include IM or oral (per os = PO). Multivalent vaccines (those containing multiple organisms) are commonly created to decrease the stress, labor, and food safety issues associated with multiple injections. Swine farm clientele expect that veterinarians will consider the costs and benefits associated with the vaccination protocols they recommend.

Pork Quality Assurance Vaccination Recommendations

Pork Quality Assurance programs strongly encourage the use of vaccines to prevent the necessity of antibiotic therapy and the potential for post therapeutic residues. They recommend the following when administering vaccines to pigs:

- Use a spot on the neck just behind and below the ear, but in front of the shoulder. Do not use a needle to inject in the ham or loin. There may be some bleeding and bruising of the muscle followed by scarring. This scar can stay in the muscle for the life of the pigs and be a blemish in the cut of meat. This standard applies to sows as well as market hogs. While sows may not be going to market soon, they are at greater risk for blemishes because of the repeated injections they typically receive over their productive life in the form of vaccinations and farrowing medications.

- Use the proper size and length of needle to ensure the medication is deposited in the muscle, not in other tissues.

	GAUGE OF NEEDLE	LENGTH OF NEEDLE (INCHES)
Baby Pigs	18 or 20	½ or ⅝
Nursery Pigs	16 or 18	⅝ or ¾
Finisher Pigs	16	1
Breeding Stock	14, 15 or 16	1 or 1½

Diseases in Swine

Diseases to vaccinate against in swine include:

- Leptospirosis
- Erysipelas
- Porcine parvovirus (PPV)
- Porcine Reproductive and Respiratory Syndrome (PRRS)
- *Mycoplasma hyopneumoniae*
- Influenza
- *Escherichia coli*
- Rotavirus
- Porcine Proliferative Enteritis (PPE)
- Porcine Circovirus Type 2 (PCV2)
- Meningitis

Leptospirosis

As in cattle, leptospirosis is a zoonotic disease, caused by bacteria of the genus *Leptospira*. There are many different serotypes of disease and prevalence varies with geographic location. Worldwide, pigs are the maintenance hosts for pomona, tarassovi, bratislava, and muenchen. Pomona causes important reproductive problems in breeding sows, spreading slowly through the herd. The skunk is a reservoir host. Once the organism is introduced into a herd, the pigs become permanent carriers with infection of the kidneys and intermittent excretion of the organism into the urine. Piglets rarely are infected. The most common manifestation is chronic low-grade disease in sows, with abortions, stillbirths, and birth of weak piglets.

Erysipelas

Swine erysipelas is caused by a bacterium, *Erysipelothrix rhusiopathiae,* that is found on most if not all pig farms. Up to half of the animals on a farm may carry it in their tonsils. It is excreted in saliva, feces, and urine, and so is common in the environment. It is also found in many other species, including birds, and can survive for long periods in the environment. The bacterium alone may cause disease but clinical disease is more common if there is concurrent infection with viral diseases such as porcine reproductive and respiratory syndrome (PRRS) virus and influenza. Disease is relatively uncommon in pigs under 12-8 weeks of age due to protection provided by maternal antibodies from colostrum. The most susceptible animals are growing pigs, non-vaccinated gilts, and young sows. Infected sows may show acute death in apparently healthy animals, fever, abortion, stillbirths, birth of mummified piglets, raised areas in the skin ("diamonds") that turn red and then black, or joint stiffness. Infertility may be a presenting concern on a farm. Infected boars with high fevers have transient decrease in semen quality, reflected as sows not getting pregnant or having smaller litters. Infected growing pigs may show acute death, fever, and the characteristic skin lesion described above.

Porcine Parvovirus (PPV)

PPV is the most common and important cause of infectious infertility in pigs. Porcine parvovirus multiplies normally in the intestine of the pig without causing clinical signs. It is worldwide in its distribution. PPV can persist in the environment for many months and is resistant to most disinfectants. Infected sows show only reproductive signs of disease. Parvovirus is associated with lack of conception, birth of mummified or stillborn pigs, and birth of live pigs with low birth weight. Sporadic disease is seen in individual females that are infected for the first time; for this reason, disease usually is seen in gilts. Once a pig is exposed, it has lifelong immunity. Reproductive problems in a herd appear about every 3-4 years if vaccination is not practiced.

Porcine Reproductive and Respiratory Syndrome (PRRS)

This is a fairly new disease; it has only been recognized in the United States since the mid-1980s and was only identified as being caused by an arterivirus in 1991. The virus has an affinity for macrophages, especially those in the lung. Up to 40% of macrophages are destroyed in a given animal, making it susceptible to other diseases. When introduced into a new herd, 90% of breeding sows will be seropositive within 4-5 months. Grower pigs shed virus for months; adult pigs shed virus for periods of time as short as 2 weeks. Nasal secretions, saliva, feces, and urine may contain virus. The virus can be airborne for up to 2 miles and can be carried between pigs and on fomites (inanimate objects) including boots, equipment, and trucks. The virus also may be carried by flies and mosquitoes. The clinical picture varies tremendously from one herd to another. As a guide, for every three herds that are exposed to PRRS for the first time, one will show no recognizable disease, the second will show mild disease, and the third will show moderate to severe disease. The reasons for this are not clearly understood. Clinical signs in sows include inappetance; fever; abortions; early farrowing with birth of mummified, stillborn, or weak pigs; prolonged return to heat after weaning of piglets; coughing; lack of milk and mastitis; lethargy; and cyanosis (blue discoloration) of the ears. This is the acute phase of the disease. Long-term, reproductive efficiency in herds in which the infection has become enzootic are associated with 10-15% reduction in farrowing rate, increased stillbirths, increased number of abortions, and inappetance in sows at farrowing. Infected piglets may show diarrhea and increase in other respiratory infections. Infected weaning and growing pigs may show other infections secondary to PRRS infection with a variety of clinical signs and mortality rate as high as 12-15%.

Mycoplasma hyopneumoniae

This is one of the most important contributors to respiratory disease in pigs. The organism damages the cilia and epithelia of the airways of the lower respiratory tract, permitting infection with other organisms, for example PRRS virus. Mycoplasma is transmitted via direct contact with infected pigs. Pigs older than 6 weeks are mainly those affected. Clinical signs include a non-productive cough, rough hair coat, and reduced growth rate and feed efficiency. With secondary bacterial infection, signs are more severe and include labored breathing, a harsher cough, fever, and prostration.

Influenza

Influenza viruses are the cause of outbreaks of acute respiratory disease. Influenza A viruses infect a wide range of avian and mammalian species, with the latter group including humans, pigs, horses, and aquatic mammals. Type A viruses are known for their ability to change their antigenic structure and create new strains. The type A viruses are further divided into serotypes, based on the antigenic nature of their surface glycoproteins hemagglutinin (H) and neuraminidase (N). Swine influenza in large herds may become endemic with intermittent bouts of disease and infertility. Different influenza strains may sequentially infect the herd. Immunity to influenza viruses is often short-lived (6 months). Outbreaks are seen throughout the year. Piglets generally are protected by maternal antibodies they receive in colostrum. Sows may show pregnancy loss secondary to fever and coughing. Weaner and grower pigs with acute illness classically are fine one day and then lying prostrate and breathing heavily the next.

Escherichia coli

Diarrhea is the most common and important disease of piglets. In a well-managed herd, there should be fewer than 3% of litters at any time requiring treatment for diarrhea and piglet mortality from diarrhea should be less than 0.5%. At birth, the gastrointestinal tract is microbiologically sterile. Organisms begin to colonize the tract quickly after birth, among them potentially pathogenic strains of *E. coli.* Ingestion of colostrum and later, of milk containing IgA, is vital for creation of immunity within the intestinal tract. If too many bacteria are present or if there are stressors present such as chilling or concurrent infection, piglets will succumb to disease. Periods of greatest risk are before 5 days of age and between 7 and 14 days of age. Weaning is another risk, as loss of sow's milk and the IgA it contains allows the bacteria to attach to the villi of the small intestines. Signs may include acute death, dehydration, and sticky feces around the rectum and tail with an accompanying characteristic sour smell.

Rotavirus

This virus is widespread in pig populations, with virtually 100% seroconversion in adult stock. It is resistant to environmental changes and many disinfectants and so persists for long periods of time in the environment. Piglets are initially protected from maternal antibodies in colostrum but become susceptible to infection by about 3-6 weeks of age. Exposure does not necessarily result in disease; it is estimated that only 10-15% of diarrheas in pigs are due to primary rotavirus infection. The virus destroys the intestinal villi, preventing fluid uptake and causing watery diarrhea.

Porcine Proliferative Enteritis (PPE)

This is a disease characterized histologically by inflammation, ulceration, and hemorrhage in the intestinal tract. The causative organism, *Lawsonia intracellularis*, is a unique obligate intracellular organism related to anaerobic bacteria. Clinical disease is characterized as an acute form common in young adults and a chronic or necrotic form in grower pigs. Carrier animals shed the organism in their feces and susceptible pigs are exposed through the fecal-oral route. Carrier sows may infect nursing pigs as early as 6 days of age. Pigs present with pallor, weakness, and rapid death. Subacute to chronic cases occur more frequently in grower pigs, which show sporadic diarrhea, wasting, and variation in growth rate.

Porcine Circovirus Type 2 (PCV2)

This is a widespread virus and essentially all pig herds are infected. However, very few have PCV2-associated disease which can include a variety of systemic disorders including clinical signs of wasting, pneumonia, enteritis, and reproductive failure. The hallmark of PCV2 infection is depletion or inflammation of lymphoid tissue. In many cases, PCV2 infection requires a trigger such as concurrent infection (PRRS virus, *Mycoplasma hyopneumoniae*) or other stressors.

Meningitis

Hemophilus parasuis and *Streptococcus suis* are two organisms associated with inflammation of the meninges in pigs. Signs of meningitis in piglets and weaned pigs include rapid onset of recumbency, shivering, nystagmus (shaking of the eyeballs), paddling, and convulsions. In older pigs (growers and adults), muscle trembling, nystagmus, and incoordination are more common clinical signs.

Vaccines for Disease in Swine

Vaccination for Reproductive Disease

Common vaccinations include:

- Leptospirosis-Erysipelas-Parvovirus combination vaccine
- Each of these components may be administered as individual vaccinations as well
- Porcine Reproductive and Respiratory Syndrome virus (PRRS) vaccine
- Modified live virus vaccine typically thought to be most effective

Common uses are:

- Typically administered twice prior to the first breeding of gilts and once before subsequent gestation periods in reproductive herd (sows and boars)

Vaccination for Respiratory Disease

Common vaccinations include:

- *Mycoplasma hyopneumoniae* vaccine
- Single dose and two dose versions exist
- Swine Influenza virus vaccine
- Normally include H1N1 and H3N2 components
- Porcine Reproductive and Respiratory Syndrome virus (PRRS) vaccine

Common uses are:

- Routine vaccinations in reproductive herds to maintain respiratory disease stability
- Acclimation of disease-negative replacement females as they enter disease-positive herds
- Growing pigs at weaning or during the nursery phase to prevent significant respiratory disease during the finisher phase

Vaccination for Gastrointestinal Disease

Common vaccinations include:

- *Escherichia coli* vaccine
- Multiple strains typically included in the vaccine

- Rotavirus vaccine
- Modified live virus, only one type included in commercial vaccine
- *Lawsonia intracellularis* vaccine
- A modified live vaccine that requires storage at -70°C and it administered orally following thawing and dilution

COMMON USES ARE:

- *Escherichia coli* and Rotavirus vaccines commonly used prior to farrowing to prevent neonatal scours in suckling piglets
- *Lawsonia intracellularis* vaccines administered in late nursery or early finisher (9-12 weeks of age) to prevent ileitis in finisher pigs OR for the acclimation of replacement females into breeding herds

Vaccination for Multi-Systemic Disease

Common vaccinations include:

- Porcine Circovirus Type 2 (PCV2) vaccine
- Currently the most common vaccine used in swine
- Considered to be highly effective in preventing a devastating disease syndrome
- Evidence that it provides effective protection in both single and two dose programs.
- *Hemophilus parasuis* vaccine
- Typically includes multiple serotypes that provide cross protection for other serotypes
- *Erysipelas rhusiopathiae* vaccine
- May be delivered IM or PO
- *Streptococcus suis* vaccine
- Efficacy is questionable
- Commonly produced as an autogenous vaccine

Common uses are:

- These vaccines are often manufactured in combination type products with respiratory specific vaccines to prevent disease in replacement females or growing pigs.

CHAPTER-5
CONTROL FOR PARASITES

PARASITE INFECTION AND TOOLS FOR DIAGNOSIS

Parasites, either internal (for example, worms) or external (for example, fleas and ticks), draw nutrients away from the host, and can cause disease. This chapter will focus on demonstration of how your understanding of the life cycle of parasites for various species in different environments will help minimize infection or infestation and help with control of the parasite in the environment. The biggest difference appears to be in overall management between large animals and small animals. In large animals, there is concern about resistance of parasites to available deworming medications and great attention is paid to minimizing development of resistant parasites. This may include leaving a small population of worms untreated, so there always are susceptible worms in the overall population and we are not just continually killing off susceptible worms and leaving behind more and more resistant worms. In small animals, where parasites can be a significant public health concern, it is a goal to kill all internal and external parasites. This does not mean there are no concerns about resistance; in 2021, resistance in hookworms, one intestinal parasite of dogs, was described.

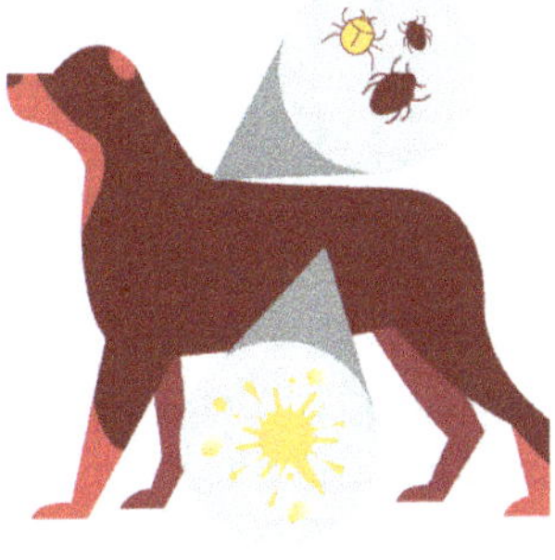

Gastrointestinal parasites are the class most commonly addressed. Some common tools used to evaluate presence of gastrointestinal parasites are fecal flotation tests and fecal egg counts. Fecal egg counts are basically quantified fecal flotations. You will also hear fecal flotations called fecal floats. Dr. Erin Burton provides the following differentiation between these two kinds of tests and how they're interpreted: A fecal flotation is a qualitative assessment of the eggs in a sample, while a fecal egg count (FEC) is a quantitative assessment. Fecal flotations are lax on the amount of solution and feces used for each float and so give at best a semi-quantitative assessment of egg burden. FECs use a measured amount of feces and solution, and then plug the number into a formula to get the egg count. FEC usually is done more than once; in order to interpret them they are performed over time and because of that they are the test primarily used to definitively define the degree of drug resistance in an animal or herd. It is also important when evaluating a fecal float or FEC to be aware of how prolific of an egg layer the nematode is. For example, one *Toxocara canis* (roundworm) can produce over 20,000 eggs each day while a whipworm only produces about 1000 per day. Thus, having larger numbers of whipworm eggs on a float or FEC is more indicative of a heavy worm burden than abundant *Toxocara* eggs on float or FEC. Finally, be aware that not all gastrointestinal parasites can be identified by fecal flotation testing. For example, tapeworm eggs generally are released within tapeworm segments, or proglottids, and because the individual eggs are not in the feces and the proglottids are too heavy to float, tapeworm infections generally cannot be diagnosed by fecal flotation testing.

BEEF CATTLE

Parasites can have potential negative effects on beef cattle that can vary from subclinical immune suppression, irritation, annoyance, appetite suppression, and decreased production, to severe clinical disease and death. The management of parasites is a component of a preventive health program that should also include immunity management (vaccinations), management procedures, handling, and nutritional considerations that reflect an in-depth understanding of not only the beef production system but farm-specific issues and goals.

Internal Parasites

Internal parasites include roundworms (nematodes), tapeworms (cestodes), flukes (trematodes) and protozoans (such as coccidia). Roundworms are considered the most economically important, and many programs revolve around their management. This section regarding internal parasites in beef cattle will focus around roundworms. Understanding the parasite life cycle and the level of parasite pressure is key to the management of internal parasites.

The following is the basic life cycle of internal (gastrointestinal) parasites in cattle:

- Adult parasites live in the gastrointestinal tract of cattle and lay eggs that are shed in the manure.
- When a parasite egg is shed on the pasture in the feces, this egg begins development, embryonating into a first stage larva (L1), then molting into a second stage larva (L2), and finally molting again into a third and infective stage larva (L3).
- During the first two larval stages in the fecal pat, the larva are fairly immobile, feeding off the bacteria and other debris found in the feces.
- During the third larval stage the larva move out of the fecal pat and onto nearby grass where they are consumed by cattle.
- L3 larvae maintain an external sheath covering that provides extra protection from environmental conditions allowing survival during winter or drought conditions. This sheath prevents feeding, thus L3 larvae have a limited life span.
- Egg development is greatly dependent upon temperature and moisture. Eggs that are passed in the middle of winter will not develop until warm weather returns in the spring. Eggs passed in the middle of a drought or other unfavorable conditions may develop into infective larvae in the feces but without moisture cannot move away from the pat where they can be consumed by a host animal when it eats grass. Eggs that are shed during favorable conditions can develop into infective larvae in just a few days if temperatures are warm and moisture is plentiful.
- Once consumed by cattle, the infective larvae mature into adults over a period of 3-4 weeks (shorter in younger cattle, longer in adult cattle) and begin to lay eggs, which are shed onto pastures to start the cycle over again.
- Some larvae can become inhibited or hypobiotic (go into hibernation) in the wall of the abomasum, sometimes referred to as L4 larvae. This process can occur during the winter in the north and in the summer in the south, with these larvae maturing and developing into adult worms when the environment for egg survival is more favorable.

Overall, the controlling of internal parasites has a significant positive return on investment for producers. The main focus of internal parasite control in beef cattle is roundworms. Diagnostics are needed to determine which specific worms are present. For beef cattle this is important because the roundworm life cycle depends on the shedding of the eggs on pasture, larvae development, and the ingestion of the larvae during grazing. Since much of beef cattle production depends on grazing of pastures, the management of roundworms is key. As long as cattle have access to grass, they will have an internal parasite challenge.

Control practices should consider the class (or age) of cattle, nutrition status, stress level, season, and likelihood of parasite contamination of the environment, and involve the use of pasture management options as well as the use of anthelmintic (dewormer) products for treatment.

Life-Cycle of Internal Parasites

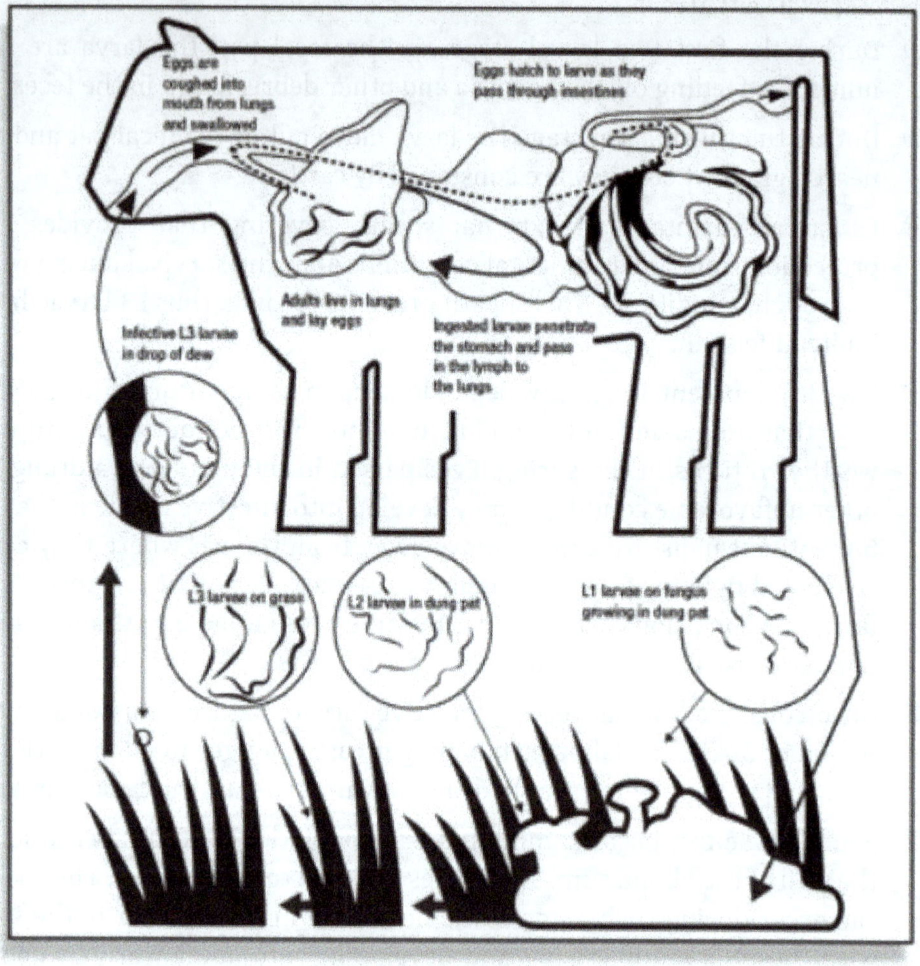

"Lifecycle of a typical roundworm", https://www.progressivecattle.com/topics/management/parasite-control-in-stocker-and-grower-cattle

- Infective L3 larvae in a drop of dew enter the cow's mouth when eating grass.
- Ingested larvae penetrate the stomach and pass in the lymph to the lungs.
- Adults live in lungs and lay eggs.
- Eggs are coughed into mouth from lungs and swallowed.

- Eggs hatch to larvae as they pass through intestines.
- L1 larvae on fungus grow in dung pat.
- L2 larvae live in dung pat.
- L3 larvae move onto grass where they again can be ingested by cows.

Parasite Contamination Susceptibility

PRIORITIZED SUSCEPTIBILITY TO PARASITES	ENVIRONMENTAL PARASITE CONTAMINATION LIKELIHOOD
Calves > Yearlings > Adult bulls > Adult cows	Spring / Early summer > Late summer (dry season) > Winter
Nutritionally challenged > Not nutritionally challenged	Continuously grazed pasture > Rested pasture > Not grazed / Hayed pasture > Recently tilled > Dry lot
Stressed (newly weaned, heat/cold stress, etc) > Not stressed	

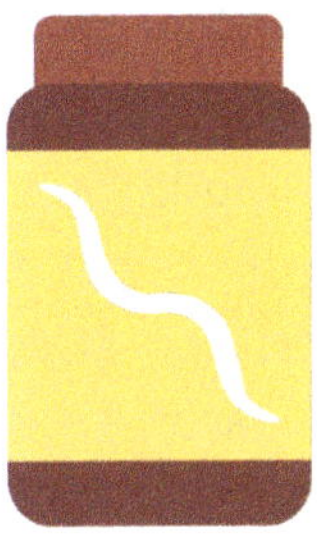

Benzimidazoles (white dewormers)

- Contain albendazole, fenbendazole, or oxfendazole
- Effective against most major adult gastrointestinal parasites

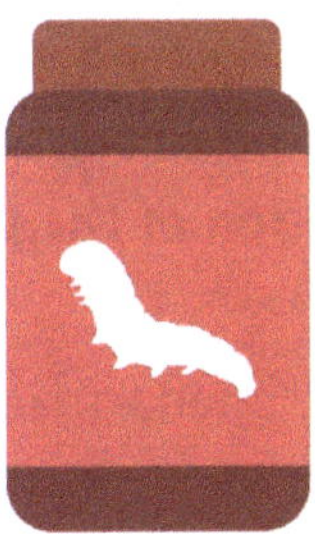

Macrocyclic lactones

- Contain ivermectin, doramectin, eprinomectin, or moxidectin
- Effective against many larval stages and many external parasites

Some pasture management activities may include leaving the pasture fallow, grazing other species, and dragging manure pats during the dry season to allow them to dry out.

Anthelmintics used to control internal parasites for beef cattle come in several forms including paste, injectable, drench, pour-on, bolus, and as a feed or mineral additive. Products have varying lengths of activity and costs, but fall into two main classes: benzimidazoles and macrocylic lactones. Benzimidazoles (white dewormers) available commercially contain albendazole, fenbendazole, or oxfendazole. Benzimidazoles are effective against most of the major adult gastrointestinal parasites and many of the larval stages. Products come in various oral formulations and have a short duration of efficacy. Macrocyclic lactones are the avermectins and milbemycins. Products in commercial use contain ivermectin, doramectin, eprinomectin, or moxidectin. The macrocyclic lactones have a potent, broad antiparasitic spectrum at low dose levels. They are active against many larval stages (including hypobiotic larvae) and are active against many external parasites as well. Products are available as oral, subcutaneous, and pour-on formulations for use in cattle. Duration of efficacy varies with the product and may be up to 35 days.

Approaches used to treat parasites in beef cattle are considered strategic deworming. This is the practice of treating cattle at times to not only get the benefit in that animal to prevent economic loss but also reduce environmental contamination for a period of time at least equal to the life cycle of the parasite removed.

Keys to strategic deworming are to place cattle that are not shedding eggs on pastures that are not infected; this is accomplished by deworming prior to spring turnout or fall treatment in the north (following killing frost). The benefit of treating in the fall is that cattle should be free of internal parasites all winter and going into the spring turnout (assuming an effective product was used). Cattle that go onto pasture at spring turnout are free of parasites, thus not shedding eggs, and will be consuming the infective larvae on the pasture if the pasture is contaminated. By consuming the infective larvae and not shedding new ones the cows will be reducing the load on the pasture (acting as vacuum cleaners). After a time the ingested infective larvae will mature and cows will start shedding eggs. Strategic deworming times the treatment so as to reduce the worm burden on the cattle and also decrease the parasite contamination of the pasture during the highest parasite period (spring/early summer).

The timing of these treatments can and should be timed with other management procedures such as summer vaccines for the calves and fall processing of calves and cows. Depending on the geographic location, such as in the south where the weather (moisture) is different, timings may be different, as well as the type of grazing program.

Calves and stockers should be considered within a strategic program while on a grazing program. Times of concern include prior to weaning while nursing the cow and while intensively grazing as a stocker. Calves should not be dewormed while being weaned. Preweaning treatment, prior to the stress of weaning, can reduce the potential negative impact on immune function as well as improve performance. Any time cattle are moving from pasture into a dry lot setting is a good time to deworm as this should clear cattle of parasite load for the time in the dry lot (similar to fall deworming) as there is no green grass to graze.

For the control of other types of internal parasites such as tapeworms (cestodes), flukes (trematodes), and protozoans (such as coccidia), similar concepts are applied. It is important to understand the different life cycles of these different types of parasites as well as the efficacy of products used to treat them.

External Parasites

The major external parasites that affect cattle include flies, grubs, lice, ticks, and mites. These external parasites feed on body tissues such as blood and skin, and in addition they cause irritation and discomfort that result in reduced weight gain and lost production. Parasites that take blood meals have the potential to serve as vectors for the transmission of diseases.

Horn Flies

Horn flies are blood-sucking flies that stay on the shoulders and backs of cattle almost continuously. A horn fly leaves the back of a cow or calf only to lay eggs in fresh manure. They take blood meals from the host 24 hours a day.

Face Flies

Face flies cluster on the faces of cattle and feed on secretions from the mucous membranes of the eyes, nose, and lips. Face flies do not suck blood. They do irritate the surface of the eyeball and may carry pathogens that contribute to pinkeye problems. They spend only a small portion of their life on cattle.

Stable Flies

Stable flies feed primarily on the legs and lower abdomen of cattle and take blood meals two to three times a day depending on the weather. After feeding they move to a resting place to digest the blood meal. Stable flies are associated with substantial economic loss in cattle from the blood loss and pain from feeding. As few as five flies per leg is economically significant in cattle.

Ticks

Ticks cause blood loss and discomfort, and can act as vectors for disease spread. High concentrations of ticks usually occur in brushy pastures and woodlands.

Lice

Lice that affect cattle are either of the biting or sucking type, and cause skin irritation and itching. The entire life cycle of lice is on the host and they are present year round but populations increase in winter months. Lice spread through contact with infested cattle. Infested cattle can experience reduced appetite and anemia, and appear unthrifty.

Mites

In cattle, mites can cause hair loss and a thickening of the skin. Infestation by mites is called mange. Mites are spread by close contact. Severe mange can weaken cattle and make them vulnerable to diseases. Certain types of mites are reportable.

Cattle Grubs (warbles)

Cattle grubs, or warbles, are the larval stage of the heel fly. The larvae migrate from the animal's heel, where the eggs are deposited by the adult fly in early summer, to the back of the animal. The larvae can cause damage to the hide (due to the breathing hole they create) and if treated during the wrong time of the year can cause paralysis due to their location near the spinal column. Cattle should not be treated with a grubicide between November 15 and March 1 if cattle grubs are a concern.

Control of External Parasites

Control of external parasites usually revolves around the use of insecticides. These usually are a pyrethrin or an organophosphate. Strategies or combinations of strategies for delivery include: dust bags, back-rubbers (oilers), animal sprays, pour-ons, and insecticide impregnated ear tags. In addition, the use of injectable products or pour-ons with systemic activity work well to control lice and mites. Larvicides can also be part of control plan for certain types of flies as well as the use of predator wasps and environmental management. The use of dust bags and back-rubbers (oilers) can provide delivery of insecticides and economic fly control if located in an area that cattle are forced to move through such as a gateway or over a mineral feeder.

Delivery of Insecticides

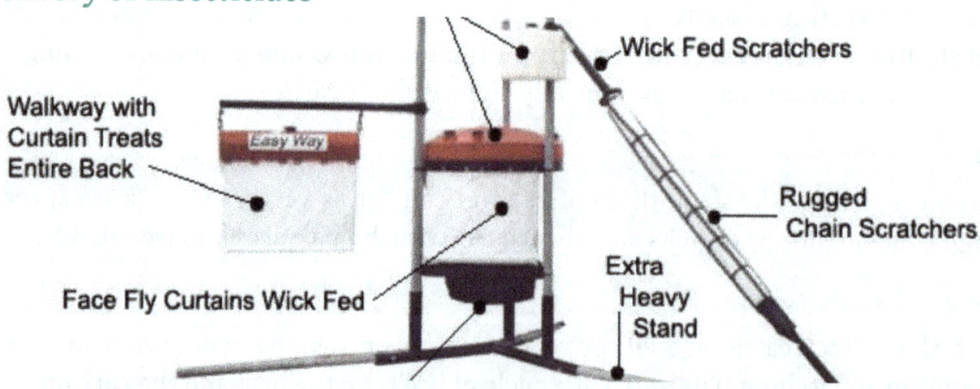

"Insecticide cattle care", http://easywaycattlecare.com/images/walkway-3.jpg

Insecticide sprays and pour-ons are effective for many different external parasites but have the drawback of increased animal handling costs and stress during the fly-season. Insecticide sprays are the only way to manage adult stable flies. Ear tags impregnated with insecticide can be effective in fly control. Maximizing control requires two tags per animal, and timing of application with peak fly numbers often requires a separate handling session of the animals. Ear tags provide good face fly control if applied properly.

Insecticide Ear Tag Fly Control

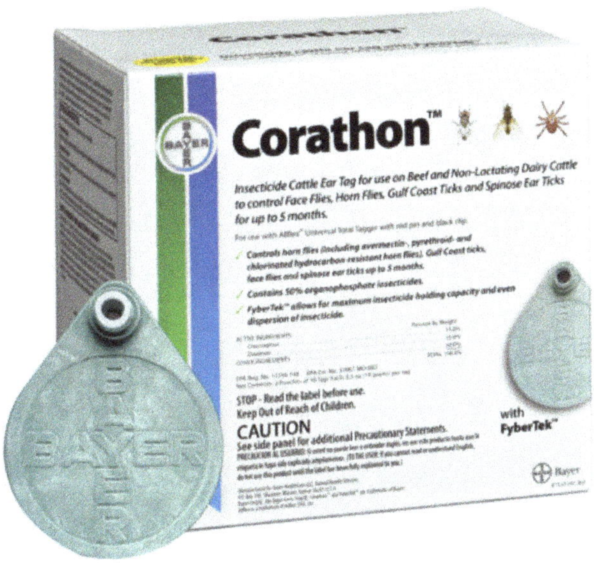

"Corathon insecticide cattle ear tags", https://www.pbsanimalhealth.com/products/corathon-insecticde-cattle-ear-tags

Larvicides prevent fly larvae from developing in to adults and are administered through free choice mineral. To be effective cattle must consume an adequate amount and not be in the proximity of untreated cattle.

Injectable products and pour-ons with systemic activity are mainly the macrocyclic lactones. These are effective against some flies as well as mites and lice. For mites and lice a second treatment may be needed in two to three weeks to kill newly hatched parasites unless using an extended duration product.

Sanitation or cleaning up of wasted feed or manure that serve as egg-laying sites for certain flies can greatly contribute to the control of certain flies locally. In addition, egg laying sites may be treated with a larvicide.

Environmental management may be a key component to tick control. The reduction of brushy areas and thick wooded areas reduces the habitat for the ticks and reduces exposure.

Certain native parasitic wasps are used as biological control agents of fly populations. Currently, farmers can buy parasitic wasps from commercial insectaries. These wasps emerge into adulthood from the pupal stage, where they develop wings. They fly from the release stations in which they have been held, hung from barn ceilings or other out-of-reach places. The wasps only target flies in their pupal stage. When the wasp finds a pupa in soil or litter, she inserts her stinger and withdraws it, drawing blood and paralyzing the pupa and inserting one egg. The egg hatches after 1 day, and the larva feeds on body fluids and organs for 2-4 weeks. Eventually, the wasp chews its way out of the dead host's puparium and flies away as an adult.

Example Strategic Control Program

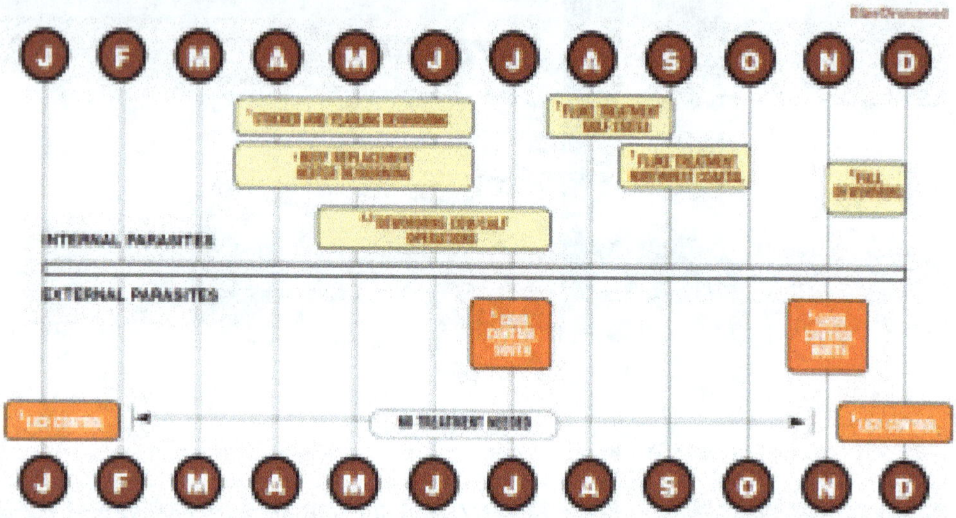

"Strategic Control: Beef Monograph", http://www.midamericaagresearch.net/documents/ BeefMonograph.pdf

- Stocker, yearling and replacement heifers dewormed at turnout, four and eight weeks after onset of grazing (0-4-8).
- Cow/calf deworming six weeks after onset of grazing.
- If cattle were not dewormed in the fall, adult cows should be dewormed at pasture turnout and again six weeks after onset of grazing.
- All cattle retained over winter should be dewormed.
- During lice season, two treatments two to three weeks apart may be necessary.
- Grub treatment three to four months after the end of heel fly season, varies south to north. Requires systemic, annual control only.

- Cattle grazed along the Gulf Coast and Northwest coast should be treated for adult and immature liver flukes.

(Horn-fly control as needed to keep populations below 200 flies per animal.)

There is increasing evidence of antiparasitic resistance in grazing species, such as cattle, small ruminants (sheep and goats), and horses, both globally and within the United States. Antiparasitic resistance is the genetic ability of parasites to survive treatment with an antiparasitic drug that was generally effective against those parasites in the past.

Many factors contribute to antiparasitic resistance, including the biology of the parasite; the immune status of the host animal; treatment practices; drug properties; and certain livestock management practices. To help combat this emerging problem, the FDA's Center for Veterinary Medicine started the Antiparasitic Resistance Management Strategy (ARMS).

DAIRY CATTLE

As in beef cattle, the overarching theme for the prevention strategy of parasitic infection is to reduce the animals' exposure to parasites and their infectious forms. Because multiple animals will be exposed, any strategy will focus on entire groups of animals rather than individuals. So far, this is similar to prevention strategies for any other infectious diseases on farm. However, when thinking about the prevention of parasite infections on farm, the veterinarian must be aware of the infectious form of the parasite (for example, eggs versus larvae) and whether or not other hosts are involved in the life cycle. Then the best parasiticide is selected and management practices, such as grazing schedule, are properly timed to avoid exposure to infectious parasite forms in the environment. In most cases, prevention strategies therefore boil down to good on-farm hygiene and use of well-timed and correctly selected dewormers, as well as pasture management as described for beef cattle. There are different forms of deworming medications for dairy cattle. For simplicity of application, many are pour-ons or feed additives; some are injectables. Oral pastes or any formulation that requires you to handle the animals' heads is rarely used because it is labor-intensive. Any product used in an animal that may be used for milk or meat has a specific withdrawal time. Withdrawal time is defined as the period from when the drug was used until the milk may be put in the bulk tank or the animal sent to slaughter for meat. How long the withdrawal time is and whether you can use a given drug in a lactating cow depends on the product. One thing that people might not be aware of – once a cow has calved for the first time, she is always considered to be a lactating animal, even if she's not being milked (dry period). Always, always, read the label to know what the product will treat for, at what dosage and frequency it should be used, by what route it should be administered, what class of animals it is for, and withdrawal times.

SMALL RUMINANTS

In general, the number of internal parasites in sheep and goats will increase with number of host animals (higher stocking rate); during warm, humid weather; and when pastures are grazed too short. The number of internal parasites will decrease in hot, dry weather; if a non-host animal (cattle or horses) grazes the same pasture; or if the pasture has been rested (no grazing, larvae die off naturally).

Some worms in a population will survive even the most appropriate drug treatments. This is due to genetic selection for resistant worms in a treated population. Modern dewormers are effective, broad in spectrum, cheap, and safe but people have relied more on drugs than on husbandry as a way to control parasites, leading to increased parasite resistance. To minimize development of parasite resistance to dewormers, use treatments specifically and selectively.

Clinical signs of parasitism in sheep and goats include diarrhea, bottle jaw (submandibular edema secondary to hypoproteinemia), anemia, and rough hair coat. Subclinical effects of parasitism include reduced weaning weight, reduced milk production, reduced reproductive performance, reduced growth rate, and increased susceptibility to disease.

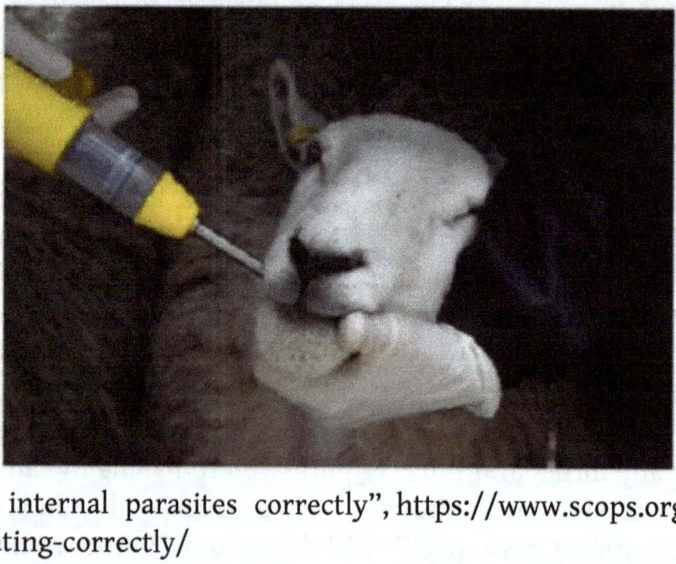

"Treating internal parasites correctly", https://www.scops.org.uk/internal-parasites/treating-correctly/

Treatment of sheep often includes drenching. The veterinarian should perform diagnostics to determine type of parasite(s) present. You may wish to perform a fecal egg count before and after treatment (fecal egg count reduction test) to determine how effective your treatment was. Weigh the sheep and prepare the dewormer based on weight. Deliver the dewormer over the tongue in the back of the throat with a drench tip or drench gun.

To determine who needs to be dewormed, veterinarians can do a fecal egg count (FEC) to measure number of worm eggs per gram of feces (epg). General class of parasites is identified (for example, strongyle-type) but the specific parasite rarely is identified (it is difficult to differentiate between *Haemonchus*, *Teladorsagia* (formerly *Ostertagia*), and *Trichostrongyles*). One recommendation for goats is to deworm bucks and dry (non-lactating) does if there are more than 2000 epg, lactating does if there are more than 750 epg, and all other animals if there are more than 1000 epg. Not all of the animals in the herd will be carrying parasites to the same extent and schemes exist that permit veterinarians to assess the animal clinically and from that, determine which individuals in the herd should be dewormed. This prevents treating animals unnecessarily, which is better for their health and less expensive for the owner, and helps prevent development of resistant parasites by minimizing use of deworming medications.

Not treating all animals also means you're leaving a certain number of untreated worms in the population; because these worms have not been exposed to dewormer, you're allowing them to persist and maintaining a more genetically diverse worm population. This population of untreated worms (called refugia) can be a valuable thing to consider when facing problems with anthelmintic resistance.

FAMACHA© is a diagnostic test to help small ruminant producers identify animals that require anthelmintic treatment and those that do not require deworming. The tool is a card that matches eyelid color to anemia levels, an indicator of clinical infection with parasites that cause anemia. A good resource about FAMACHA testing and general information about parasite control in small ruminants is the American Consortium for Small Ruminant Parasite Control.

As in cattle, pasture management is another important component of parasite control. To stop the parasite life cycle, remove sheep and goats from pastures for 3-6 months to allow worm larvae in the pasture to die off. Alternate or co-graze pastures with horses or adult cattle. Maintain stocking rates of no more than 6-8 sheep or goats per acre.

General considerations for parasite control include:

- Do not overgraze pastures; the vast majority of infective nematode larvae are on the first 2" of vegetation for a given plant.
- Spread manure in hot, dry conditions to kill worm eggs and larvae that may be in the feces.
- Rotate crops and livestock.
- Ensure a high plane of nutrition for ewes/does and lambs/kids.
- Use body condition score and other clinical signs to monitor flock health.

SWINE

Management and housing techniques used in modern commercial pig production, as well as the prudent use of anti-parasitic products, has dramatically reduced, and in many cases, eliminated the disease and animal welfare issues associated with parasite infections in pigs. Although parasites are no longer a significant challenge to the majority of pigs being produced in North America, they continue to play a role in some types of pig production, primarily in those animals exposed to outdoor environments. Therefore, a solid understanding of their types and prevention are important.

Internal Parasites

Categories of internal parasites include nematodes (roundworms), thorny-headed worms, tapeworms, and protozoa. *Ascarus suum* (a nematode or roundworm) and coccidia (a protozoan) are the most common internal parasites in commercial pig production at this time.

External Parasites

Categories of external parasites include ticks, mites, lice, mosquitoes, and flies. Mosquitoes and flies continue to be common challenges in both indoor and outdoor pig production while ticks, mites, and lice are primarily limited to pigs that are raised outdoors. Mosquitoes and biting flies are known to mechanically spread important diseases between groups and premises.

Prevention of Parasite Infections

Key factors to consider for the prevention of both internal and external parasite infections include:

- Source negative pigs
    - Knowledge of negative parasite status of replacement breeding stock prior to purchase and the prevention of moving positive stock into negative herds
- Minimize dose or eliminate exposure completely
    - Indoor production eliminates access to normal source of infection
    - All in-all out production: regular emptying of facilities between production groups
    - Sanitation: regular cleaning of facilities using appropriate detergent and disinfectant between production groups
    - Eliminate areas where external parasites can breed and develop (e.g. elimination of standing water reservoirs decreases mosquito levels)

- Monitoring program to insure early identification
  - A good monitoring program allows the early detection of a parasite challenge and the early application of intervention strategies.
  - This may include a routine fecal sampling program, observation of clinical signs, and gross signs on routine post mortems or slaughter checks.
- Therapeutic prevention programs
- Strategic preventive therapy programs are commonly used to treat parasite infections so that the challenge to the individual and challenge to herd mates (via shedding) is minimized.

HORSES

The internal parasites of greatest importance among North American horses are small strongyles (cyathostomes), large strongyles, ascarids (roundworms), tapeworms, and bots. Strongyles and ascarids are transmitted via a direct fecal-oral route, tapeworms have a more indirect fecal-oral transmission pattern involving the orbatid mite as intermediate host, and bots are transmitted when horses ingest fly eggs deposited on the hairs of their front legs. Small strongyles, ascarids (in young horses under 2 years of age), and tapeworms are the main focus of an equine parasite control program, as they have the greatest potential to cause disease. Bots rarely cause disease and are generally well controlled as a side benefit of the control program used to control strongyles and ascarids.

Ascarids (*Parascaris equorum*) are a significant health risk for foals, weanlings, and yearlings, but not for adult horses due to development of age-related immunity. Adult horses within a given herd can vary greatly in their susceptibility to parasite infestation, especially with respect to small strongyles. A small percentage of horses in the herd tend to harbor the majority of worms, and these horses are targeted for more frequent deworming.

Factors contributing to gastrointestinal parasitism in the horse are similar to those in other species: animal age; stocking density; geography and climate; presence and abundance of intermediate hosts; whether the animals are on pasture or dry lot; and pasture/paddock management practices.

Light parasite burdens are not associated with clinical disease, but heavy burdens can result in disease and death. Clinical signs of heavy parasitism include weight loss, stunted growth in juvenile horses, anemia and hypoproteinemia, colic (abdominal pain), acute or chronic diarrhea, and pulmonary injury. Young horses and immunodeficient geriatric horses are most susceptible to heavy parasite burdens and disease, but all horses are susceptible under the right conditions and in the absence of an effective parasite control program.

The goals of an equine parasite control program are to:

- Minimize the risk of parasite-related disease.
- Limit the extent of parasite shedding into the environment.
- Preserve the effectiveness of anti-parasitic medications.

As with vaccination programs, there is no such thing as a "one-size-fits-all" parasite control program that is appropriate for use in all horses!

Anti-Parasitic Medications

Over the past 30 years, widespread frequent use of over-the-counter oral anthelmintic products has resulted in excellent control of parasite-related disease across the population, but also accelerated the development of drug resistance among parasites. It was not uncommon to see that every horse on a farm was getting dewormed every 8 weeks, and often more frequently than that! In other words, too rigorous and indiscriminate an approach was taken. Resistance issues are of great concern because there are no new parasite control products in the drug production pipeline.

Current recommendations strive to avoid development of further resistance problems while still providing adequate protection from parasite-related disease. Compared to historical approaches, we now recommend a more strategic and targeted approach that results in much less frequent deworming for the majority of horses.

Horses are dewormed using over-the-counter commercial oral paste products that are dosed on the basis of body weight. Available medications include the macrocyclic lactones (ivermectin and moxidectin), pyrantel pamoate and tartrate, benzimidazoles (fenbendazole and oxibendazole), and praziquantel (available only in combination with ivermectin or moxidectin). To date, most parasite resistance is related to the benzimidazole and pyrantel products, but some resistance to the avermectins has also begun to appear recently. The parasite species most likely to exhibit resistance are small strongyles and ascarids.

A variety of herbal and organic deworming products are available and widely promoted among horse owners and managers, but there is no scientific evidence that these products are effective. They have not undergone formal testing for safety and efficacy, and are not approved or licensed as drugs by the FDA. Because non-drug products are allowed much more leniency in labeling, manufacturers can make almost any claim they want without having to substantiate that claim.

Design of Parasite Control Programs

In adult horses, decision-making about which horses to deworm, and with what products, is guided by serial quantitative fecal egg count (FEC) surveillance.

Determination of the number of strongyle eggs per gram (epg) of manure helps owners and veterinarians to (i) estimate individual parasite burdens; (ii) identify the horses with moderate or heavy parasite burdens that will benefit from deworming; (iii) identify the specific horses within the herd that serve as the major long-term parasite reservoirs and require more frequent deworming; and (iv) determine which specific deworming products are effective against parasites on that farm.

On the basis of FEC, horses are categorized as low shedders (0-200 epg), moderate shedders (200-500 epg), or high shedders (> 500 epg). In a well managed herd it is common for 70-90% of adult horses to fall in the low-shedding category; these horses require as few as 2 deworming treatments per year (spring and fall). Management of moderate shedders varies by region, but these horses typically require at least one additional deworming treatment during the parasite transmission season. In Minnesota, for example, these horses generally receive one additional treatment for strongyles between April and October, with the timing dictated by the egg reappearance period (ERP) for the dewormer used in spring. Heavy shedders require treatment throughout the spring/summer parasite season, though never any earlier than the expected ERP for the deworming products used.

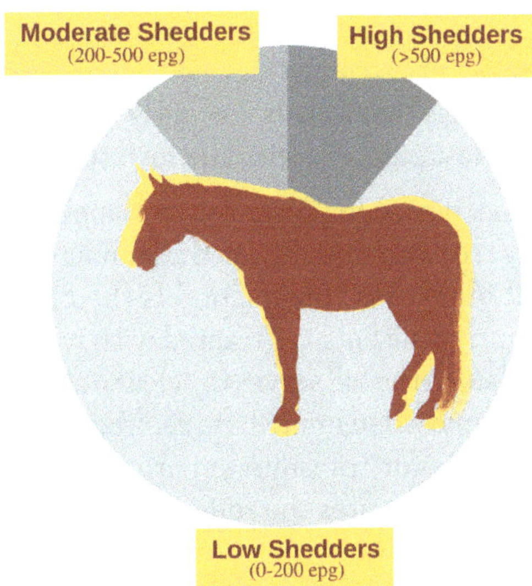

Fecal egg count reduction tests (FECRT) are used to evaluate the efficacy of specific deworming agents against both strongyles and ascarids. This entails running FEC tests immediately prior to worming and then 14 days after worming, and then calculating the percent reduction in fecal egg counts due to treatment. Specific cut-offs for suspicion of resistance vary between medications and parasites, but in general a dewormer should be dropping egg counts by 90-95% or more if the parasite is susceptible to its killing effects.

Under this type of program, adult horses with innate resistance to parasitism that carry low worm burdens are dewormed only 1-2 times per year. This ensures that many of the worms in the population are able to avoid the frequent exposure to deworming medications that selects for development of drug resistance. By contrast, horses with high worm burdens that are at greater risk for disease and contribute most to environmental contamination are selected for more frequent dosing. This applies some selection pressure for development of resistance, but is counterbalanced by the larger population of worms that remain genetically susceptible (refugia). The higher the proportion of worms in refugia, the more slowly resistance develops!

Foals, weanlings, and yearlings are approached differently due to their high level of susceptibility to parasitism in general, and ascarids in particular. Current recommendations are to treat them a minimum of 4 times in the first year of life, with the first treatment at 2-3 months of age using a benzimidazole (for example, fenbendazole). A second deworming is recommended just prior to weaning at approximately 6 months of age, prior to which an FEC is performed to determine whether worm burdens consist primarily of ascarids or of strongyles. The third and fourth treatments are administered at approximately 9 and 12 months of age, and should target primarily strongyles. One of those treatments should also include praziquantel to address tapeworms. Recently dewormed weanlings should be turned out into the cleanest pastures with the lowest worm/egg burdens.

Fecal egg counts are *not* useful for diagnosis of tapeworm or bot infestation, so most horses are simply treated annually for these in late fall on the assumption that a significant infestation exists. Praziquantel is the only medication licensed for treatment of tapeworms, while bots are treated with ivermectin or moxidectin. Timing this treatment for late in the fall serves to "clear out" the existing population of bots and tapeworms at a time when immediate reinfection is not possible because the flies and mites responsible for transmission are no longer active. Horses will begin to re-accumulate those parasites the following spring when flies and mites appear to resume transmission.

Environmental Management

As in other species, periodic administration of anthelmintic drugs is only one element of an effective control program and environmental sanitation and management are also important. The most effective approach is removal of manure from paddocks and pastures; twice-weekly manure collection is recommended. Dragging or harrowing paddocks and pastures to break up manure pats is much less effective, and only recommended for geographic regions in which spread manure will dry rapidly. Composting of manure and soiled bedding generates enough heat to kill parasite larvae and eggs. Non-composted manure should never be spread on pastures as this will serve to increase the level of parasite contamination. Reducing animal numbers, reducing stocking density, and avoiding overgrazing will reduce parasite exposure, as will rotating pastures and grazing other types of livestock on rested pastures. New horses should have an FEC on arrival, and be dewormed if warranted, before being turned out with resident horses.

SMALL ANIMALS

This is an excerpt from a book for pet owners (Root Kustritz MV (ed), The University of Minnesota Guide to Dog and Cat Wellness, ASIN: B00GCC0YN8).

Most puppies and kittens are born carrying some internal parasites, even if they are born into excellent breeding facilities. Your veterinarian can check the puppy or kitten's feces for evidence of the parasites, but many infected puppies and kittens will test negative. Your veterinarian may recommend routine worming for your puppy or kitten several times when they are young, to ensure they are not carrying internal parasites. Adult dogs also may carry these parasites. If worm eggs in the feces hatch outside, the young worms may live in your lawn and infect humans, especially children, and other animals. Because of this, all feces should be picked up and disposed of immediately.

Intestinal parasites are treated with specific anti-parasitic drugs. *Note from Dr. Root for Preventive Medicine course – classes of wormers commonly used are those described for beef cattle (benzimidazoles and macrocyclic lactones) with some specific wormers for other classes used for things like tapeworms. Each type of worm is treated with a specific drug so it is important that the specific type of parasite present in your animal is identified. Over-the-counter wormers generally are not as effective as those available from your veterinarian. Some medications must be dosed more than once to destroy both juvenile and adult worms.

Heartworm is a form of internal parasite that infests the circulatory system. Young worms are injected by infected mosquitoes into the dog or cat. These young worms eventually lodge in the heart as adults where they mate and produce young worms that circulate in your dog or cat, infecting mosquitoes that feed on other animals and continuing the life cycle. Your dog or cat can contract heartworm anywhere they encounter mosquitoes, including indoors. The adult heartworms cause severe and potentially fatal damage to the heart, lungs, and other vital organs. Clinical signs of heartworm disease include coughing, fatigue, loss of appetite, and possibly episodes of fainting. Many infected dogs and cats show no signs of disease. Your veterinarian will test your dog yearly for this disorder; cats should be tested as well. Treatment is difficult so prevention is preferred. There is no treatment available for cats, so prevention is critical. Fortunately, cats are more resistant to heartworm disease than are dogs, so incidence of heartworm disease is lower in cats than in dogs. Your dog should be tested yearly and preventative medications given monthly. Heartworm prevention can be instituted in puppies as early as 6-8 weeks of age. Be aware that many heartworm medications also protect your pet against intestinal parasites described earlier.

Common Intestinal Parasites of Dogs and Cats

COMMON NAME	APPEARANCE	CLINICAL SIGNS	HOW TRANSMITTED
Round-worms	3-12″ long, spaghetti-like	Usually do not cause clinical signs; may see worms passed in feces, young animals may show poor weight gain. Most common in dogs and cats less than 6 months of age.	Eggs in feces, across the placenta or while nursing from the dam
Hookworms	Very small, thread-like	May see anemia, digested or frank blood in feces.	Eggs or young worms in feces, on the ground, nursing from the dam, penetration of larvae through skin
Whipworms	Very small, thread-like	Usually do not cause clinical signs; may occasionally be associated with diarrhea.	Eggs in feces, on the ground
Tapeworms	Very long and flat, made up of segments that look like grains of rice caught in the hair around the anus	May cause weight loss.	Eating rabbits, rodents, or eating fleas containing the worm.

External parasites of most concern are ticks and fleas. Fleas feed on blood and can transmit disease, including tapeworms. Fleas are primarily an environmental concern; 95% of the flea population (eggs, larvae and pupae) live in the environment and only 5% (adult) live on animals. Outside areas exposed to sunlight in summer or extreme cold in winter are unlikely to harbor fleas. Inside the home, flea populations will be concentrated where the animal spends the most time resting or sleeping. Fleas are the most common external parasite in small animals; cats are twice as likely as dogs to have fleas when examined by veterinarians. Successful flea control requires treatment of the animal and the environment. There are excellent flea control products available. Not all are safe for use in puppies and kittens.

Ticks can transmit disease to dogs including Lyme disease, anaplasmosis, ehrlichiosis, and Rocky Mountain Spotted Fever. Safe and effective tick products are available but there is no tick preventative that is 100% effective; dogs and outside cats should be checked and ticks removed by hand at least once daily in the warmer months.

Fleas and Ticks in Small Animals

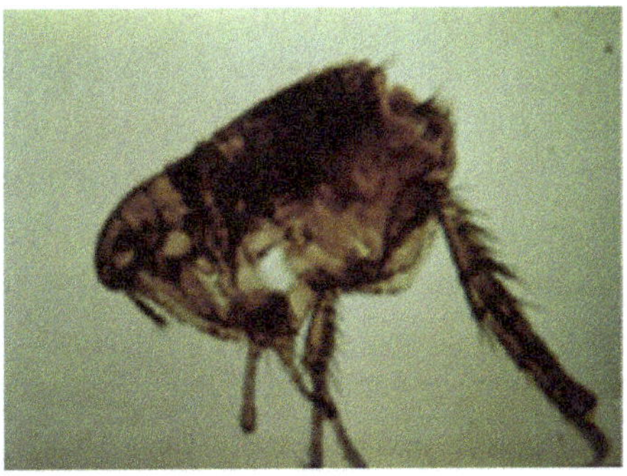

Flea (Ctenocephalides canis) enlarged, (photo courtesy of Drs. Sheila Torres and Laura Molgaard)

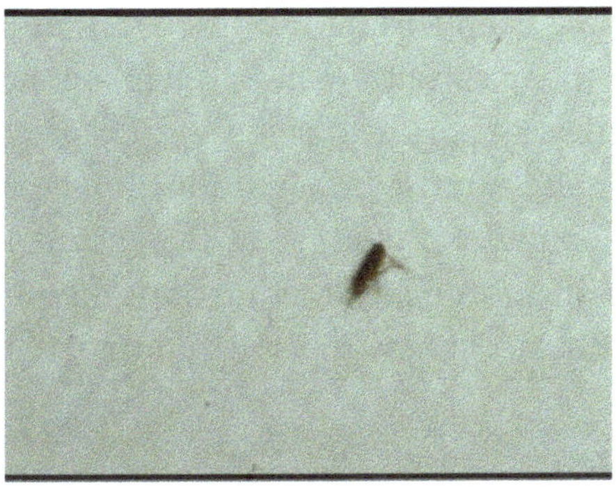

Flea near actual size, (photo courtesy of Dr. Sheila Torres)

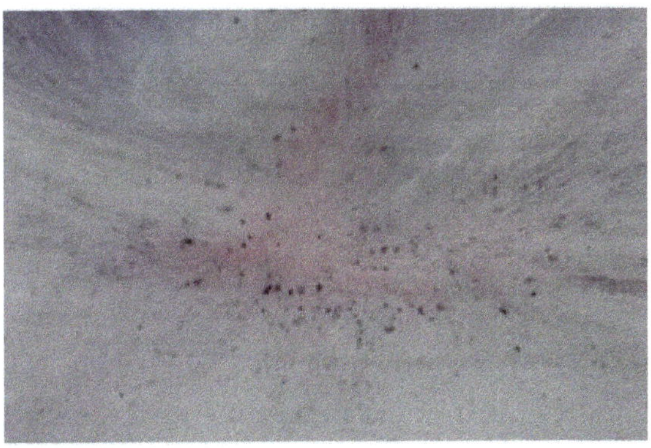

Flea dirt on the skin at the base of the hairs (photo courtesy of Dr. Sheila Torres)

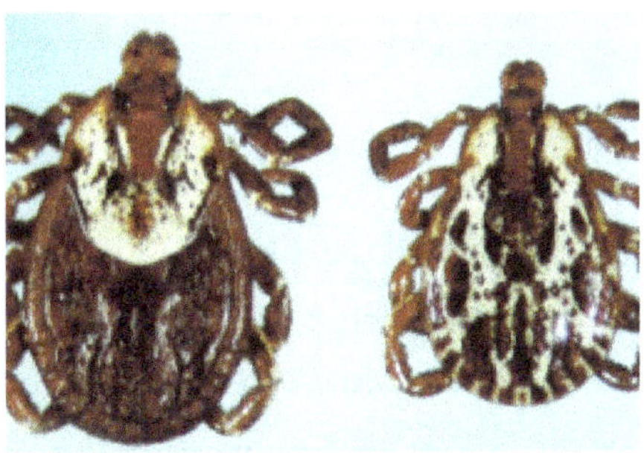

Common dog tick (wood tick; Dermacentor variabilis) enlarged, (photo courtesy of Dr. Bert Stromberg)

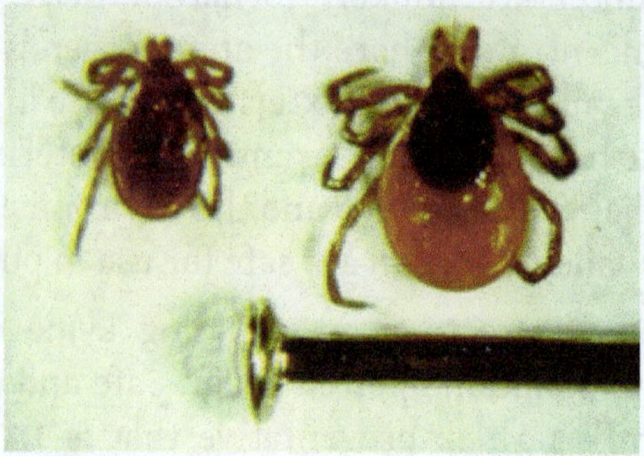

Deer tick (Ixodes scapularis) enlarged, (photo courtesy of Dr. Bert Stromberg)

Control of small animal parasites in shelter / rescue operations

It is estimated that as many as 40% of owned dogs and cats in the United States have been through some sort of animal shelter. Animals entering shelters may be in poor condition and are closely housed, which increases risk of exposure. Many internal parasites release eggs or cysts that are impervious to disinfecting agents. Shelters must be rigorous about prompt removal of feces and regular complete cleaning of facilities to decrease overall exposure. Animals commonly are treated with appropriate medications for control of roundworms, hookworms, whipworms, and coccidia, with repeated treatment every 2 weeks if needed.

List your five (5) take-home points – What are things you want to remember from this chapter as you progress through the curriculum and into your career?

EXTRA RESOURCES

Flea products: https:// todaysveterinarypractice.com/ practical-parasitologythe - flea-infested-pet-overview-current-products/.

Managing fleas on the pet and in the environment: https://todaysveterinarypractice.com/practical-parasitologythe-flea-infested-pethow-manage-pet-environment/.

Fly control products and approvals: http://entomology.unl.edu/livestock.

Applicability of the Antiparasitic Resistance Management Strategy (ARMS) to cattle: https://www.fda.gov/animal-veterinary/safety-health/antiparasitic-resistance.

American Consortium for Small Ruminant Parasite Control: www.acsrpc.org.

Internal parasite categories in swine: https://thepigsite.com/disease-guide/endoparasites-internal-parasites-worms-nematodes

External parasite categories in swine: https://thepigsite.com/disease-guide/ectoparasites

Fleas in small animals: https://www.banfield.com/state-of-pet-health/skin-allergies/overview

CHAPTER-6

CONTROL OVER REPRODUCTION

REPRODUCTIVE PHYSIOLOGY OF THE FEMALE

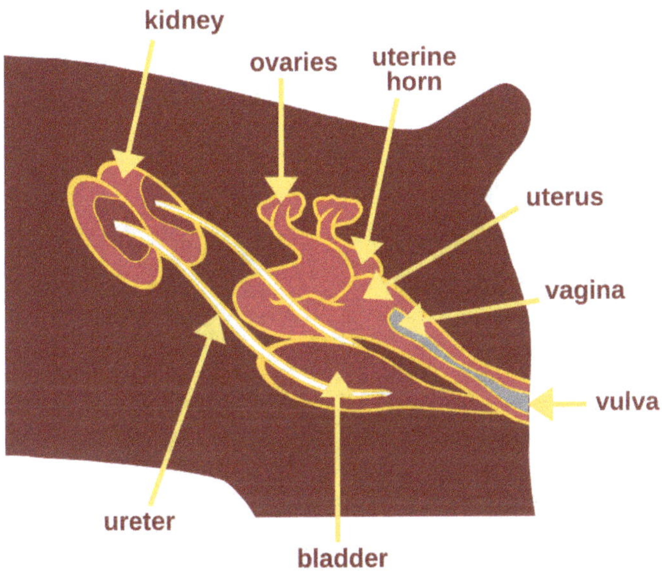

The ovaries contain thousands of follicles, each of which contains an egg or ovum. As each estrous cycle begins, a cohort of follicles is selected to begin development. Development is promoted by release of hormones from the hypothalamus (gonadotropin releasing hormone [GnRH]) and pituitary (follicle stimulating hormone [FSH] and luteinizing hormone [LH]). As the follicle develops, it secretes estrogen, which causes the physical and behavioral signs of early heat, or proestrus. Estrogen concentrations fall about 9 days after the onset of proestrus; at this time, the bitch will stand to be bred (standing heat or estrus) and a surge of LH is released, causing ovulation. This is spontaneous ovulation. Queens are induced ovulators. In this species, copulation is the most common trigger for release of GnRH and subsequent ovulation. In either spontaneous or induced ovulators, the eggs are released from the follicles into the uterine tube, where fertilization occurs.

The egg is surrounded by a thick capsule, the zona pellucida, and by a layer of cells from the follicle. Spermatozoa introduced into the reproductive tract of the bitch undergo capacitation, a process involving the acrosome reaction on the head of the spermatozoon and achievement of hypermotility. Capacitated spermatozoa digest the layer of cells surrounding the egg and invade the zona pellucida. As soon as one spermatozoon gets to the inner layer of the zona pellucida, entry of other spermatozoa is blocked by an electrochemical reaction so only one spermatozoon fertilizes each egg. Cell division begins immediately. The developing embryos move into the uterus within days but do not implant in the uterine wall and develop placentas until about 12 days after the LH surge in cats and about 16-18 days after the LH surge in dogs.

REPRODUCTIVE PHYSIOLOGY OF THE MALE

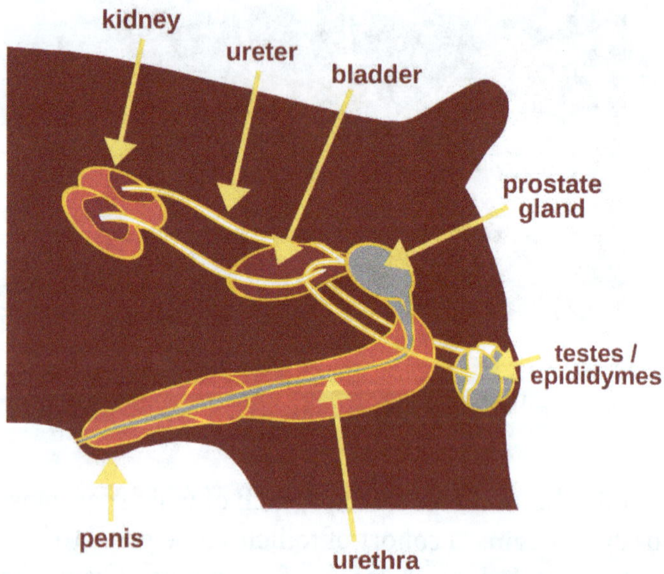

Testes of male dogs should be descended into the scrotum by 8-14 weeks of age and must be descended by 6 months of age for the dog to be considered normal. Testes usually are descended at birth in male cats but may not be palpable until 6-8 weeks of age. The testes contain spermatogonia, which will divide to form spermatozoa under the influence of the hormone testosterone. Testosterone secretion from testicular Leydig (interstitial) cells is stimulated by GnRH and LH release from the hypothalamus and pituitary, respectively. Spermatozoa are manufactured in the testis but are neither motile nor capable of fertilization until after they pass through the adjoining tissue, the epididymis. Spermatozoa ejaculated at the time of semen collection come from the epididymis.

REPRODUCTION CONTROL

Contraception

Any procedure that prevents reproduction for a time but is reversible such that the individual may be capable of reproduction in the future.

Sterilization

Any procedure that makes an individual permanently incapable of reproduction.

Research into non-surgical methods for sterilization of dogs and cats is ongoing and no products are available at this time.

Surgical Sterilization

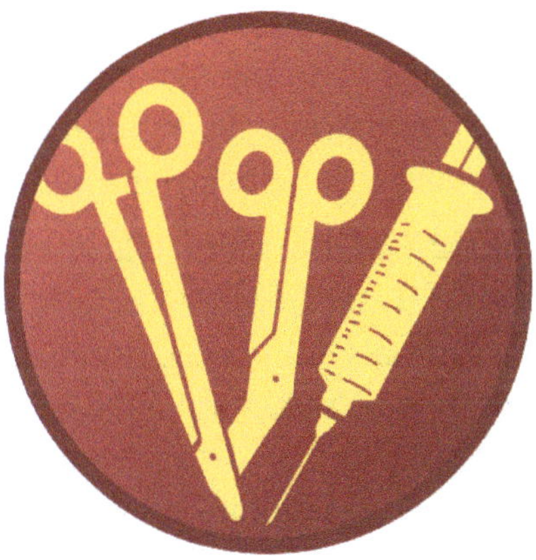

Ovariectomy (surgical removal of the ovaries), hysterectomy (surgical removal of the uterus, also called 'ovary-sparing spay'), ovariohysterectomy (surgical removal of the ovaries and uterus) and tubal ligation (tying off the uterine tubes) are the techniques described in the literature for sterilization of bitches and queens. Tubal ligation is not commonly used for contraception of bitches or queens anywhere in the world.

Ovariectomy is commonly used in Europe and appears to offer the same benefits and concerns as does ovariohysterectomy (OHE or spay). Ovariectomy is reported to be less time-consuming and less invasive then OHE. In one study of 264 dogs, 126 of which had undergone ovariectomy and 138 of which had undergone OHE, no significant differences were reported in incidence of urogenital problems during a follow-up period of 8-11 years after surgery. Urinary incontinence was a reported finding in both groups; difference in incidence between the groups was not statistically significant. Ovary-sparing spay requires complete removal of the uterus to the level of the cervix and is not quicker or less-invasive than OHE. In the United States, OHE still is the most common surgical sterilization method.

In male dogs and cats, castration (surgical removal of both testes) and vasectomy (tying off the spermatic cord) are reported sterilization techniques. Castration is the most common surgical sterilization method.

Optimal Age for Surgical Sterilization of Dogs and Cats

Optimal age at which to perform OHE or castration of dogs and cats is not defined by the veterinary literature. In the United States, most veterinarians recommend cats and dogs be spayed or neutered when about 6 months of age, prior to puberty, which is defined as acquisition of normal breeding behavior and semen quality in males and first estrus in females. In other countries, veterinarians recommend that dogs and cats be spayed after their first estrus, or do not recommend elective surgical sterilization be performed at any age. Indeed, in some countries, elective gonadectomy is considered unethical and is either strongly discouraged or illegal. For this discussion, it is assumed that the veterinarian is comfortable with the ethics of elective gonadectomy and practices in a country in which such surgery is considered acceptable by professional associations and the society at large.

Dogs and cats can be considered as part of a larger population of animals or as individuals. Recommendation for age at which to perform elective gonadectomy must take this into account. Animals at humane organizations should be evaluated as part of the larger population as those animals are not yet associated with a responsible owner or guardian. Dogs and cats with an owner or guardian may be considered either as part of a larger population or as an individual.

Sterilization of Dogs and Cats With No Owner or Guardian

In the United States, a serious problem with pet overpopulation exists, such that millions of unowned dogs and cats are euthanized yearly. Some of these are feral animals, some are abandoned and brought to the humane association as a stray, and many are relinquished. Intact animals are much more likely to be relinquished than are spayed or neutered animals and animals that are adopted out from the humane association while still intact may either be returned or may repopulate that shelter with their offspring. While most intact animals are adopted out with a spay-neuter contract, compliance with such contracts has been demonstrated to be less than 60%. There is a significant lack of knowledge among pet owners regarding normal reproductive physiology among dog and cats owners; studies have demonstrated that up to 57% of bitch owners were unaware that bitches cycle at least twice yearly, up to 83% of queen owners were unaware that queens are polyestrous from spring to early fall, and up to 61% of dog and cat owners were unsure or believed that their animal would somehow be "better" after having had at least one litter. In one survey of dog- and cat-owning households, 56% of 154 canine litters and 68% of 317 feline litters were unplanned, with the majority of those owners reporting that they did not know the female had been in heat. While everyone would like to believe that better education of pet owners would lead to more responsible pet ownership, and while increasing education is a worthy goal that should be pursued, gonadectomy of dogs and cats prior to adoption is one weapon in the fight against overpopulation that should be employed at this time. Multiple studies have been published demonstrating safety of gonadectomy in puppies and kittens as young as 7 weeks of age. To that end, I recommend that all male and female dogs and cats should be spayed or castrated prior to adoption from humane organizations.

Sterilization of Dogs and Cats With an Owner or Guardian

Pros and cons of spay/castration can include behavioral and medical concerns. Here are some definitions you may find useful:

Incidence = the number of new cases in a population over a period of time

Morbidity = extent of illness among those having the condition

Mortality = death due to the condition

Male Cats – The normal behavior of most intact male cats is incompatible with their living as house pets. Breeding behavior in cats is aggressive and intact male cats show that behavior readily. Urine from intact male cats is used for territorial marking and has a very distinct, strong odor. Incidence of obesity after castration is high, and is due to decreased metabolic rate in cats after gonadectomy. There are virtually no other health conditions reported to be increased or decreased in association with gonadectomy in male cats. Because of this, I recommend that any male cat not intended for breeding be castrated.

- **Female Cats** – Benefits of OHE in female cats include decreased incidence of mammary neoplasia, ovarian or uterine tumors, and pyometra. Of these, the most significant is mammary neoplasia. Mammary neoplasia is the third most common tumor of female cats, with a reported incidence of 2.5%. Incidence is increased with number of estrous cycles in the cat's life and is increased in the Siamese and domestic Japanese breeds. Greater than 90% of cases are malignant adenocarcinoma.

Detriments of OHE in female cats include possible complications of surgery, obesity, increased incidence of feline lower urinary tract disease (FLUTD), and increased incidence of diabetes mellitus. Reported incidence of post-surgical complications in cats is 2.6%, with most reported complications mild and self-resolving. Incidence of obesity after OHE is high, and is due to decreased metabolic rate in cats after gonadectomy. Obesity can be controlled by use of a proper feeding regimen. Finally, increased incidence of FLUTD and diabetes mellitus has been reported after OHE in queens, with the Burmese breed especially prone to development of diabetes mellitus. Incidence of these two conditions is 0.6% and 0.5%, respectively.

Because the incidence and morbidity of mammary neoplasia are much higher than are the incidences of FLUTD and diabetes mellitus, and because morbidity associated with obesity can be controlled by the owner or guardian of the cat, I believe that female cats not intended for breeding should be spayed as early in their life as possible.

- **Male Dogs** – Benefits of castration in male dogs include decreased incidence of testicular neoplasia and non-neoplastic prostate disease, and possible increased lifespan. Testicular neoplasia is a common tumor of aged, intact male dogs, with a reported incidence of 0.9%. Morbidity generally is low. Benign prostatic hypertrophy (BPH) is a very common disorder of male dogs, with reported incidence of 75-80% in dogs aged 6 years or more. Again, morbidity generally is low. Finally, several studies have documented increased lifespan in castrated male dogs compared to intact males. This may be due to greater care by owners after the "investment" of surgery has been made in that animal, or may be due to a decrease in sexually dimorphic behaviors that put the animal at increased risk, such as roaming.

Detriments of castration in male dogs include complications of surgery; increased incidence of prostatic neoplasia, transitional cell carcinoma, osteosarcoma, lymphosarcoma, and hemangiosarcoma; increased incidence of anterior cruciate ligament (ACL) injury and hip dysplasia; obesity; and possible increased incidence of diabetes mellitus. Some reports also suggests increased incidence of behavioral disorders, such as fear of storms. Reported incidence of post-surgical complications in dogs is 6.1%, with most reported complications mild and self-resolving. Prostatic neoplasia, transitional cell carcinoma, osteosarcoma, and hemangiosarcoma generally are low in incidence but high in morbidity and mortality. No breed predisposition has been identified for prostatic neoplasia, but does exist for the other cancers noted. Incidence of ACL injury in dogs is relatively high, at 1.8%, and morbidity may be high, although this is generally considered to be a curable condition with surgery. Again, some breeds, most notably large and giant breeds, are predisposed to ACL injury. Obesity is high in incidence but morbidity can be controlled by the owner or guardian.

Appropriate recommendation for castration of male dogs is less readily evident than is that for male cats. While a given male dog can produce many more offspring than can a given bitch, suggesting that castration is necessary for population control, the significant morbidity associated with castration as a possible predisposing cause of the conditions described above suggests that castration is not recommended when considering the animal as an individual. I believe this recommendation must be made on a case-by-case basis, evaluating the breed of the dog, his intended working life or activity level, and the owner's wishes regarding use of that animal for breeding. Many owners choose castration for male dogs to control normal male reproductive behaviors that we have deemed to be inappropriate, such as mounting.

- **Female Dogs** – Benefits of OHE in bitches include decreased incidence of mammary neoplasia, with greatest benefit if spayed before the first heat; decreased incidence of ovarian or uterine neoplasia and pyometra; and possible increased lifespan. Mammary neoplasia is the most common tumor of female dogs,with reported incidence of 3.4%. It is the most common malignant tumor in female dogs, with 50.9% of mammary tumors reported to be malignant; metastases are found in about 75% of cases of mammary carcinoma with the lung the most common site of metastasis. Exact cause-and-effect relationship has not been defined, although a hormonal basis for malignant transformation of mammary cells and progression of neoplasia is hypothesized based on the decreasing benefit of OHE with increasing number of estrous cycles in the dog's life prior to surgery. The other very common disorder in female dogs when aged is pyometra, reported to occur in 15.2% of dogs by 4 years of age and in 23-24% of dogs by 10 years of age. Morbidity is high, although OHE at the time of clinical presentation is curative; reported mortality ranges from 0-17% in dogs.

Detriments of OHE in female dogs include complications of surgery; increased incidence of transitional cell carcinoma, osteosarcoma, lymphosarcoma, cutaneous mast cell tumors, and hemangiosarcoma; increased incidence of ACL injury and hip dysplasia; obesity and diabetes mellitus; a possible increase in aggression in at least one breed and reactivity in one breed; and increased incidence of urethral sphincter mechanism incompetence (estrogen-responsive urinary incontinence). Reported incidence of post-surgical complications in dogs is 6.1%, with most reported complications mild and self-resolving. As in male dogs, incidence of tumors reportedly associated with gonadectomy is low but morbidity with these tumor types is high. Breed predispositions exist for many tumor types. Incidence of obesity is high after OHE but morbidity can be controlled by the owner. Incidence of ACL injury in dogs is relatively high, at 1.8%, and morbidity may be high, although this is generally considered to be a curable condition with surgery. Again, some breeds, most notably large and giant breeds, are predisposed to ACL injury. Aggression after OHE has been reported in English Springer Spaniels; there is some suggestion that this effect may be more likely in bitches that demonstrated aggressive tendencies prior to surgery. Urethral sphincter mechanism incompetence is a problem of spayed female dogs, especially those weighing more than 20 kg. Morbidity is low and this is a disease easily controlled with medical therapy in most female dogs. Evidence exists suggesting incidence can be decreased by spaying bitches when greater than 3-5 months of age.

Appropriate recommendation for OHE of female dogs is less readily evident than is that for female cats. Certainly mammary neoplasia and pyometra are of high incidence and high morbidity, and are greatly decreased in incidence by OHE. However, possible predisposition to very high morbidity tumor types or ACL injury must be evaluated. As with male dogs, I believe this recommendation must be made on a case-by-case basis, evaluating the breed of the dog, her intended working life or activity level, and the owner's wishes regarding use of that animal for breeding.

Much information and misinformation about this topic is available to the owners, guardians, and breeders of dogs and cats. It behooves us, as veterinarians, to be familiar with the current veterinary literature and to base our recommendations on science, rather than on anecdote or tradition.

Benefits and Detriments of Spay / Castration Surgery in Dogs and Cats

Bold indicates high incidence, *Italic* indicates high morbidity or mortality

	MALE CAT	FEMALE CAT	MALE DOG	FEMALE DOG
Undesirable physical or behavioral manifestations of reproduction	↓	↓	↓	↓
Ovarian **/ Uterine disease (pyometra)**		↓		↓
Mammary cancer		↓		↓
Benign prostatic hypertrophy			↓	

Testicular cancer	↓		↓	
Risks of anesthesia / surgery	↑	↑	↑	↑
Bone cancer			↑	↑
Genitourinary cancer			↑	↑
Anterior cruciate ligament injury			↑	↑
Urinary incontinence				↑
Obesity	↑	↑	↑	↑

Non-Surgical Reproductive Control

What about non-surgical sterilants? Are there contraceptives available for dogs that would control reproduction without completely removing the possibility of fertility in that animal later in life?

Pharmacologic Reproductive Control

Drug therapy affects normal hormone secretion, decreasing estrous cycling. Examples include:

- **Progesterone** – Megestrol acetate (Ovaban™). This is the only drug that was ever FDA-approved for estrus suppression for breeding dogs in the United States. It is not available as a veterinary product but can be dispensed through human pharmacies. Ovaban can be given either during anestrus (0.25 mg/lb once daily per os x 30 days) to prolong time until the next proestrus begins, or within the first 3 days of proestrus (1.0 mg/lb once daily per os x 8 days) at which point the bitch will go out of heat in 5-6 days and will not ovulate at that cycle. If used properly, megestrol acetate should not cause uterine disease or impact fertility in bitches. Possible side-effects of treatment with any form of progesterone in dogs include weight gain, predisposition to mammary neoplasia and uterine disease, and induction of diabetes mellitus. These same side-effects are seen in queens with administration of progesterone, as is mammary hypertrophy. Current research describes use of progesterone within silastic implants, reported to suppress estrus for up to 2 years in bitches with no side-effects.

- **Androgens** – The only androgen that was FDA-approved for use in female dogs (Cheque™) was never approved for use in breeding animals and is no longer available from the manufacturer. The active ingredient, mibolerone, is available through compounding pharmacies. Other androgens described for estrus suppression are forms of testosterone, which are effective in a dose-dependent manner and have been reported to be only 66% effective at suppressing estrus in Beagle bitches. Possible side-effects include vaginitis, hypertrophy of the clitoris, and liver disease. Androgens cannot safely be used for estrus suppression in queens, in which they are hepatotoxic and thyrotoxic.
- **GnRH agonists** – These drugs mimic the action of GnRH, causing release of FSH and LH. Initially this will cause estrus but continued treatment with the drug will shut down the system, with no further estrous cycling. These drugs have been demonstrated to prevent estrus in bitches for up to 27 months and have not been associated with decreased fertility. Similarly, in males initially administration of these drugs will cause increased release of LH and testosterone but will eventually shut down the system, decreasing testosterone secretion and spermatogenesis. GnRH agonists have been demonstrated to suppress fertility for up to 27 months in dogs with subsequent return to normal fertility. These drugs are not approved for use in dogs or cats in the United States. In queens, GnRH can be used to induce ovulation (GnRH; 25 mcg/cat IM). Luteinized follicles will be maintained an average of 40 to 50 days, giving the owner a respite from estrous cycling in the queen. Ovulation induction by physical means also has been described but in the author's experience is less effective than is pharmacologic induction of ovulation.
- **Estrogen** – Estrogen compounds can be used to induce azoospermia (lack of spermatozoa in the ejaculate) in dogs. However, toxic effects of estrogen include induction of squamous metaplasia in the prostate and pancytopenia. I do not recommend the use of estrogens in male dogs.

Immunologic Reproductive Control

Immunologic approaches to contraception work by vaccinating the animal against one of the tissues or hormones described above. When an animal is vaccinated against a tissue, for example, it will create antibodies against that tissue that will either destroy the tissue or prevent its normal function. There is no commercially available contraceptive vaccine for dogs or cats at this time. Compounds that are being investigated include:

- **Zona pellucida** – Vaccinated bitches and queens may or may not continue to cycle and time until re-vaccination is required varies much between individuals. This technique may or may not be reversible; ovarian pathology described after immunization of bitches against porcine zona pellucida proteins include ovarian atrophy and polycystic disease.
- **GnRH** – This is a compound against which animals do not develop antibodies readily. Immune response in tested animals has been variable, however, this vaccine may be the best candidate for commercial availability in the near future.

The search for the elusive "spay vaccine" has been ongoing for decades. Recently, a concerted effort has been made to gather like-minded scientists and to ensure sharing of ideas and materials. These collaborative efforts by the Alliance for Contraception in Cats and Dogs and the Found Animals Foundation have served to increase the number of research studies performed in field of dog and cat contraception and sterilization. Current concepts under investigation include immunocontraception, targeted cytotoxins, and gene silencing. No such products are commercially available as of this writing. Products approved for use in other species show great promise in dogs and cats and it is hoped that some sort of injectable reproductive control agent will be available within the next 10-5 years.

Sclerosing Agents for Reproductive Control

Sclerosing agents are drugs or compounds that are injected into the testes or epididymes to cause localized inflammation and destroy or scar testicular or epididymal tissue, preventing formation and movement of spermatozoa. Testicular tissue does not regenerate so if that tissue and the spermatogonia within it are destroyed, sterility may be achieved. Many compounds have been investigated.

In 2002, the FDA approved one compound, Neutersol™, for use in puppies aged 3-10 months with testicular width between 10 and 27 mm. This compound was most recently available under the brand name Zeuterin™; as of this writing, no product is commercially available in the United States. The compound (zinc gluconate with arginine) is injected directly into each testis, with dose dependent on testicular width. Sedation may be required but most dogs are reported to tolerate the injection well. Immediate side-effects include transient swelling of the testes or scrotum, and vomiting. Zeuterin™ cannot be used in cryptorchid dogs and should not be used in dogs with scrotal irritation or malformation of the testes or epididymes. In a field study of 224 dogs treated with Neutersol™, 223 were considered to be completely sterilized by 6-12 months after injection, based on inability to collect normal semen from these males. Testosterone secretion was decreased but not to as great an extent as with castration. Studies are ongoing for evaluation of safety of the product, efficacy as a contraceptive or sterilant, and effect of decreased testosterone concentrations on prostate disease and on behavior.

Non-Surgical Sterilization Techniques Currently Under Investigation

	DEFINITION	EXAMPLE
Immunocontraception	Induction of humoral (antibody) and cellular immunity to destroy proteins or tissues specific to reproduction	"Vaccination" against zona pellucida (outer layer of ova) to prevent conception by inducing antibodies that block sperm-binding sites
Targeted Cytotoxins	Attachment of toxins to carriers that will bind to and destroy cells specific to reproductive function ; analogous to chemotherapy for cancer treatment	Exotoxin A from **Pseudomonas aeruginosa** bound to a ligand that binds to the receptor for FSH, selectively destroying cells that require FSH to function, such as granulosa cells lining ovarian follicles
Gene Silencing	Introduction of short strands of RNA that block transcription of homologous segments of DNA and effectively abolish expression of that gene	Use of interfering RNA to block production of kisspeptin in neurons, subsequently altering section of GnRH and FSH

EXTRA RESOURCES

Non-Surgical Reproductive Control: Dr Bob Weedon – pdf presentation

Alliance for Contraception in Cats and Dogs: (www.acc-d.org)

Found Animals Foundation: (http://www.michelsonprizeandgrants.org/)

CHAPTER-7

TAKING GOOD CARE OF THE YOUNG

COLOSTRUM NEED BY SPECIES

Specific actions may be taken to promote health in young animals. Amount of veterinary intervention varies by species. You will note that there are no notes for small animal; that is because there is little routine prenatal care provided and after giving birth, the bitch and queen care for their puppies and kittens with virtually no veterinary intervention associated with preventive healthcare. Notes for this course will review preventive healthcare in foals, calves, and piglets.

One overarching theme when discussing care of any young animal is the need for them to ingest colostrum. Colostrum is the primary route by which most young animals get maternal antibodies (passive transfer) to protect them from disease before they have a functional immune system. How much antibody transfer occurs is dependent on placentation in that species. There are six possible layers in placentas. Three are always present (fetal endothelium, fetal connective tissue, and fetal epithelium, also known as the chorion). The chorion abuts the uterine tissue of the dam, with varying degrees of penetration into that tissue. In an epitheliochorial placenta, the chorion abuts the dam's epithelium (6 layers). This is the type of placenta in cattle, horses, and pigs. In some species, cells from the chorion fuse with maternal epithelial cells, creating intermittent or continuous areas with 5 layers. This used to be called a syndesmochorial placenta. Now it is understood that this is a variant of the epitheliochorial placenta, sometimes called a synepitheliochorial placenta. This is seen in sheep and goats and may be seen in cattle. In an endotheliochorial placenta, the chorion abuts the dam's endothelium (4 layers). This is the type of placenta in dogs and cats. In a hemochorial placenta, the chorion is bathed in the dam's blood (3 layers). This is the type of placenta in primates and rodents. The big picture is that animals with thicker placentas have reduced access to maternal proteins through the placenta, including antibodies, and are therefore more prone to failure of passive transfer, making them dependent on colostrum to a larger extent than other species. Failure of passive transfer (lack of antibodies needed to protect newborn animals against infectious disease) can occur either because a newborn animal didn't get antibodies through the placenta while *in utero* or because they did not get colostrum, the antibody-rich first milk, immediately after birth.

CARE OF SMALL ANIMALS

Veterinarians do not provide routine veterinary care for puppies and kittens immediately after birth as they do in other species. The chart below provides you with information regarding normal developmental milestones in puppies and kittens. Extensive information about physical examination and common disorders of puppies and kittens is available in the resources folder for this module of the course.

Timing of Significant Events in Pediatric Development of Puppies and Kittens

EVENT	AGE AT OCCURRENCE
Umbilical cord dries and falls off	2 to 3 days
Eyelids open	5 to 14 days
External ear canals open	6 to 14 days
Extensor dominance	5 days
Capable of crawling	7 to 14 days
Capable of walking, urinating and defecating spontaneously	14 to 21 days
Hematocrit / RBC number stabilize near that of adult	8 weeks
Renal function nears that of adult	8 weeks
Hepatic function nears that of adult	4 to 5 months

CARE OF FOALS

The level of care and degree of intervention for any neonate will vary with the management type and philosophy, and to some extent with the value of the individual offspring. In this section we'll look at fairly typical care of neonatal foals. Good management of the foal starts prior to birth, with care of the dam integral to optimizing postnatal foal health, and continues with common management procedures and veterinary examination of the neonate.

MANAGEMENT OF THE PREGNANT MARE TO OPTIMIZE FOAL HEALTH

Maximizing Colostral Quality

Even though they become immunocompetent during gestation, while cocooned in the uterus foals are generally not exposed to environmental and common disease-causing pathogens that they will be exposed to after birth. Due to their type of placentation, antibodies from the mare are not transferred prior to birth so the foal is born agammaglobulinemic and naïve regarding protection against potential pathogens they will encounter once born. Their initial circulating antibodies are absorbed from the mare's colostrum so it is important that the antibody content of colostrum is high in quantity and quality – that is to say that it is directed against organisms the foal is likely to encounter. Two strategies are generally employed to ensure this:

- If the mare is to be moved to a different farm for foaling (this often happens either to have her at a location with more supervision/experience in foaling mares or to have her at the farm where she will be re-bred for the next season), this move should occur at least 4-6 weeks prior to birth. This allows the mare to be exposed to the local microflora and to make use of gut-associated lymphoid tissue (GALT) to push antibodies against local flora into colostrum and later to create IgA in milk for continued protection against invasion.
- Vaccinate the mare 4-8 weeks prior to parturition to boost colostral antibodies.

This is a time to use vaccines that will give a systemic (IgG) response in the mare versus a local (IgA) response because we want the serum IgG available for transfer into the colostrum.

Typical vaccines used include those against:

- Tetanus
- Rabies
- Western and Eastern Equine Encephalitis (WEE/EEE)
- West Nile Virus
- Herpes Virus 1 and 4 – or just use EHV-1 and hope for cross-protection
- Influenza

Additional vaccines occasionally used depending on locale/farm conditions and likely pathogen exposure may include:

- Botulism
- Rotavirus
- *Streptococcus equi*

When giving large numbers of vaccines to a mare it is often considered good practice to give no more than four antigens at one time and to have a 2-4 week break before giving the next group, until the administration of all those desired has been completed. To accomplish this, the vaccines against diseases of lower risk and the vaccines resulting in the most robust antibody response are given earlier, and the "weaker" antigens are given later, usually about 4 weeks prior to foaling. Of those listed above, both tetanus and rabies vaccines are known to give a robust response and thus can be moved to the earlier time. Note that a mare in her first pregnancy may need an initial series of vaccines she has not had previously; in subsequent pregnancies it is most often just a single booster.

Measuring Colostral Quality

As foaling is imminent or immediately following birth of the foal, many larger farms will measure the quality of the colostrum. This is done by measuring specific gravity using a colostrometer or by measuring total solids using a sugar refractometer as a proxy for IgG concentration (Note: regular clinical refractometers used for plasma protein or urine specific gravity DO NOT work). Foals from mares with poor quality colostrum may be targeted for early supplementation from a frozen colostrum bank. Mares with excellent quality colostrum have some stripped out (250-300 ml) and frozen to deposit in the bank.

Mare Anti-RBC Antibody Screening

On larger farms and particularly for mares that have previously had a foal with neonatal isoerythrolysis (antibody-associated break down of red blood cells by the foal shortly after birth and colostrum ingestion), a blood sample is taken from the mare in the last two weeks of gestation to screen for antibodies directed against red cell antigens. Like other animals, horses have blood types and if the mare has antibodies against red cell antigens her foal has inherited (from the sire) it can result is severe red cell lysis once the foal has suckled. These antibodies are concentrated in colostrum and absorbed by the foal. In cases where a mare comes up positive the foal is NOT permitted to suckle her initially but is given colostrum from a safe source. The mare is milked out and the colostrum discarded. This is repeated and the foal not permitted to suck until about 24 hours of life (when the colostrum is gone and the foal's gut has closed to antibody absorption).

Anthelmintic (dewormer) Administration

On or about the day of parturition the mare is given an anthelmintic (usually ivermectin) to reduce passage of parasites to the foal. A particular parasite targeted by this is *Strongyloides westeri*, which is transmitted through the milk.

Management and Care of the Newborn Foal

If pregnancy and delivery were normal, the farm staff will observe the foal for normal behaviors and "milestones". If everything is going well, you, as a veterinarian, will probably see the foal for the first time when it is 12-18 hours old. If things were abnormal at birth or are not progressing as usual, you can expect a call earlier, and in the case of a high risk pregnancy, may be in attendance at birth.

Normal parameters for farm personnel to watch for are:

- Following birth the foal should be vigorous, have good muscle tone, and attain sternal recumbency within 2 minutes (i.e. not stay in lateral).
- A suckle reflex should be present in 10-15 minutes.
- The foal should attempt to stand in 15-30 minutes and achieve standing within 1 hour.
- The foal should nurse the mare's udder within 2 hours – Note that it is normal for it to try a few other places before it locates the udder!
- Normal behavior is for the foal to nurse about 7 times an hour for about 90 seconds/bout. They should gain about 2-3 lbs/day in weight.
- The foal should pass meconium (first poop, sticky dark tan/orangy stuff) within 4 hours.
- The foal should first urinate in about 4 hours and then keep on doing so. The urine should be pale, not distinctly yellow.

What the farm personnel will/should do:

- Dip the umbilical stump to help prevent ascending infections
    - Generally done with dilute chlorhexidine (0.5% = 1 in 4 dilution) or dilute iodine
    - Usually repeated several times in the first 24 hours
    - Use a syringe case or soaked gauze – they need to dip the umbilical remnant, not the entire ventral abdomen
- Weigh the foal
- Save the placenta for veterinarian to examine
- Plastic bag inside a clean 5 gallon feed pail with lid
- This avoids the common pathological artifact lesionae doggus chewus
- On many farms it is usual to give the foal an enema either prophylactically or if no meconium has passed in a few hours. Usually warm soapy water or a commercial "Fleet" enema is used.

Important Newborn Foal Milestones

Some of the vital milestones are summarized as the 1-2-3 rule:

- The foal should be standing within 1 hour
- The foal should have suckled from the mare within 2 hours
- The mare should have passed the placenta within 3 hours

Assuming all this happens and there are no other issues, then the first time the foal is seen by a veterinarian is for the well foal examination.

Well Foal Examination

Usually occurs at 12-18 hours of age (but may be out to 24-36 hours on a distant farm), and the veterinarian will:

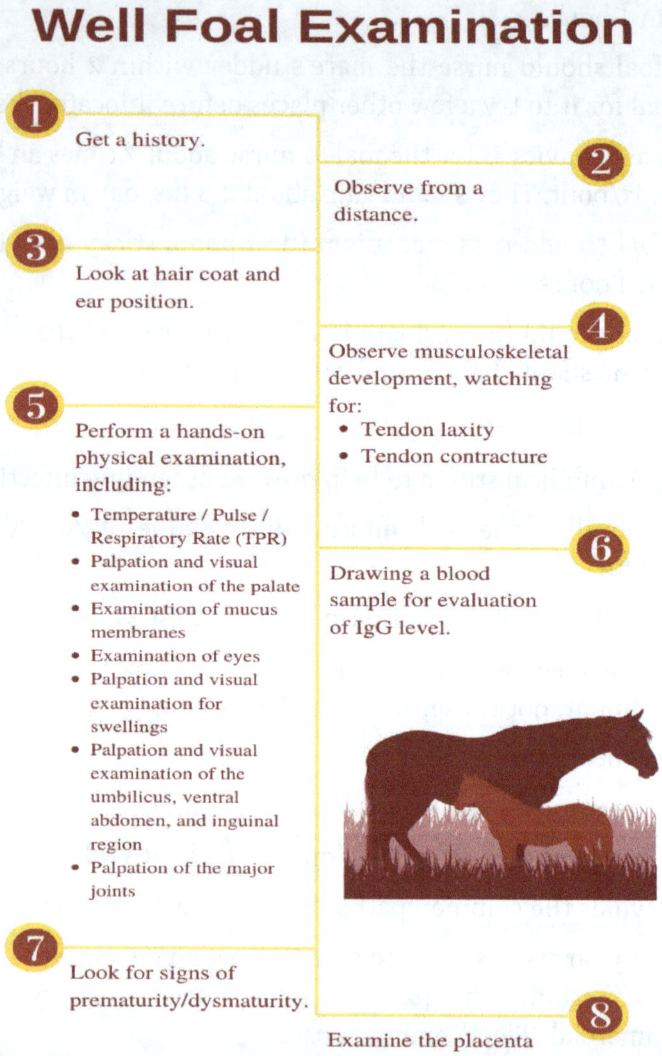

- Get a history including length of pregnancy, time and length of delivery, and the parameters listed previously (time to stand/nurse/pass meconium)
- Observe from a distance for normal behavior and respiratory effort and character
  - Normal foals are active between naps and have slightly jerky movements. Reduced activity and somnolence are signs of a problem

as is a distended udder in the mare – usually an indicator that the foal is not nursing.

- Look at hair coat and ear position (silky coat and/or floppy ears are a sign of prematurity/dysmaturity).
- Observe musculoskeletal development, particularly of the limbs, watching for:
    - Tendon laxity – fetlocks near/on the ground, toes tipped up, carpus hyperextended
    - Tendon laxity is another sign of prematurity/dysmaturity
    - Tendon contracture – club foot, upright fetlocks, flexed carpi
    - Limb deviations in the mediolateral plane when viewed from in front or behind
    - Valgus and varus
- Perform a hands-on physical examination particularly including:
    - Temperature / Pulse / Respiratory Rate (TPR)
    - It is normal to auscult a heart murmur for 1-2 days following birth; murmurs or arrhythmias present beyond 4 days after birth need investigating
    - Palpation and visual examination of the palate (for cleft palate – additional sign may be milk coming from the nostrils)
    - Examination of mucus membranes for normal color and refill and no petechiation (petechiation is a sign of sepsis)
    - Examination of eyes for cataract, corneal ulcers or entropion (rolled in eyelashes rubbing on cornea)
    - Foals don't have a reliable menace response (blink as you poke toward their eye) until about 2 weeks of age, so they have to learn to be scared of getting poked in the eye by stuff
    - Palpation and visual examination for swellings over the ribs and "clicks" indicative of fracture (birth in the horse is a fairly violent event)
    - Palpation and visual examination of the umbilicus, ventral abdomen, and inguinal region for evidence of swelling or herniation
    - Palpation of the major joints (carpus, stifles, fetlocks) for effusion
    - Joint effusion is usually related to infection in the joint, secondary to septicemia; this would be early to pick it up

- Drawing a blood sample for evaluation of IgG level (to assess adequacy of passive transfer of colostral antibodies – VITALLY IMPORTANT).
    - This is usually performed as a stall side test using a rapid ELISA kit
    - Foals with less than adequate levels (<800 mg/dL) get supplemental IgG, usually in the form of IV plasma, because sepsis is a leading cause of foal mortality and foals without adequate IgG levels are much more likely to become septic.
- Look for signs of prematurity/dysmaturity.
    - Foals with these signs that are otherwise doing okay should have carpi and tarsi radiographed to check for cuboidal bone ossification (the small bones that make up the carpus and tarsus), and have activity restricted if these are incompletely formed to avoid crush injuries.
- Examine the placenta
    - Is it complete?
    - Bits left in the mare promote uterine infection with resultant endotoxemia and laminitis – a very bad deal.
    - Are there abnormalities that indicate the foal may deserve a more thorough examination, closer observation or even some prophylactic treatment?
    - Placentitis, evidence of premature placental separation, reduced placental size.

Expected Vitals for Newborn Foals

AGE (hours)	HEART RATE (/min)	RESPIRATORY RATE (/min)	TEMPERATURE (°F)
0-2	120-150	60-80	99-100.5
2-36	90-120	20-40	99-101.5
48+	60-80	20-40	99-101.5

Other Things People May Do to Neonatal Foals Prophylactically

- Prophylactic antibiotics
    - On farms that have particular problems with septicemia or other neonatal bacterial infections, foals may be placed on antibiotics for the first 3-5 days of life. There is evidence in some studies of a significant reduction in serious infections when this is done.
- Hyperimmune plasma
    - Plasma from donor animals specifically vaccinated to provide high antibody titers against certain diseases is commercially available (e.g.

against clostridial organisms) and is used as an IV infusion, usually in the first day of life, on farms that have particular problems.

  - Some may also be administered by stomach tube to provide high levels in the gastrointestinal tract to prevent toxin absorption or bacterial adhesion (depending on whether you give an antitoxin-based antibody or one against the bacteria itself)

- Blood sample for complete blood count (CBC)/chemistry
  - People who have had sick foals previously may have a blood sample submitted for a CBC and serum chemistry panel as another early indicator of any possible infection (the earlier you can detect and treat the better it usually goes).
  - If the foal is being insured, a CBC may be part of the insurance company requirement prior to issuing a policy.

Physical Exercise for Newborn Foals

Foals have a fairly large surface area to volume ratio and not much in the way of insulating adipose tissue, so they depend on food intake and movement to generate heat. Provided the foal is normal and the weather and footing reasonable they can start life outside right away; obviously, that is the way they were designed. However, since we often modify the breeding season for economic reasons so birth is close to January 1st, conditions are often less than ideal. In particularly cold weather the mare and foal are usually housed inside, ideally with turnout a couple of times a day in an indoor arena or at least hand walking.

Foals with abnormalities of the musculoskeletal system (identified by management or on the veterinary examination) are more restricted:

- Premature and dysmature foals with incompletely ossified cuboidal bones are kept in a stall and often non-weight-bearing (i.e. lying down) as much as possible to avoid crush injury until ossification is complete (monitored by serial radiographs).
- Foals with tendon laxity are given controlled exercise, usually turnout in a small area so they don't try to get up too much speed until the tendons strengthen.
- Foals with tendon contracture have fairly heavy bandages or even casts put on their legs which actually encourage tendons to relax (you restrict something on a foal and it tends to respond by getting floppy), with some very controlled exercise to encourage stretching, and pain control (e.g. a non-steroidal anti-inflammatory like ketoprofen).

Other treatments for these can include frequent foot trims, corrective shoeing (glue on at this age), and medical and surgical options for those that are more severe or are not responding to conservative management.

CARE OF CALVES

Disease in dairy calves is not uncommon, with incidence of pre-weaning mortality reported as 5.6% and incidence of post-weaning mortality reported as 1.9%. Common causes for pre-weaning mortality include scours (gastrointestinal disease), respiratory disorders, and calving problems. The most common cause of post-weaning mortality is respiratory disease.

Calfhood disease is associated with short-term losses (labor to manage calves, drugs, calf mortality) and long-term losses (decreased rate of gain, increased risk of death before achieving goals as an adult such as increased risk of culling before first calving or increased age at first calving). Specific goals are set by the Dairy Calf and Heifer Association; these standards give farmers and their veterinarians goals to shoot for in disease management. For example, the goal for a given farm for pre-weaning mortality is less than 3%.

Key Management Areas for Pre-Weaned Dairy and Beef Calves and Specific Management Strategies

Late Gestation

In the last trimester, nutrition, immunity, and environment/housing of cows must be managed. Be aware that dairy cows are bred and calve year-round and that beef cows are bred and calve seasonally, with calving seasons in spring and fall. Late gestation nutrition includes feeding a diet balanced for energy, protein, vitamins, and minerals. Food must be palatable and may be available free choice. Free choice fresh water must be available. Body condition score should be at or just above average (3.0 to 3.5 on a 5-point scale for dairy cows, 5 to 6 on a 10-point scale for beef cows). Poor nutrition is associated with lower birth weight of calves; difficulty calving, especially in fat cows; lower production of colostrum and milk; slower calf growth; and overall lower calf survival. Cows are often vaccinated late in gestation to ensure high antibody concentrations in colostrum to protect the calf. In the time just prior to calving, dairy cows should be housed on clean, dry bedding and should not be overcrowded. Control heat in the summer (shade, fans, sprinklers) and provide protection from wind and precipitation in the winter. Beef cows are tough but do require a wind break, access to bedding, and access to feed.

Calving Environment

The calving area must be well-bedded and draft-free. It is important to keep it as clean and dry as possible by frequently removing dirty bedding and adding clean bedding. The calving area must be well away from pens for sick animals in the facility. Animals should be handled in a calm manner. Try to keep the cow from standing in mud, which is made up of manure, urine, and dirt. Her udder and the ground will be the first things to which the calf is exposed and both should be as clean as possible. An example of a pasture rotation system used in beef cattle to ensure calves are born on clean, parasite-free pasture is the Sandhills Calving System – The Sandhills Calving System uses larger, contiguous, pastures for calving, rather than high animal-density calving lots. Cows are turned into the first calving pasture (Pasture 1) as soon as the first calves are born. Calving continues in Pasture 1 for two weeks. After two weeks the cows that have not yet calved are moved to Pasture 2. Existing cow-calf pairs remain in Pasture 1. After a week of calving in Pasture 2, cows that have not calved are moved to Pasture 3 and cow-calf pairs born in Pasture 2 remain in Pasture 2. Each subsequent week cows that have not yet calved are moved to a new pasture and pairs remain in their pasture of birth. The result is cow-calf pairs distributed over multiple pastures; each containing calves within one week of age of each other. Cow-calf pairs from different pastures may be comingled after the youngest calf is four weeks of age and all calves are considered low-risk for neonatal diarrhea.

Care of the Newborn Calf

For beef calves, calving should be monitored and assisted if needed. The calf's umbilicus should be disinfected with 7% tincture of iodine. The calf is assessed to ensure good vigor and a protected area with or without a heat lamp and other supportive care is provided if needed. The calf is individually identified with an ear tag and will remain with the cow until weaning. For dairy calves, calving should be monitored and assisted if needed. The calf's umbilicus is disinfected with 7% tincture of iodine. The calf is immediately removed from the cow (within 30-60 minutes of birth) and is raised separately from her. Immediately post-partum, the calf is dried in a warming box, with a heat lamp, or in a warm room if the calf is born during cold winter months. Calf blankets may be used and the calf is individually identified with an ear tag.

Colostrum

Cows have an epithelichorial placenta with six complete layers (three each from the fetus and dam). There is virtually no movement of antibodies across this placenta so all calves are born without protective circulating antibodies. Colostrum, the first milk secreted after parturition, is rich in immunoglobulins (IgG, IgA, IgM), cytokines, and nutrients. Colostral antibodies are absorbed across the gut early in the calf's life and so help the calf develop circulating concentrations of antibodies that provide temporary immune protection until the calf's immune system develops. Blood can be drawn from calves between 24 hours and 7 days of age to determine if they have had sufficient antibody transfer; normal values are greater than 10 mg/mL of serum IgG and/or greater than 5.2 gm/dL of serum total protein. Dairy calves are presented with colostrum by the farmer in the first days of life. Beef calves get colostrum directly from the dam; if the cow is not a good mother or the calf if not nursing for some other reason, the calf may need to be fostered onto another cow or handfed to ensure it receives colostrum. It is reported that up to 14% of dairy calves in the United States have insufficient transfer of antibodies ("failure of passive transfer") and that 31% of deaths in the first 3 weeks of life are associated with failure of passive transfer.

Specifics of colostrum management include:

- **Evaluation of quality** – The goal is to have greater than 50 gm/L of IgG in colostrum. Factors that impact colostrum quality include late gestation (dry cow) vaccinations, dry cow nutrition, avoiding stress in dry cows (heat, crowding), and ensuring the dry period is of adequate length (not shorter than 21 days). Antibody concentration is measured on a colostrometer or Brix (sugar) refractometer (22% total solids = 50 gm/L IgG).
- **Ensure calves are receiving the right quantity** – The goal is to feed 150-200 gm of IgG. This usually is done by providing 10% of the calf's body weight (usually 3-4 liters or 4 quarts) within 6 hours of birth. Dairy calves can be fed using a nippled bottle or an esophageal tube feeder.
- **Ensure time to first feeding is as quick as possible** – The gut loses ability to absorb large proteins like antibodies by 24 hours of life so the goal is to provide colostrum orally within the first 1-2 hours of life if possible.

Beef calves are left to nurse off of the cow and to receive colostrum with less oversight. Someone should verify that the cow has colostrum (thicker and yellower than regular milk), that the cow's teats are patent, that the calf is up and trying to nurse, and that the dam is allowing the calf to nurse. If a dairy or beef cow has no colostrum, calves can be fed frozen colostrum from storage, or colostrum replacement products. As in foals, blood can be drawn from calves within the first week of life to determine if they have received adequate colostrum.

Pre-Weaning Nutrition

See Nutrition-Herbivores chapter.

Housing and Sanitation

The goal when housing dairy calves prior to weaning is to avoid contact of that calf with older animals or their environment, including air, water, bedding, feed, and pasture used by older animals. Calves also should not directly contact each other. The housing may be individual calf hutches or other individual enclosures. If producers do group dairy calves prior to weaning, then introduction to the group should be delayed until the calf is 12-14 days old, and group sizes should be kept as small as possible (< 8 calves/group) in order to reduce disease risk. The enclosure should be draft-free but well ventilated and bedded with abundant clean, dry bedding. Enclosures should be well cleaned and sanitized between uses. The setup should be such that calves can be managed and moved with minimal stress and decreased risk of injury. Calves are not in solitary confinement when in calf hutches; a study published in Applied Animal Behavior Science in 2015 demonstrated that calves that had gentle interactions with handlers up to three minutes per day as they received their normal feeding and care gained more weight in the first two weeks of life. Research has shown some benefits of allowing pre-weaned calves to socialize (i.e. have a buddy). Pair housing (groups of 2 calves) is a viable compromise to allow socialization between pre-weaned calves while still minimizing the increased disease risk that occurs if we group pre-weaned calves. Since early weight gain is associated with increased milk production as an adult, this has behavioral benefits for the calves and benefits for the producer as well.

Health Procedures

Which procedures are performed depends on the farm, with the program determined by the farmer and veterinarian. Examples include ear tag application and dipping the umbilicus as described above, testing serum protein concentrations to assess for failure of passive transfer, tests for specific diseases, vaccination, dehorning, and castration.

Disease Detection and Treatment

This again varies by farm. Early detection and treatment of disease improves success and may help prevent spread of disease in the facility. Veterinarians may be involved in helping develop protocols and in training farm staff.

CARE OF PIGLETS

The following notes are largely excerpted from: http://extension.missouri.edu/p/G2500.

The most critical period in the life cycle of a pig is from birth to weaning. On the average, about 1-2 piglets per litter are lost during this period, with an average pre-weaning mortality of 12%. As number of piglets per litter increases, birth weights of individual piglets decreases. Piglets that weigh less than 2.2-2.4 pounds (1 kg) at birth have more than a 50% chance of dying before weaning. Other common causes of mortality are crushing, starvation, and dehydration due to diarrhea.

Weaning large litters of thrifty, heavyweight pigs is a key factor for a profitable swine herd. This publication attempts to outline management practices that help keep pigs alive and profits high.

Farrowing

Preparation for Farrowing

The average gestation period for sows is 114 days. To prepare for farrowing, producers should know when sows are due. Producers should be ready for delivery prior to the due date because of individual variation in gestation.

Newborn piglets have a better survival chance if they arrive in a clean, warm, and sanitized farrowing facility. Research has shown that a break between farrowing reduces disease buildup. Many producers, however, only allow for a one-day break between groups of sows to maximize use of expensive facilities. If the facility is used continuously, cleaning and sanitation must be optimized to control spread of disease.

In addition, it would be beneficial to wash the sow with soap and warm water immediately prior to being put into the farrowing stall; this is rarely done for practical reasons.

Care at Farrowing

Three basic requirements for newborn pigs:

- A good environment
- Adequate and regular nutrition
- Safety from disease and crushing

Individual attention from the producer at this point pays off with more live pigs. The amount of labor available may determine how much time you spend in the farrowing house. One dedicated team in charge of the farrowing works well in larger operations. The table below indicates the scope and causes of piglet mortality.

Causes of piglet death (Leman and Knudson, 1972)

CAUSE	PERCENTAGE AFFECTED
Crushing	30.9
Starvation	17.6
Born Weak	14.7
Chilling	5.5
Transmissible gastroenteritis	3.9
Other diarrheas	12.9
Pneumonia	1.4
Others	13.1
TOTAL	100

Management — First Few Days After Farrowing

There are many essential chores to be done shortly after pigs are born. The navel should be disinfected the day pigs are born using tincture of iodine. If possible, match the number of piglets to the number of functional mammary glands. If several sows are farrowing within a 24-hour period, pigs can be transferred successfully from one sow to another if piglets are moved within the first 3 days of life and have received colostrum before transfer. Transfer bigger pigs in the litter, not the runts. Transfer of piglets may not be recommended during a disease outbreak; for example, pork producers were working through emergence of the new disease Porcine Epidemic Diarrhea (PED) in 2013 and veterinarians were recommending not moving piglets as a biocontainment measure.

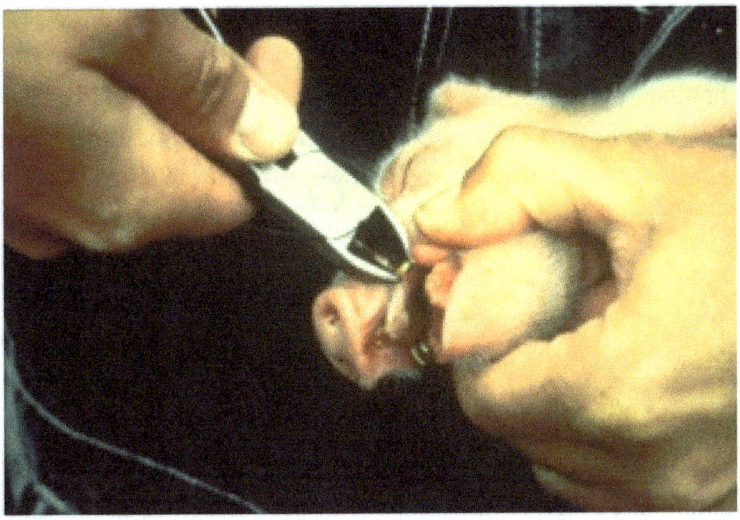

"Newborn Pig: Clipping Needle Teeth", http://animalbiosciences.uoguelph.ca/~gking/Ag_2350/farrow.htm

Clip needle teeth, being careful not to crush the teeth or cut the gums. "Pigs are born with eight needle (sometimes called wolf) teeth located on the sides of the upper and lower jaws. Historically, needle teeth were clipped in newborn pigs to prevent potential damage to the sow underline and consequentially, a reluctance to allow nursing. Clipping needle teeth was also seen as a means for preventing injuries to the faces of littermates when fighting occurred. Some producers have totally abandoned the procedure or clip needle teeth only when sows are not milking well or if disease is present in the herd. [Based on a study performed at Virginia Tech], they suggest that "clipping needle teeth may be warranted on some farms to prevent pig and teat injuries, and that the process has no positive or negative impact on pig and sow performance." (Excerpt from Virginia Tech Extension) A controlled study comparing litters with clipped or intact needle teeth showed no difference in weight gain and mortality but demonstrated that piglets with intact needle teeth were more likely to have facial injuries. One of the students in the class of 2019 shared that she worked at a farrowing unit where they chose to stop clipping needle teeth for a time. They decided to start clipping needle teeth again because they found that when they were clipped, the piglets had fewer facial swellings and infections from biting each other and the sows were more comfortable and less likely to jump up and interrupt nursing of piglets because their underlines were not being traumatized by the needle teeth when piglets were suckling.

At the same time needle teeth are clipped, tails can be docked. Tail docking is performed to prevent tail biting and cannibalism among pigs later in life. Leave a stub on the tail about 1/4-inch long. Tail-docking is best done when the pigs are one day old. Ear-notching is practiced in some smaller herds. This identification helps select replacement animals from top litters and gives a check on age when pigs reach market weight. An evaluation of welfare implications of teeth clipping, tail docking, and permanent identification of piglets is available from the AVMA.

Iron deficiency develops rapidly in nursing pigs reared in confinement because of:

- Low body storage of iron in the newborn pig
- Low iron content of sow's colostrum and milk
- Elimination of contact with iron from soil
- The rapid growth of the nursing pig

Iron deficiency is associated with inability to produce hemoglobin and subsequent anemia. There are many good sources of iron that can be used to prevent anemia. Iron-dextran injected in the muscle is an effective method. Injections are done in the neck. Common levels are 150-200 milligrams of iron as iron-dextran, usually given the first 2 days after birth. Don't give overdoses of iron because it may induce shock. Iron also can be mixed in the feed or in the drinking water. Supplying uncontaminated soil in the pig area is another method of supplying iron but is not used much in today's confinement systems.

Management During Lactation

Baby Pig Scours

Baby pig scours are major ongoing problems for swine producers. Most common diarrheas are caused by various strains of *E. coli*. The symptom of *E. coli*-induced diarrhea is a watery, yellowish stool. Pigs are most susceptible from 1-4 days of age, at 3 weeks of age, and at around the time of weaning. Although pigs are born with little disease resistance, this resistance increases as they absorb antibodies from their mother's colostrum. Because pigs' ability to absorb antibodies decreases rapidly from birth, it becomes important that they feed on colostrum soon after birth. Colostrum provides the only natural disease protection they will have until their own mechanism for antibody production begins to function effectively at 4-5 weeks. Disease resistance is lowest at 3 weeks. It is wise to avoid unnecessary stress (castration, vaccination, worming) at this time. In treating common scours, orally administered drugs are usually more effective than injections. You should use a drug effective against the bacterial strain on your farm. It is important to remember that many viruses also can be the cause of baby pig scours. A dry, warm, draft-free environment is of primary importance in reducing scours. Sanitation is also very important in reducing the incidence of baby pig scours.

Castration

Boar pigs can be castrated any time before they are 4 weeks old. In most states, it is legal for the farmer to perform this surgery in pigs and it is done before the piglets are one week old.

EXTRA RESOURCES

Clipping of needle teeth: http://www.sites.ext.vt.edu/newsletter-archive/livestock/aps-01_11/aps-0431.html

Valgus and varus: www.acvs.org/large-animal/angular-limb-deviation

Pediatric course information from Dr. Peggy Root: https://sites.google.com/a/umn.edu/margaret-v-peggy-root-kustritz/home/archived-courses/cvm-6451—pediatrics

CHAPTER-8

INTRODUCTION TO DENTISTRY

SMALL ANIMAL PREVENTIVE DENTISTRY

Puppies and kittens are born with no visible teeth. The deciduous (baby) teeth erupt over about the first 6 weeks of life and then are replaced by the permanent teeth by about 4-6 months of age. The incisors are lost first, then the premolars and finally, the canine teeth. The canine teeth are reliably lost at about 6 months of age and this

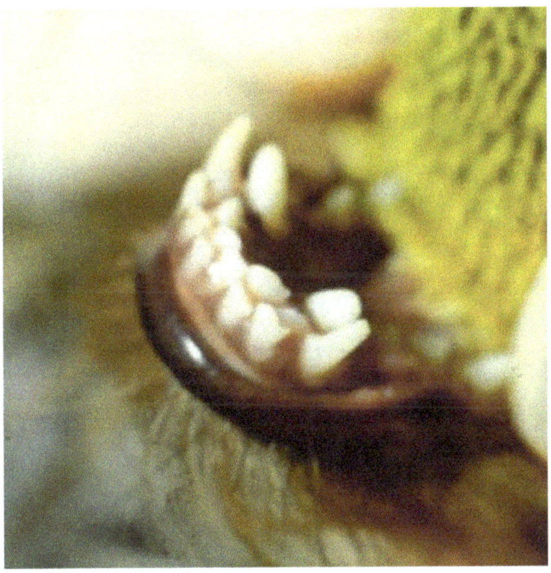

Retained deciduous teeth in a dog (Photo courtesy of Drs. Gary Goldstein and Kevin Stepaniuk)

Knowledge can be used to judge age of puppies or kittens. Most teeth are lost when the animal is eating and so are swallowed. This does not harm the puppy or kitten. Some dogs will grow in their adult teeth next to their deciduous teeth, without the deciduous teeth falling out. Those deciduous teeth should be removed as soon as possible as they may cause or worsen an abnormal bite and predispose the animal to dental disease.

One year, students found a chart on DVM 360 that stated that the sequence of eruption of adult teeth in small animals was incisors followed by canines followed by premolars. I checked with a veterinary dentist for clarification. When talking about animals losing their baby teeth, you have to differentiate eruption from complete replacement. Incisors always are first. Premolars and canines may erupt through the gum near the same time but because canines take longer to completely erupt, they are the last to be completely replaced in the mouth. So the sequence to remember for small animals is incisors - premolars - canines.

Determining Age of Cats and Dogs Through Their Teeth

Animal Sheltering "HOW TO" SERIES

How to Determine a Cat's or Dog's Age

Shelters are depositories for animals of all types and ages, from the cute, unweaned kitten whose eyes are barely open to the graying, noble 17-year-old shepherd mix who can hardly stand on his own. How can you figure out the age of an animal who falls somewhere in between these two extremes? Start by looking at the teeth.

Examining teeth is one of the best ways to determine the approximate age of a cat or dog. Look at the degree of *growth* to determine the ages of kittens and puppies, and look at the degree of *wear* to determine the ages of adult cats and dogs. The diagram and chart below can help.

Be aware of two things that can throw off your estimate. First, an animal who has received dental care will have better-looking teeth than an animal who has not received such treatment. Second, variations exist among animals, even two from the same litter. Teeth are only a rough indicator of any animal's actual age.

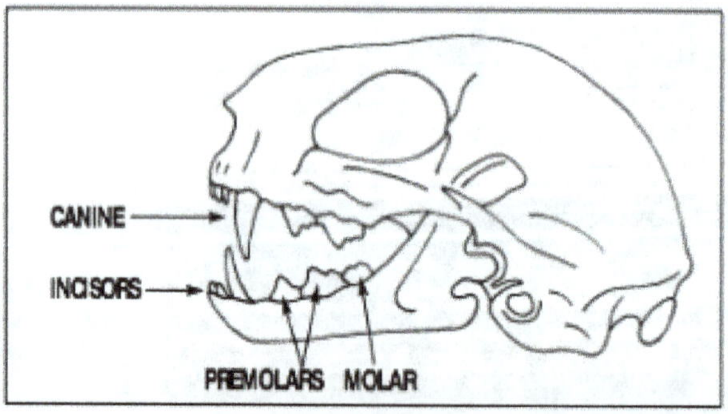

Note: The location of teeth in a dog's jaw is similar to the cat's jaw shown here.

"Determining age by examining teeth", https://www.goldenacresdogs.com/dog-teeth-by-age.html

ESTIMATED AGE	CAT'S TEETH	DOG'S TEETH
2-4 weeks	Deciduous (baby) incisors coming in	No noticeable tooth growth
3-4 weeks	Deciduous (baby) canines coming in	Deciduous (baby) canines coming in

ESTIMATED AGE	CAT'S TEETH	DOG'S TEETH
4-6 weeks	Deciduous (baby) premolars coming in on lower jaw	Deciduous (baby) incisors and premolars coming in
8 weeks	All deciduous (baby) teeth are in	All deciduous (baby) teeth are in
3 1/2 – 4 months	Permanent incisors coming in	No noticeable permanent tooth growth
4-5 months	Permanent canines,premolars, and molars	Permanent incisors coming in; some growth coming in of premolars and molars
5-7 months	All permanent teeth in by 6 months	Permanent canines, premolars, and molars coming in; all teeth in by 7 months
1 year	Teeth white and clean	Teeth white and clean
1-2 years	Teeth may appear dull with some tartar build-up	Teeth may appear dull with some tartar (yellowing) on back teeth
3-5 years	Teeth show more tartar build-up (on all teeth)	Teeth show more tartar build-up (on all teeth) and some tooth wear
5-10 years	Teeth show increased wear and disease; pigment	Teeth show increased wear and disease visible on gums
10-15 years	Teeth are worn and show heavy tartar build-up	Teeth are worn and show heavy tartar; some teeth may be missing

Periodontal disease in small animals is caused by plaque and formation of pockets. On clean teeth, a biofilm develops in minutes and plaque in hours, with that plaque maturing over weeks and eventually mineralizing into calculus (tartar). Plaque is composed primarily of bacteria, and also contains water, saliva, minerals, and food particles. As the host's immune system responds to formation of plaque, inflammation and disease develop under the gum line. This is gingivitis, inflammation of gingival tissue resulting from build-up of plaque and calculus and secondary accumulation of bacterial by-products and endotoxins. Gingivitis is reversible. If the process is not stopped, inflammation affects the periodontium and the supporting structures of the teeth. This is periodontitis and it is irreversible.

Periodontal Disease in Small Animals

STAGE OF DISEASE	CLINICAL SIGNS	PATIENT/CLIENT RECOMMENDATIONS
Healthy	No evidence of disease, gums are coral pink, gingival margins are razor sharp	Brush teeth daily, provide dental toys and chews, present the animal for an oral examination every 6-12 months, plan for the first professional dental cleaning at 1 year of age (small dogs, cats) or 2 years of age (larger dogs)

STAGE OF DISEASE	CLINICAL SIGNS	PATIENT/CLIENT RECOMMENDATIONS
Stage 1	Inflammation of gingival margins, halitosis, gum edema, some bleeding upon probing of gums	Professional dental cleaning (consider full mouth dental radiographs), continue to brush teeth daily and provide dental toys and chews
Stage 2	Moderate gingivitis, probing may show loss of attachment at tooth of up to 25% and pockets 3-5 mm in depth with more bleeding with probing, halitosis, teeth are stable	Professional dental cleaning (full mouth dental radiographs), continue to brush teeth daily and provide dental toys and chews
Stages 3 and 4	Severe inflammation, bleeding gums and exposed tooth roots with tooth instability, severe halitosis	This is a level of disease requiring extensive dental treatment. The goal of preventive dentistry is to keep this level of disease from developing.

BRUSHING DOGS' OR CATS' TEETH: FOR PET OWNERS

Here is an excerpt from a text for pet owners regarding how to brush their dog's or cat's teeth: To slow the development of dental disease, you can brush your pet's teeth. If possible, you should accustom them to this practice when they are young, however pets of any age can be trained to accept brushing of teeth. Plaque usually accumulates on the surface of the teeth against the cheek. Only toothpaste specific for dogs and cats should be used. A soft, nylon-bristle toothbrush designed for dogs and cats, or a pediatric human toothbrush can be used. Brush once daily and do not worry about rinsing. Your animal will require a professional cleaning and polishing under general anesthesia periodically over its life. Your veterinarian will examine your animal's teeth every time they do a physical examination and can give you advice regarding dental care.

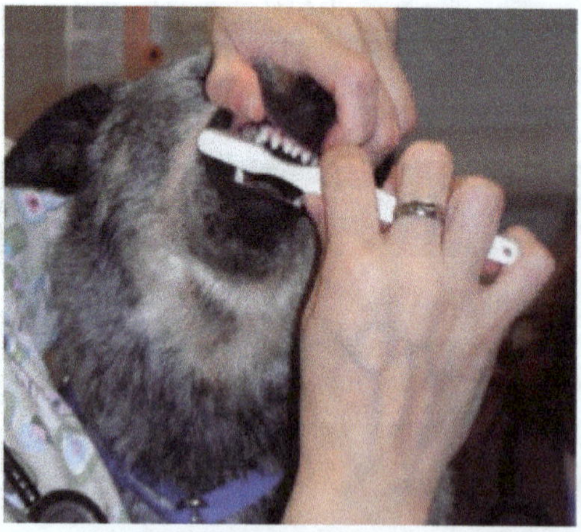

Brushing a dog's teeth, (photo courtesy of Marie Kustritz)

Many products are marketed as means of maintaining good oral health in dogs and cats. These include foods, chews, oral rinses, and products to be dissolved in the drinking water. Some products have been proven to show some benefit, as described by the Veterinary Oral Health Council.

What procedures constitute a professional dental cleaning? Controversy exists regarding use of anesthesia for dental cleanings in dogs with minimal dental disease. The American Animal Hospital Association recommends that all dogs and cats undergoing a dental cleaning be maintained on an inhalant anesthetic with a properly cuffed endotracheal tube in place. A complete oral examination usually is best done with the dog or cat under general anesthesia.

Dental prophylaxis (commonly called a "prophy") is performed on animals with a healthy mouth or very mild to moderate gingivitis. A thorough oral examination is performed. The teeth, including subgingival areas, are scaled with an ultrasonic scaler and curettes, and are then polished. This is the goal of preventive small animal dentistry. The 2013 AAHA article by Holmstrom et al outlines current recommendations for high-quality small animal dentistry in practice.

Conversation Points to Help Pet Owners Understand Preventive Dentistry

- Periodontal disease and infection are common; 91% of dogs and 85% of cats have some degree of dental disease. Dental disease can be painful and may cause the animal to change eating and drinking behaviors or other behaviors in ways that affect their overall health and how they interact with other animals and family members.
- Periodontal disease is preventable. Just looking at your own pet's teeth is not enough, because gum disease starts beneath the gum line.
- Preventive dental care can slow or stop the progression of periodontal disease.

EQUINE DENTISTRY

Basics of Equine Dentistry

- Horses have deciduous (baby) teeth that are lost as the permanent teeth begin to erupt. There is a chart in the Extra Resources folder demonstrating timing of loss of deciduous teeth in the horse if you're interested. Once permanent teeth begin to erupt, they continue to erupt over the horse's life. There is a link to information in the Merck Manual about how to use examination of teeth to estimate age in horses.
- General anesthesia is induction of complete unconsciousness through the use of drugs. Horses (or any animal) under general anesthesia cannot stand. Specifically with horses, there are concerns about getting the horse

down as you induce anesthesia and getting the horse up as it awakes from anesthesia. As you might imagine, as the horse loses and gains consciousness, it has abnormal balance and to have something that big lurching around is a danger to the animal and to the humans working with it. Outside of injury, horses also undergo a decrease in gut motility while under general anesthesia, which may be associated with colic after the anesthetic episode is done. For these reasons, we try not to induce general anesthesia and instead more commonly try to do standing sedation in horses, where they are given drugs that decrease anxiety and pain but do not induce complete unconsciousness.

- Floating is the term used to describe the removal of sharp points and small abnormalities of bite to make the horse more comfortable. The float is a rasp and as such, smooths and levels as it is used. Horses, as herbivores, need the occlusal surfaces of their teeth to be rough. You would never purposefully float the occlusal surfaces of teeth on a horse.

EXTRA RESOURCES

2017 WSAVA Dental guidelines: https://www.wsava.org/WSAVA/media/Documents/Guidelines/Dental-Guidleines-for-endorsement_0.pdf

Estimation of age by examination of the teeth in horses, cattle, and dogs: https://www.msdvetmanual.com/digestive-system/dental-development/estimation-of-age-by-examination-of-the-teeth

Products that benefit oral health in dogs and cats: www.vohc.org

Procedures for a professional dental cleaning: https://www.aaha.org/aaha-guidelines/dental-care/dental-care-home/

Current recommendations for small animal dentistry in practice: https://www.ncbi.nlm.nih.gov/pubmed/23443202

Basics of equine dentistry: https://pressbooks.umn.edu/app/uploads/sites/7/2019/08/8_Equine-Dentistry_Dr.-Linn.pdf

Normal equine dentition: https://sceniccityvet.com/veterinary-services/dental-care

CHAPTER-9
BEHAVIOR: AN OVERVIEW

This chapter does not include information about assessing behaviors or moving and handling cattle.

BEHAVIOR OF BIRDS

The big take-home point from this chapter is that all behavior has function.

Birds physically have a different brain from mammals with a much smoother surface. Historically, people though that meant that birds had a less complex brain and were, therefore, less capable of high level thought ("bird brains"). We now know that is not true.

Research into behavior has demonstrated that behavior in birds, as in many species, is a blend of genetics and physical adaptations to environmental change. Long-term evolutionary change to adapt to the environment in birds includes physical adaptations such as wings, beaks, and vocal structures to permit communications. Long- and short-term adaptations also occur in learning. People have addressed the science of understanding learning and behavior through three models. The ethological approach is species-specific and focuses on genetic adaptations through natural selection. The medical approach considers behavior to be a symptom of something we can diagnose and potentially treat or cure. The behavioral approach looks at the interaction between the observable behavior and the observable condition and asks how this specific animal is responding to this specific environment. All three models have their place.

Birds adapted over millennia to take advantage of specific niches in the environment. Their free-ranging (natural) behaviors include foraging, social interactions, self-maintenance (grooming), and resting. Some natural behaviors are not conducive to life in captivity.

If you consider domestication, dogs have been selected by humans for years for their value as companions and part of that is their ability to "read" humans. Birds (except for chickens) are not domesticated and there are so many species that it's difficult for any one person to know the specific set of behaviors common in that bird species. Birds will therefore show maladaptive behaviors, which are normal behaviors expressed in an abnormal setting. These may include things like calling out (birds need to call loudly to be heard in noisy tropical environments), personal space boundaries (different species of birds have widely differing natural territories), wood chewing (making nest cavities), and flinging of food (birds in the wild have abundant food and can be messy eaters). Birds also may show truly abnormal behaviors, such as feather destructive behaviors, biting, excessive vocalization, excessive egg-laying, and perch potato syndrome. Birds may show these behaviors because they have too little control or too little mental stimulation in their captive environment, in their perception, or because they are truly malfunctional, with abnormal physiology, neurochemistry, or brain development.

A brief history in aviculture may help our understanding of current behavior concerns with caged bird species. Prior to the 1970s, birds were captured in the wild and imported. Captive breeding began in the 70s and 80s and was required after the Wild Bird Importation Act was passed in 1992, which banned importation of captured wild birds. Birds can be very long-lived so you may still see some birds that were wild caught but most of the birds we see were captive bred and raised by humans. In an attempt to do the best possible for these birds, we raised them in environments with good biosecurity, and wing-clipped and weaned them early, so we could hand feed them and they would bond to humans. This was not the best strategy. Some birds are reproductive R-strategists (lay many eggs and provide little parenting) and some are reproductive K-strategists (lay few eggs and provide a lot of parenting, often in flocks) and we did not have enough information to let us know how to raise these varying types of birds. This created many birds with the equivalent of "orphanage syndrome", which is seen in primates that fail to thrive despite having received all necessary physiological needs because of lack of emotional attachment. The current gold standard for raising birds is to choose healthy parents with good behavioral traits; leave young birds with the parents as long as possible; habituate them to humans by vocal signals, gentle massage, and light contact; allow them to develop curiosity, socialization and exploration; and allow them to develop flight.

Investigating Behavior Problems in Birds

Problems in birds may develop because their captive lifestyle does not mimic their natural lifestyle in any respect. Birds reproduce, molt, migrate and then start that cycle over in the wild. These are all energy-intensive behaviors that occur due to environmental triggers and hormonal cues. With constant lighting and temperature of indoor environments, presence of potential "mates" (including humans), abundant food, and nest box availability, birds may show normal reproductive behaviors that are maladaptive in the captive environment. Examples include pair bonding, courtship regurgitation, cavity seeking, nest building, and territorial defense. Birds may also undergo hormone toxicity, which is early onset of sexual maturity or prolonged triggering of reproductive behaviors.

A multidisciplinary approach is needed where medical conditions are investigated and a functional behavior analysis is performed. Some definitions to guide this discussion are:

- **Behavior** – what an animal does under certain conditions that can be observed – it is something an animal does, not something an animal is, and it can be observed and measured.
- **Construct** – a label or interpretation.

It is important to separate behavior from constructs. If a bird bites, you may think he's mean. Biting is a behavior. Being mean is a construct. Constructs are not useful because they lead to circular thinking (he bites because he's mean and I know he's mean because he bites), they give you a false sense of having explained the behavior and so provide an excuse to give up, they can be self-fulfilling, and they can predispose you to trying harmful strategies to change the behavior.

To promote new behaviors, you need to empower the learner and give them a choice. You need to create a situation where the good behavior is more functional for the bird.

The ABCs of Behavior

A = antecedent (environment: what makes the bird show the behavior)

B = behavior

C = consequence

Predicting Behavior

Identifying the antecedent, resultant behavior, and consequences that follow does not always allow one to predict future behavior. Here is a checklist:

- Define the target behavior.
- Does the antecedent set the occasion for the behavior to occur?
- Does the consequence depend on the behavior? Are they functionally related?
- Does the consequence maintain, increase, or decrease the behavior?
- Can it predict future behavior?

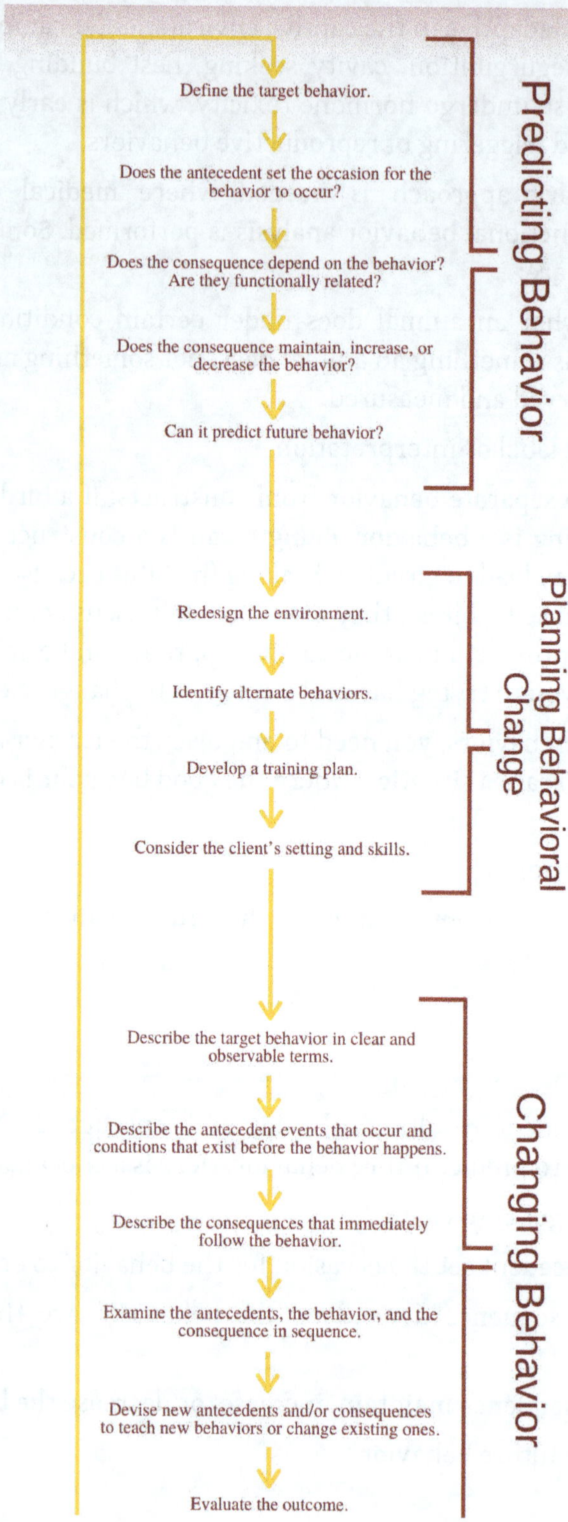
Define the target behavior.
Does the antecedent set the occasion for the behavior to occur?
Does the consequence depend on the behavior? Are they functionally related?
Does the consequence maintain, increase, or decrease the behavior?
Can it predict future behavior?
Predicting Behavior
Redesign the environment.
Identify alternate behaviors.
Develop a training plan.
Consider the client's setting and skills.
Planning Behavioral Change
Describe the target behavior in clear and observable terms.
Describe the antecedent events that occur and conditions that exist before the behavior happens.
Describe the consequences that immediately follow the behavior.
Examine the antecedents, the behavior, and the consequence in sequence.
Devise new antecedents and/or consequences to teach new behaviors or change existing ones.
Evaluate the outcome.
Changing Behavior

As in other species, reinforcers increase behaviors and punishers decrease behaviors. Effective reinforcement has contingency (it always happens) and contiguity (it always happens immediately after the behavior) and is highly individual. It is the bird who decides if a reward is reinforcing (leading to an increase in that behavior) or not. Something you may think is a great reward may mean nothing to that bird. Begin by reinforcing a behavior already exhibited by the bird. Once the bird has mastered it, withhold reinforcement. This will lead to an "extinction burst", which is an increase in behavior seen when rewards go away. Punishment decreases behaviors but may be associated with learned helplessness, generalized fear or phobias, withdrawal from the training relationship, or apathy. If you want a bird to stop a behavior, try reinforcing an acceptable substitute behavior or an incompatible behavior (for example, to stop biting, reinforce something else that occupies their beak).

When Making a Plan to Change Behavior

- Redesign the environment
- Identify alternate behaviors
- Develop a training plan
- Consider the client's setting and skills

Six Steps to Behavior Change

- Describe the target behavior in clear and observable terms.
- Describe the antecedent events that occur and conditions that exist before the behavior happens.
- Describe the consequences that immediately follow the behavior.
- Examine the antecedents, the behavior, and the consequence in sequence.
- Devise new antecedents and/or consequences to teach new behaviors or change existing ones.
- Evaluate the outcome.

Specific Problem Behaviors

Feather destructive behavior is self-inflicted damage where birds break and/or pull out feathers. It is not a diagnosis, it is a sign and causes are multiple. It has a relationship to neurological development and to lack of enrichment. It is most common in big parrots and those species that bond most strongly to humans. It is thought to be related to syndromes in non-human primates (who, like birds, are intelligent, social, and altricial (immature) at birth) who injure themselves as a consequence of having been reared in isolation. This is similar to psittacine (parrot-like) birds that were taken from their parents at an early age, reared by humans, and individually caged at weaning or as juveniles. The self-wounding is a physiological positive reinforcer of the behavior and acts as a coping strategy. Enrichment may be beneficial (see below). Other behavioral interventions include distracting the bird from the destructive behavior, positively reinforcing for a different, non-destructive behavior, and using preventive measures by trying to identify cues that the bird is about to start picking. Drug therapies are rarely helpful.

Enrichment is about simulating activities in the wild and redirecting energy away from reproductive behaviors and toward survival behaviors. Chewing activities are good for enrichment. If food is part of enrichment, avoid high fat and high sugar foods, and refined carbohydrates.

For enrichment, provide both non-destructible and destructible items. Rotate them regularly and do not overload the cage. Examples include chew toys, climbing toys, foot toys, and puzzle toys. This may include things to shred (phone books, paperback books, catalogs, junk mail, paper cups), things to hunt for (toys filled with food), alternate perching sites, coils and ropes for climbing, play stands and gyms, an outdoor aviary, and opportunities to forage. In one study, foraging in the wild was shown to occupy 4-6 hours per day and foraging birds in the wild ate a large variety of fruits, seeds, nuts, berries, blossoms, and leaf buds, from up to 60 plant species. Caged birds generally eat for 30-72 minutes per day and expend no energy getting the food. Foraging toys can be used to make birds "hunt" for their food as they would in the wild. Good examples of enrichment can be found in The Parrot Enrichment Activity Book by Kris Porter.

Dr. Ponder's Myths About Bird Behavior

- Height dominance (birds want to be higher than you no matter what and will bite if you try to get them down): This does not occur and is actually a bad choice for birds, as they would be more likely to be attacked by aerial predators if they chose to perch very high in the wild.
- Parrots must obey: This is the same idea as the need to exert dominance in dogs and is equally untrue.
- Flock dominance (one bird in the flock is at the top of the pecking order): There is nothing to support this theory.
- If it's green, it's mean: This is a construct!
- Punishment doesn't work: Punishment may cause a decrease in behavior but also may have undesirable side-effects as described earlier.
- Positive reinforcement takes too long: Positive reinforcement takes patience but is a good training tool.

BEHAVIOR OF HORSES

Horses are prey animals. They are precocial, which means they are born in an advanced state and are able to feed themselves almost immediately. They are able to run within hours of birth. All horses have an extremely reactive flight response. We must learn how to help them modify this response in order to effectively and safely train the horse to offer acceptable behaviors.

Their main response is flight. If they are unable to flee, they will fight (kick, strike, run over handler). Anyone within 10 feet of a frightened horse is at risk of serious injury.

In horses, the corpus callosum, which connects the right and left hemispheres of the brain, is underdeveloped. This means that horses may learn to do something on their right side and need to be trained also to do it on their left side, or that they may see something with their right eye and be unfamiliar with it when they see it with their left eye.

Horses have laterally placed eyes. This means that they have a panoramic field of vision with a narrow window of binocular vision and blind spots directly in front and directly behind them. They have monocular vision with poor depth perception from their nose to their hip on each side. They see few colors. They will tilt or turn their head toward an object, raise their head to see forward, and tuck their nose down to move their field of vision downward.

Horses have very acute hearing, especially for higher frequency sound waves. They can independently turn their ears toward sounds so you can monitor to what a horse is paying attention by watching where it is aiming its ears. When working with a horse, you want to encourage it to keep one ear on you at all times. If a horse has its ears pinned back, do not push it further as it is already uncomfortable and/or irritated and may lash out.

Certain areas on horses are very sensitive to touch. Horses frequently groom each other (allo-grooming). They prefer a stroking motion to slapping as we approach them. The areas most sensitive to touch are the ears, girth region, flanks, perineal region, nose, and legs. They enjoy forehead rubs and scratching of the withers.

Anatomy of a Horse

"Horse Anatomy 101", https://www.ponydreams.com/horse-anatomy-external/

Horses communicate mainly through body language and tension, not vocalization. They readily pick up on the body language of humans. It has been shown that people who are nervous when handling horses make those horses more nervous. It is important to have a calm demeanor around horses and to breathe deeply to help relax nervous horses.

Restraining Horses

Restraining frequently will be necessary when working with horses, and is used for the following reasons:

- Safety! No matter how sweet a horse it, every horse will react to something if it is scared or painful enough. Anyone within 10 feet of a horse is at risk of injury.
- Time is money for a veterinarian. We do not have time to train the horse so restraint often is necessary.

Be aware that all forms of restraint have pluses and minuses. There is no "one size fits all" approach to restraint as it varies with horse, procedure, and handler. Most veterinarians prefer to use the least restraint possible. You may need to complete some components of the physical examination before the horse is restrained, so you know you are seeing true responses and not those induced by the restraint used. This is especially true for sedation and other kinds of chemical restraint.

Types of Restraint

- Twitches – Rope or chain twitches can be applied to the end of the nose. This is supposed to cause release of endorphins and calm the horse but some horses will rear as it is released. A skin twitch is pinching of the skin and can be effective just before vaccination. Ear twitching, where the base of the ear is twisted, is rarely used and may make horses head-shy.
- Lip cords or chains – A cord (shoe-lace often is used) or chain is run across the inside of the lip. This prevents the horse from backing up or rearing.
- Chemical restraint – A variety of sedative drugs may be used for restraint.
- Hobbles – These join the legs together. They are uncommonly used but may be seen in mares during breeding, to prevent the mare from kicking a valuable stallion.

Training Horses

Operant conditioning is training the horse to respond consistently to signals through positive reinforcement and negative reinforcement. Timing of reinforcement is critical to success of the training used. Horses, as prey animals, respond well both to negative and positive reinforcement. Incorrect use of punishment can lower a horse's motivation to try offering a response (the horse shuts down, often seen in abused horses) or create fear or desensitize the horse to the instruments of punishment (spur or whip, for example).

Negative Reinforcement

Negative reinforcement involves the use of pressure. Pressure (tactile, visual, auditory) is applied until the horse offers the desired behavior at which point the pressure is immediately released. Start with light pressure, then slowly increase the amount and frequency of the pressure. Pressure should be firm and steady, not abrupt or harsh. This can be used to teach horses to stand still, lower their head, step forward, back up, move laterally, allow handling of sensitive areas, and accept use of clippers or other instruments. Keys to negative reinforcement are to apply pressure initially lightly, then gradually increasing with ongoing training; to hold pressure steady; to wait for the horse to respond – patience is a virtue; to release as the reward; and to praise the horse afterward.

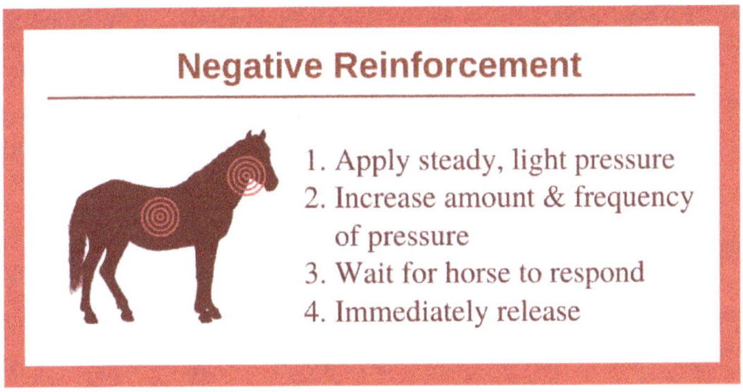

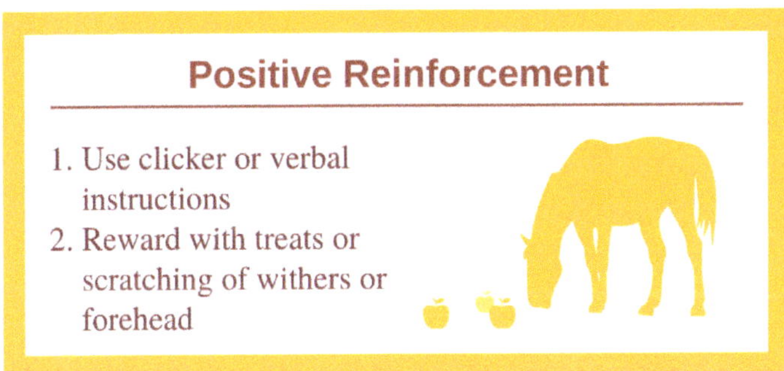
Positive Reinforcement
1. Use clicker or verbal instructions
2. Reward with treats or scratching of withers or forehead

Positive Reinforcement

Positive reinforcement may involve clicker training or some other verbal marker followed by rewards as in the dog, or scratching of the withers or forehead instead of giving treats. This kind of training is difficult to do when mounted on the horse (also called being under saddle) and is better for ground work. Be wary of horses who are inclined to nip or bite – use a bucket instead of offering treats directly from your hands. This can be used to help desensitize needle-shy horses or to allow use of clippers around the head.

All horses learn best when they are relaxed. A nervous or fearful horse cannot focus attention on training. By going slowly with training, you will accomplish more in a shorter time. If you start to lose your ability to remain calm, it is time to stop the training session.

Methods for Training Horses

	DEFINITION	EXAMPLES
Positive Reinforcement	The **addition** of a pleasant stimulus (reinforce) to reward the desired response and thus make the response more likely in the future (Skinner, 1953; McLean, 2003)	Clicker training – Food treats
Negative Reinforcement	The **subtraction** of something aversive (such as pressure) to reward the desired response and thus lower the motivational drive (Skinner, 1953)	Release tension on a lead rope to reward taking a step forward
Positive Punishment	The **addition** of an aversive stimulus to make a particular response less likely in the future	Yanking on the nose chain when a horse tries to bite you
Negative Punishment	The **subtraction** of a reinforcing stimulus to make a particular response less likely in the future	Walking away from a horse that paws at a stall door to get out

Good Horsemanship and Performing Veterinary Work

As a veterinarian working with horses, you will be required to assess the general demeanor of the horse, do a complete physical examination, take a rectal temperature, auscult the heart and lungs, take a pulse rate and respiratory rate, auscult the GI tract, do a dental examination, do a lameness examination, perhaps do a rectal examination and pass a nasogastric tube (for example, if assessing a horse for colic), and know how to load a horse into a trailer so it can be transported for emergencies or referrals.

Keys to Good Horsemanship

- Be mentally present, with no distractions.
- Project a quiet, confident demeanor.
- Be patient and fair in your contact with the horse.
- Be the leader.
- Move slowly and deliberately, with no quick or jerky movements.
- Be firm but kind.
- Avoid invoking the fight or flight response! Never allow the horse's stress levels to escalate.

Performing Veterinary Work

Right or wrong, clients often equate good horsemanship with good veterinary skills where horses are concerned. Steps are:

- Introduce yourself to the horse. Horses communicate through body language. You must address the whole horse, not just the area of concern. Approach the shoulder at a 45 degree angle. Divert your eyes downward and have a calm, quiet demeanor. Stroke the neck and shoulder. Wait for the horse to relax – the horse's eyes will soften, he will drop his head, he will chew, he will cock one hind leg. Stroke with the stethoscope from neck to shoulder and then down into the axilla and wait a minute to assess the heart and take the pulse rate; heart rate will increase with initial contact.
- To approach the head, stand off to one side, never directly in front of the horse. Rub the neck and slowly advance upwards. Retreat to a "safe zone" if the horse raises his head. Rub the forehead and withers as a reward.
- To do an oral examination, rub the side of the mouth and insert one finger into the interdental space. Reward the horse by removing the finger. Slowly make more contact with the mouth and tongue. Stay to one side as much as possible and do not hold him tight but instead move as he moves.

To do an ocular examination, sedation may be required and local anesthesia may be required if an injury is present. Evaluate ocular reflexes (pupillary light response [PLR], menace, and dazzle) before sedating the horse. PLR is closure of both pupils in response to light in one eye. Direct PLR is in the eye in which light is being shown; indirect PLR is in the other eye. Indirect PLR testing is difficult to do without standing in front of the horse. Use an assistant if possible to help manage the horse and be cautious. Menace is flinching or blinking as the eye is approached physically. Dazzle is flinching or blinking with sudden bright illumination of the eye.

- Nasogastric intubation is passing of a semi-rigid tube through the nose to access the GI tract of a horse. This can be done with minimal restraint. Desensitize the nostril to the presence of your finger in the ventral meatus about three times, releasing pressure of your finger as a reward. Then introduce the tube. The most resistance will be met in the first 3-4 inches of insertion. A nose twitch, lip cord, or sedation may be necessary in some horses.

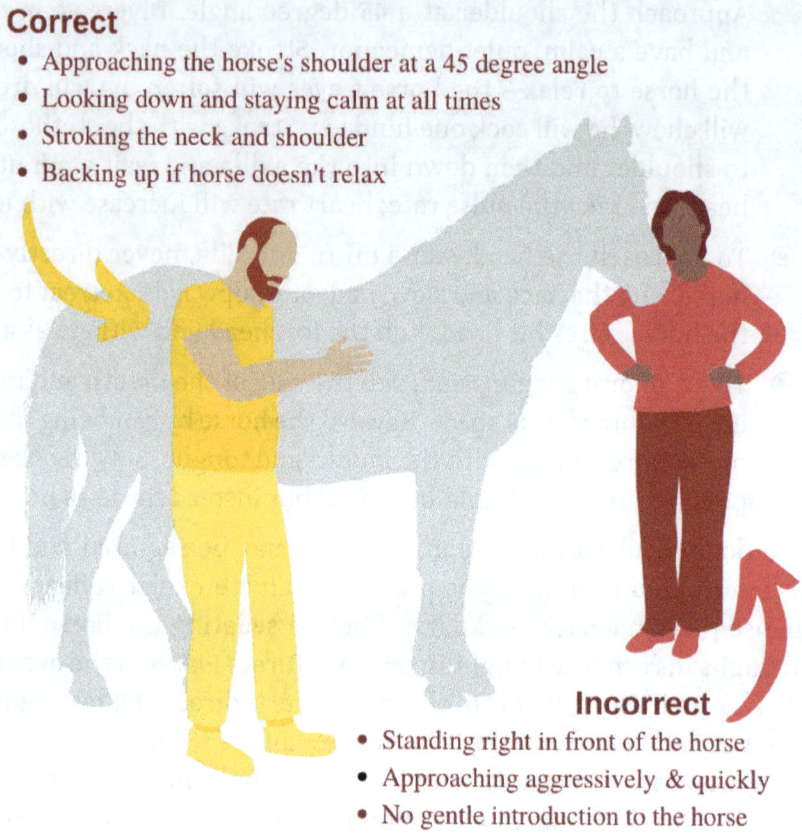
Correct
• Approaching the horse's shoulder at a 45 degree angle
• Looking down and staying calm at all times
• Stroking the neck and shoulder
• Backing up if horse doesn't relax
Incorrect
• Standing right in front of the horse
• Approaching aggressively & quickly
• No gentle introduction to the horse

- To take a rectal temperature, the handler of the horse should be on the same side of the horse as the veterinarian. Stand as close to the hip as possible. Be prepared to move quickly. Keep one hand on the hip as you approach the tail. Massage the underside of the tail; many horses will raise their tail as you do this. Gently touch the anus with the thermometer and insert with a rotating motion.
- Rectal palpation is a dangerous technique because you are in a danger zone for being kicked and are in the horse's blind spot. Try to stand slightly to one side and make sure the handler is on the same side of the horse as veterinarian. Use lots of lubrication. Insert one finger at a time and do not force entry or exit.
- To perform limb palpation, for example for a lameness examination, make sure the handler is on the same side of the horse as the veterinarian. Stand

parallel and next to the limb. Feel down the limb as the horse is standing, feeling for heat, swelling, and pain. As you approach the lower part of the leg, give a verbal cue to the horse ("ask for the limb"). Gently squeeze the flexor tendons or pinch the chestnut to get the horse to lift the leg. When the limb is elevated, gently palpate the tendons and ligaments. Hold the limb until the horse relaxes and then release it.

- For horses that are needle-shy, here are some things to try:
  - Have the handler cover the horse's eyes.
  - Have the handler or assistant distract the horse with a large treat that they spend some time working on.
  - Rock the horse back-and-forth on its feet while inserting the needle.
  - Rub the skin vigorously, then pinch it, then slide the needle in.
  - Use oral sedation if the horse is truly dangerous.
  - Help the owner train (desensitize) the horse between appointments.
- To load a horse on a trailer, use a trailer that is as open as possible. Make sure you are in a well-lit area with no obstructions. Reward any attempt the horse makes to step forward toward the trailer, and consider use of lip cords.

SMALL ANIMAL BEHAVIOR

Dog Topics

How Dogs Learn

Dogs do what works for them! They learn by consequences; what is reinforced will occur more often and what is punished will occur less often. Reinforcers = if provided immediately at the time of behavior, make the behavior more likely – examples are food, toys, play, attention, petting, movement. Punishers = if provided immediately at the time of behavior, make the behavior less likely – examples can be physical, verbal, auditory, removal of a valued resource, removal of attention, or anything the dog finds unpleasant. Reinforcers and punishers must come within 1-2 seconds of the behavior in order to be effective. It is the animal who decides what is a reinforcer and what is a punisher.

Dogs don't understand the concept of being punished for past behavior, as is described below under house-training. Behavior that happens when the owner is absent frequently is misinterpreted as spite. Usually this occurs when the owner has accidentally trained the dog to perform the behavior when the owner is not present. The dog looks "guilty" but is actually exhibiting behavior meant to "cut off" aggressive behaviors from other members of their pack or group. He looks guilty to you but really he's just frightened of being punished for no apparent reason.

For many years, people adhered to a theory that all dogs were vying for the "top" or "alpha" position, and must be lowered in rank to eliminate problem behavior. Traditional suggestions were for humans to exert their dominance by rolling the dog on its back, shaking its scruff, going through doors first, eating first, and not allowing dogs on the furniture. We now know that dominance describes a relationship that sorts out who gets what and at what time. It is about resources and is a fluid trait, not a fixed or personality trait. It is not necessarily related to social status and depends on the resources and individuals in question. For us, this means that dogs are looking for a clear, humane, fair leader, not an alpha wolf. Most of the behaviors we consider to be problem behaviors have nothing to do with status or dominance and are just normal dog behaviors. Our goal is to teach our dogs how to behave rather than to dominate them.

Training the Dog to Do What You Want

Training generally is done with positive reinforcement. Make it fun for the dog do things correctly. The goal is to prevent wrong behaviors from starting and to keep the dog from practicing wrong behaviors. Try to avoid fear and pain when training. These may cause aggression, anxiety, creation of new problem behaviors, and confusion, and are hard to use appropriately. It is impossible to predict how dogs will respond to fear and pain when training and punishment doesn't tell dogs what they should do. Dogs naturally repeat behaviors that benefit them, just like people. It is easier, faster, and less stressful to reward what we want instead of punishing what we don't want.

Responding to Unwanted Behavior

- Ignore (turn your back, look away, walk away)
- Redirect (offer the puppy a toy to chew instead of the table leg)
- Give an instructive command ("sit" or another obedience command generally is better than "no")
- Remove any reinforcement (stop the game, walk away, remove the treat, take away the toy, etc.)
- Use training tools to interrupt the behavior (use a Gentle Leader to close the dog's mouth, hold a mouthing puppy away from you with a leash, put a puppy in a crate or away from you for a time out)
- Make sure you're not unintentionally rewarding a wrong behavior – allow a 4-5 second delay between wrong and right behavior before rewarding the right behavior

Tools of the Trade

- **Rewards** – Examples of rewards include clickers and food rewards (chicken, cheese, lamb lung, hot dogs, food rolls, all cut into small pieces). With clicker training, the dog is taught to associate the "click" sound with a food reward. The handler clicks when the desired behavior occurs, then gives the dog a treat. Timing is important – the click marks the behavior and the treat comes after the click. The click must immediately follow the behavior and then the treat appears up to several seconds later. When the behavior is solid, the click is phased out and a verbal cue replaces the click.
- **Collars** – Head halters include the Gentle Leader and Halti collars. Both allow control of the dog's entire head. The Gentle Leader permits the handler to gently close the dog's mouth and reduces pulling, barking, mouthing, and jumping. This is a great tool to prevent puppy biting. Use of these collars depends on the user recognizing when the dog is doing what you want and leaving some slack in the leash; it is release of pressure from around the nose and behind the neck that is the reward for good behavior. Martingales are wide collars that connect to a leash in a way that tightens the collar to prevent it from slipping over the head. These are commonly used in sighthounds (for example Greyhounds), which often have a neck that is wider than the head. This performs the same function as a choke collar but with pressure spread out over the neck by the width of the collar. The limited slip design prevents escape and the collar can be fitted so as not to fully close. Buckle collars are those that are most commonly used. They may have a quick-release clip or an actual buckle. Dogs can back out of these if they are fitted too loosely. Prong or pinch collars, choke collars, shock collars, and citronella collars generally are not recommended by behaviorists. These can be used by experienced people in appropriate situations.
- **Harnesses** – Easy-Walk and Halti are some brand names for harnesses. These fit around the chest of the dog and clip in the front, which makes pulling by the dog less efficient. These give handlers more control over the dog. These should be removed when not in use. The Freedom harness is a halter that clips over the back and can have two leashes attached; this harness also is used to control pulling when walking a dog.
- **Leashes** – Leashes that are 4-6 feet in length are recommended for training. They may be made of nylon or leather. A lightweight leash with a small clip is recommended for use with the Gentle Leader. If a dog chews the leash, one can be made of tie-out material covered in rubber or made of small-link chain. Leashes can be used as drag lines, as described below for

housetraining. If the puppy / dog is wearing a leash in the house, the owner can walk the dog off furniture or through doorways without physically touching them, which the dog may perceive as a reward.

- Retractable leads generally are not recommended. They can be useful in wide-open areas with little to no traffic but are not recommended for use in crowded venues, near bike paths, for dogs not yet trained to walk well on a loose leash, for children to walk dogs, or for people to walk dogs while multi-tasking (for example, while texting). Retractable leads offer too little control and too much freedom of movement for the dog and are difficult to hold onto if the dog is out of control. The lock can fail and fingers can be severely injured if they become entangled in the leash cord.
- **Crates and kennels-** Crates / kennels are described below, under housetraining. To train a dog to enter a crate, toss treats into the crate and let the dog eat and exit at will. Then feed meals in the kennel and put in things that teach the dog that spending time in the kennel is good, for example Kong or food puzzle treats that the dog has to work at to get the reward. Gradually increase the time the dog spends in the kennel. If the dog does not want to be in the crate and is making noise, wait until the noise stops before opening the door. **Gates** – Gates can be made of plastic, metal, or wood. They are great for multi-dog households and households with dogs and children. They can be used to prevent dogs from dashing through open doors but must be properly installed (or they can be knocked over) and of an appropriate height (or they can jump or crawl over them).

Management Techniques

Puppies are always learning, even if we're not present. It is better not to let them practice doing things incorrectly, because they will get really good at whatever they practice. It is easier to prevent problem behaviors than to eliminate them once the animal is showing them. Management is about setting puppies and adult dogs up for success and requires us to be thinking about how best to keep the animal on track when it is not being supervised. Often, this involves changing behavior of the owners to ensure good behaviors on the part of the dog.

Housetraining

Housetraining is a necessity for all dogs, young and old. Young dogs need to be trained if they are to live inside as house pets and older dogs should be re-trained every time they move to a new home location. It is unrealistic to expect dogs of any age to readily understand our expectations of them regarding housetraining as we travel with them or move to new residences. When training, proper and consistent management is crucial to success and expectations must be age-appropriate.

Basics of Housetraining

- Take the puppy / dog out every hour on a leash – Do not let them run free outside until after they have urinated or defecated.
- Take the puppy / dog out immediately after it finishes eating, after it has been playing, and after it wakes up.
- Reward the puppy / dog immediately after it urinates or defecates, not after they get back in the house – you want them to learn that the reward is for eliminating, not for going back in the house.
- Keep the puppy / dog on a leash when indoors and use it to keep the animal physically attached to someone at all times.

Confine the puppy / dog to a crate or enclosure (ex-pen (see below) or small room) when supervision isn't possible.

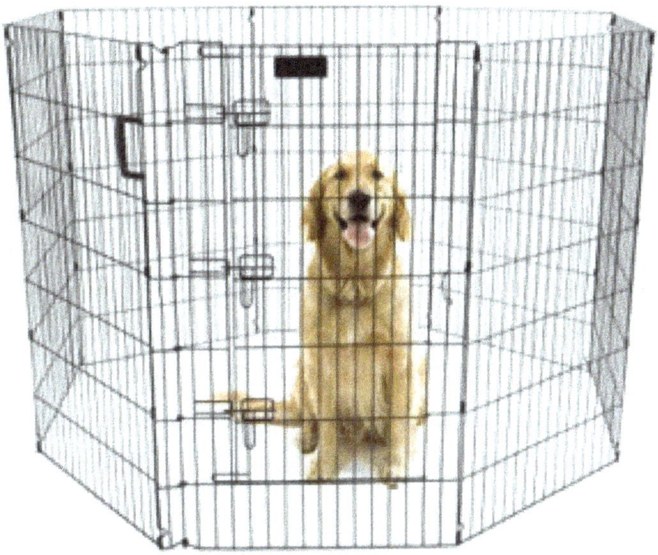

"Precision Pet Ultimate ExPen", https://www.amazon.com/Precision-Pet-Ultimate-ExPen-Black/dp/B00028IX7M

If you're going to use a crate, crate-training requires use of a crate that is big enough for the dog to stand up and move around and to lie down comfortably, but not so big that the animal can urinate or defecate in the back of the crate and lie in a dry spot away from that area. You may, therefore, need to purchase more than one crate as your puppy grows, or to put something in the back of a large crate to decrease the usable space for a time. You may or may not choose to put something on the floor of the crate. Newspapers may stain dogs, especially if they get wet, and dogs may chew on towels or other soft bedding. The maximum number of hours a puppy should be in the crate is its age in months plus one – for example, a 2-month-old puppy should not be left in the crate for more than 3 hours at a time. For adult dogs, start with shorter durations (for example, 3-4 hours) and gradually increase duration. People are often eager to get puppies to sleep through the night very quickly but that is not a realistic goal; their urinary bladder is only so big. If they do sleep through the night, you should not expect them also to be able to hold their urine for that same length of time during the day. The crate should not be used as a punishment. It is a safe place for the dog and can be used not just for housetraining but also to control chewing; to manage multiple animals in a household, especially as they're first being introduced; and when traveling.

Accidents will happen while you're housetraining a dog. All should be cleaned with an enzyme-based cleaner, which will biologically break down the urine and feces and remove the smell. Smell is a strong indicator to animals that they should use that spot for elimination again. Remember that their sense of smell is much stronger than ours; just because you can't smell it, that doesn't mean they can't smell it. If you are worried you're not seeing all of the places where the dog has urinated, a blacklight flashlight can be used to help locate stains. Be aware that the blacklight is picking up protein so it also will identify places where the dog has drooled.

Puppies / dogs should not be punished for accidents you find after the fact. Punishment at that point is not associated in their mind with having urinated or defecated. If you catch them in the act, scoop them up and hurry them outside and if they do even one drop out there, heavily reward them. Do not punish them if you catch them in the act; it may teach them to urinate or defecate where no one can see them and it does not help them learn what we want them to do.

Other tools that may be used for housetraining are potty pads and belly bands. Potty pads are useful for those dogs that have limited mobility or live in places where it is hard to get outside (for example, high-rise apartments or houseboats). The puppy / dog is taken to the potty pad instead of being taken outside and is rewarded for urinating or defecating on that surface. All other aspects of housetraining are the same as above. Owners can purchase commercial potty pads or use newspaper; if you use newspaper, you need many layers to keep urine from soaking through. Belly bands wrap around the prepuce and penis of male dogs and are intended to prevent leg-lifting accidents and marking with urine on vertical surfaces. They should only be used when the dog is supervised and must be removed when the dog is taken outside or placed in a crate.

Choosing a New Puppy

Recommended sources for new puppies are shelters or humane societies, rescue organizations, and reputable breeders. You will see below that it is not recommended to purchase puppies from pet stores; this does not include pet stores holding adoption days for local humane or rescue organizations. Reputable breeders do genetic and infectious disease testing on their bitches and stud dogs before breeding, use best practices for socialization and care of young pups, and screen prospective owners to ensure the new owners understand the personality and adult size of the chosen breed. The American Kennel Club has a quiz available to help perspective owners understand various dog breeds and which breed is best for them and their situation. In general, it is not recommended to get a new puppy from a pet store, which may be receiving their animals from puppy mills and other unregulated breeders, or from "backyard breeders" and from those offering puppies "free to good home", who often do not do genetic and infectious disease testing of sires and dams and may, therefore, produce pups with significant congenital defects and/or disease.

The average family wants a dog who:

- Likes men, women and children
- Enjoys being petted and touched
- Is relatively easy to walk and train
- Will settle down during family downtime

Red flag phrases do not describe bad dogs but dogs that may be the wrong fit for the average dog owner or families with children, as it suggests it may be a dog that is anxious around strange people or new situations, has far more energy than the owner is ready for, or may require extensive work and training to prevent problem behavior. Red flag phrases for many family pets are:

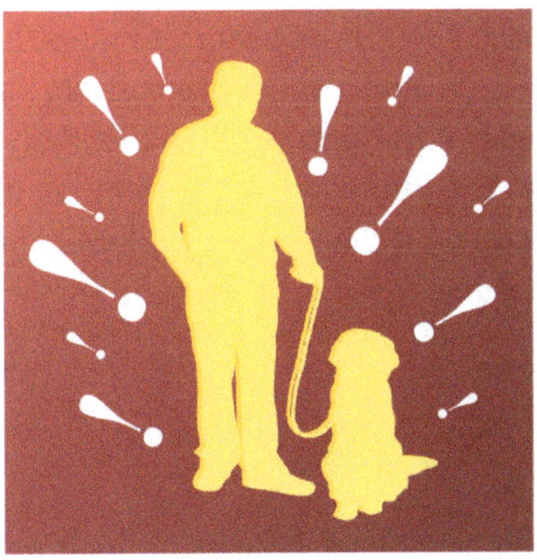

- Takes a while to warm up to people
- A one-person dog
- **Very protective of me** – Dogs with any of the above designations may be fearful or shy, may be reactive or aggressive, or simply may be a less social breed.

- **Field bred or working lines** – These suggest dogs that are very focused on having a job (herding, for example) and who will be bored and likely destructive in many home settings.

Should I get a dog for protection? The answer is "no". Dogs are already hard-wired for caution toward strangers and will spend more time with our friends and families than with intruders. The dog decides what is scary and that can be unpredictable. Aggression brings a lot of liability and can be difficult (if not impossible) to resolve. A watch dog is not the same as a guard dog – watch dogs, also called alarm dogs, warn their owner that something is not right, usually by barking, but do not engage with the threat.

Socialization Guidelines

The American Veterinary Society of Animal Behavior states the following: "The primary and most important time for puppy socialization is the first three months of life. During this time puppies should be exposed to as many new people, animals, stimuli and environments as can be achieved safely and without causing overstimulation manifested as excessive fear, withdrawal or avoidance behavior. For this reason, the American Veterinary Society of Animal Behavior believes that it should be the standard of care for puppies to receive such socialization before they are fully vaccinated". Good socialization venues for puppies are "puppy kindergarten" classes, often held at training facilities and humane organizations; "puppy parties"; supervised play groups; trips to safe and approved human environments (family and friend's homes for example); and places where puppies can be introduced to gentle, socially appropriate dogs. Socialization venues to be avoided include dog parks, which can be unsanitary and contain uncontrolled and untrained dogs; anywhere the pup would be roughly handled, for example by young children; anywhere the pup would get too much exercise, for example on a long hike; anywhere the pup would be overstimulated and stressed; and anywhere the pup would find frightening.

Preventing Dog Bites

To prevent dog bites and to be able to teach people how to prevent dog bites, you must know the following:

- What dog should I choose? What are you looking for in a dog? Remember that a dog cannot be trained automatically to know who is a "good" person and who is a "suspicious" person – people may believe they need a "protection" dog without knowing what that might mean.
- Learn behavior basics. Can I identify warning signs (body language)? Can I recognize signs of aggression?
- Learn and teach others how to greet a dog and what to avoid.

Aggression is a behavior, not a personality trait. Any dog or cat will show aggression if sufficiently stressed. Approaching a dog can be a source of serious stress and danger, so it's important to know how to properly greet a dog. Determining the dog's triggers is key to maintaining safety. Finally, no dog is guaranteed not to bite, just as no human is guaranteed never to yell at or shove another person.

Dog Body Language

Colleen Pelar has created a simple system to help us all remember what some body language of dogs means:

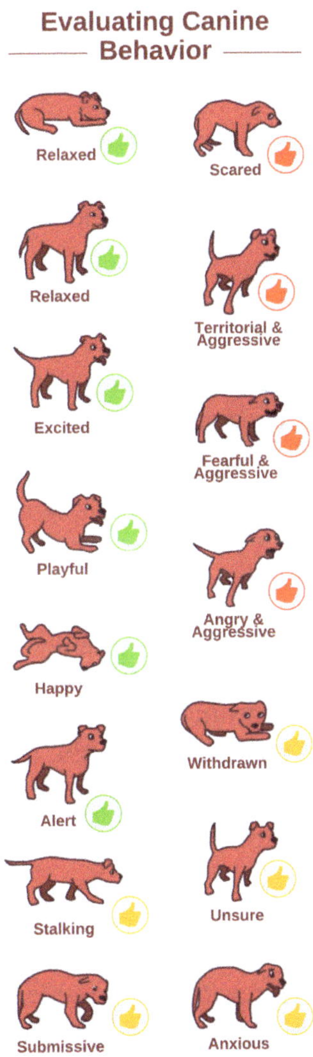

- "Enjoyment" is associated with the dog having a loose body, open mouth, and squinty eyes – there is no need to intervene.
- "Tolerance" is associated with the dog having a closed mouth, still body, ears back, and the whites of the eyes showing – try to improve the situation to calm the dog and you may need to intervene if a human is threatened.
- "Enough already" is associated with stiff body, teeth displayed, staring, freezing, growling, snapping, and trying to flee – the dog must be removed from the situation immediately without punishment. If the dog has reached this point, we have already missed several warning signs and we do not want to punish the dog and teach it not to show us those warning signs.

Helping Dogs Cope with Stressful Events

- Keep the environment as predictable as possible. If the dog is crate-trained, bring the crate. Bring familiar chew toys and items with family members' scent. Limit unnecessary handling and stress.
- Pair new or frightening things with good things. If it is a noise, try introducing it at a low volume or at a distance (for example, thunder). If it is a new place, do it in stages (first is the car ride, then the ride and walk in the parking lot, then the ride and through the parking lot into the vet clinic). Pair any new experience with a high-value reward and remove the reward when the trigger is not present.
- Prevent stress as much as possible. Use medications if necessary. Do not try anything new when the dog is already stressed (for example, training procedures).
- Comfort the animal as necessary. Comforting dogs and cats does not reward fear! Fear is an emotion, not a volitional behavior. Soothing will either reduce the fear or do nothing; it will not increase it. The comforter's body language and stress levels are key – the dog can sense if you're saying it's okay with your mouth but your body is tense.

Cat Topics

Litterbox Management

Most behaviorists will recommend uncovered litter boxes that are of a size appropriate for the cat(s) – they should be able to easily get in and out and to scratch to cover whatever they produce. Uncovered boxes are preferred by many cats because they can easily escape them if feeling threatened and foul odors are not readily trapped within the area of the box. There are many types of litter available. Most behaviorists will recommend unscented clumping litter that is deep enough that the cat can scratch and not expose the bottom of the box. Cats will definitely have preferences for the type and amount of litter they want to use and the size and placement of the box.

Number of cat boxes in the household should be number of cats plus one. So if you have one cat, you should have two boxes and if you have four cats, you should have five boxes. People may complain that they don't have enough room for multiple boxes. Cats are particular about how they use the box and some will want to urinate in one box and defecate in another. Cats also may guard boxes and prevent other cats in the household from using them, so there have to be enough boxes so everyone can use one.

Boxes should be placed away from where food and water are provided, in a semi-private location away from disturbances and high traffic, in an area that is somewhat open so the cat does not feel cornered or trapped (do not put litterboxes in a closet, for example), and should be spaced out into different parts of the home to prevent the guarding problem described earlier. It is not valuable to have three boxes if they are all placed right next to each other.

Feces and clumped urine should be scooped out at least once daily. Avoid use of deodorizers, cat box liners, and perfumed litter – this is designed for humans, not for the cats. Use of these products can mask the smell of the box but may lead to owners cleaning less frequently. Cats also may be bothered by these smells and textures. All litter should be dumped out, the box completely cleaned with warm water and mild detergent, and new litter placed in the box every 2 weeks. Do not add new litter to a dirty box. A good way to remind clients of the need to clean the box is to let them know that cats don't like a dirty toilet any more than we do, and we certainly would not be content if toilets only flushed every couple of days.

So what causes litterbox problems?

- Insufficient cleaning
- Not enough boxes
- Wrong size (too small or too large)
- Tension between pets
- Substrate preference (clay, sand, newspaper, etc.)
- Stress (change in routine, new furniture)
- Medical problem (constipation, urinary tract infection)
- Litterbox location suddenly changed
- Not enough privacy and/or escape routes

- Stress, outdoor intruders

What doesn't cause litterbox problems?

- Spite
- Anger
- Jealousy
- Stupidity

If a cat is presented for the problem of inappropriate urination / defecation (not using the box), it is valuable to take a very detailed history about the number and size of the box(es), where they're placed, what kind of litter is used, how the box(es) are cleaned, and if any changes have been made in the litterbox routine. Empathize with the client and then educate.

Introducing a New Cat

A single indoor cat generally enjoys only about ¼ of what would be its natural territory if it lived outside. Each addition of a new cat increases the likelihood of stress and behavior problems. Before you get that second (or third or fourth) cat, ask yourself if you're getting the cat to be a buddy for your current pet(s) or if you're getting it for yourself – are you grieving the loss of a pet, or are you bored or lonely? Those are not bad reasons to get a cat but you have to consider how your needs may impact stress levels in your current pets. You also need to be ready for the extra time, energy, and money required, and to be prepared for all outcomes, including possibly having to find a new home or to permanently separate the cats within your home if they can't learn to get along.

Make sure you have enough litterboxes for the new number of cats, toys, bowls, beds and perches, and maybe a calming spray, such as Feliway. Make sure you have some hiding places. These will reduce stress, prevent conflicts, and allow escape from other pets. Examples are cat condos, tunnels, paper shopping bags, and visual barriers, such as screens.

When selecting a new cat, don't worry too much about the gender of the cats involved. Age and temperament are the most important factors. Adult cats will usually accept a new kitten much more easily than they will accept a new adult cat. Cats are territorial, and your cat may resent an adult feline intruder. If you're able to choose from a group of kittens, avoid a kitten that's hissing, growling or engaged in serious battle with his mates. If owners prefer to adopt an adult cat, success depends largely on the personality of your present cat; if he's easygoing and the new cat is also laid back, you may have little trouble if you introduce them slowly and correctly.

When introducing a new cat, first impressions are really important. Keep them separated for about one week and make sure the new cat has been examined by a veterinarian before being brought into the home. Feed the cats on opposite sides of a door. Slowly move the bowls closer to the door over the week and gradually crack the door open for a moment while they're eating. In the second week, switch which room each cat is in or swap their bedding. In the second to third week, supervise time when they're together for 15-30 minutes. During that time, give them equal attention and create good associations with them being together and getting play time and affection. Giving them this gradual introduction sets the tone for the relationship (letting them "work it out" or "fight it out" can seriously damage the relationship). They may be wary of each other at first and it will take time to determine if they're going to be best buddies, roommates, or enemies. As they're working this out, they may be stressed and stop using the litterbox or may do territorial spraying, which is spraying of urine on vertical surfaces. If they really hate each other, try re-introducing them gradually, seek help from a professional, permanently separate them in the home, or find a new home for the new cat.

When introducing cats to dogs, do not force interactions. Keep the dog leashed whenever the cat is in the area and let the cat approach the dog at its own pace. Reward the dog with treats whenever the cat is visible. Always make sure the cat has plenty of escape routes. If the dog attempts to chase the cat, move him further away. Keep them separate if they cannot be supervised.

Dogs vs. Cats

Similarities between dogs and cats are that they both:

- Attach strongly to their human families
- Enjoy interactive play with humans
- Primarily use body language to communicate with those around them
- Are natural predators
- Respond to the laws of learning (behavior that is rewarded gets stronger)

Dissimilarities between dogs and cats are:

- Cats generally tolerate less physical contact than dogs
- Cats receive far less socialization and environmental stimulation than dogs
- Cats are carnivores, dogs are omnivores
- Cats are nocturnal, dogs are crepuscular (active at dawn and dusk)
- Cats climb and perch in high places to feel safe
- Body language – see below

Small Animal Body Language

	DOG	CAT
Tail	Wagging tail usually indicates pleasure	Lashing tail indicates arousal and aggression
Exposed Belly	Cut-off or calming signal	Social discomfort, potential defensive aggression (can use claws on all four feet) – if a cat's belly is exposed while it's sleeping, that is a sign of relaxation
Self-Licking	Anxiety or physical discomfort	Normal grooming behavior

Carrier Training

To train a cat to enter a carrier, first place the carrier next to the cat's food dish. Leave it in this location for a few days. When the cat no longer appears afraid of the presence of the crate, feed the cat inside the crate with the door open. You can also throw treats for the cat into the carrier and let the cat run in and out. Once the cat is comfortable doing that, add a verbal cue (for example, "kennel up"). When the cat is very comfortable, close the door and feed treats or the regular diet through a gap.

EXTRA RESOURCES

Puppy socialization position statement: https://avsab.org/wp-content/uploads/2018/03/Puppy_Socialization_Position_Statement_Download_-_10-3-14.pdf

Puppy parties for socialization: https://dogtime.com/puppies/1206-dunbar-puppy-parties

How to properly greet a dog: https://drsophiayin.com/app/uploads/2017/08/How-to-Greet-a-Dog-Poster.pdf

CHAPTER-10

BASICS OF NUTRITION

GENERAL NUTRITION INFORMATION

Nutrients are chemical substances obtained from food and are used to provide energy, to build structure (bone, muscle, etc.), and to regulate growth, maintenance, and repair. There is an optimal amount of intake of any given nutrient; if too little it taken in, the animal is deficient and if too much is taken in, toxicity may occur.

- **Water** – Water acts as a solvent for transport of dissolved substances through the body, it is required for hydrolysis reactions of other nutrients, it helps maintain normal body temperature, and it provides shape and resilience to the body. Young animals have a higher percentage of total body water. The body in animals ranges from 40 to 80% water. Water requirements vary with age, body surface area, ambient temperature, state of health, amount of exercise, and life stage (growth, maintenance, pregnancy, lactation, etc.). Water is taken in directly (drinking) and indirectly (eating and in some species, through the skin).
- **Energy** – Energy is not a nutrient but is what is generated as nutrients are broken down. The energy in food is chemical energy. The body converts chemical energy to mechanical, electrical, or heat energy. Gross energy (the full amount taken in) is higher than digestible energy (gross energy minus energy lost in feces), which is higher than metabolizable energy (digestible energy minus energy lost in urine and gases from the GI tract). Net energy is metabolizable energy minus the heat increment, which is the amount of energy lost in fermentation and in metabolic processes. Net energy is what is available to the animal to use and it is not used with the same efficiency for all processes.

Besides water, animals take in vitamins, minerals, fats, proteins, and carbohydrates. Fats, proteins, and carbohydrates are the nutrients that are broken down to provide energy.

- **Fats** – Fats are one type of lipid. Lipids include fats; sterols (for example, cholesterol); mono-, di-, and triglycerides; fat-soluble vitamins (A, D, E, K); and phospholipids. Lipids provide energy and are a structural component of cell membranes. Fatty acids are made from acetyl CoA and NADPH in the cytoplasm of the cell and are a linear chain of an even number of carbons with hydrogens along the length and on one end (the methyl end) and a -COOH group on the other (the -COOH is what makes it an acid). Fatty acids with no double bonds are "saturated", those with one double bond are "monounsaturated" and those with multiple double bonds are "polyunsaturated". Those fatty acids denoted as "omega 3" fatty acids have a double bond three carbons away from the methyl end and those denoted as "omega 6" fatty acids have a double bond six carbons away from the methyl end. Phospholipids make up the cell membrane, preferentially permit substances to cross the cell membrane, and when added to foods, act as an emulsifier. Cholesterol is a base lipid that is the precursor to many other substances in the body including bile acids in the GI tract, sex hormones, adrenal hormones, and vitamin D.

When ingested, fats remain separate from fluid components in the stomach until they are emulsified. Bile has affinity both for water and fat. Exposure to bile in the small intestine breaks up large fat globules, exposing more surface area to enzymes in the digestive fluid. Glycerol and small lipids move directly into the bloodstream. Large lipids combine with bile to form micelles that are water-soluble and move directly into cells. Most of the bile released into the small intestine is reabsorbed and sent back to the liver (= enterohepatic circulation of bile). Some bile moves through the GI tract and is excreted in feces.

The fat-soluble vitamins are A, D, E, and K. All fat-soluble vitamins are effectively stored in the body and so need not be taken in daily. Because they are stored, toxicity is possible if they are consumed in excess. Water-soluble vitamins are not stored and toxicity is rare. Vitamin A is also called retinol acetate and supports vision, cell differentiation, and reproduction and growth. It is available in plants as beta-carotene; not all species can readily convert beta-carotene to vitamin A. Vitamin D is also called calciferol. It can be synthesized by the body and functions in calcium metabolism. Synthesis is stimulated by exposure to sunlight; not all species readily can synthesize vitamin D even with sunlight exposure. Vitamin E is also called tocopherol. It is an anti-oxidant. Vitamin K is also called menadione. It is a component of the blood-clotting cascade.

The terms "fat" and "triglyceride" are synonymous, as fats are made up of three fatty acid chains and glycerol. Fats in the diet efficiently provide energy, transport and store fat-soluble vitamins, increase palatability and satiety, and reduce dustiness of feed. Fats produce energy by being broken down to acetyl CoA, which then enters the Krebs cycle (also called the citric acid cycle or tricarboxylic acid cycle [TCA]), where it is oxidized to produce CO_2 and ATP. As a general rule of thumb, lipids contain 2.25 times more gross energy than protein or carbohydrate (9 kcal/gm for fat versus 4 kcal/gm for protein and carbohydrate). Fats are considered energy-dense nutrients.

- **Proteins** – Proteins are made up of amino acids and are required in the diet both to provide essential aminoacids that cannot be synthesized by the body and to provide the nitrogen needed for other essential compounds such as heme, nucleic acids, and creatinine. Essential (also called indispensable) amino acids are those that cannot be produced by the body quickly enough to meet demands for normal growth; these vary by species. There generally are 10 essential amino acids (threonine, tryptophan, valine, arginine, histidine, lysine, phenyalanine, leucine, isoleucine, methionine) that can be remembered using these mnemonics – These Ten Valuable Amino acids Have Long Preserved Life In Man or PVT TIM HALL. Most true carnivores (for example cats), also require taurine so the mnemonics can be changed to – These Ten Valuable Amino acids Have Long Preserved Life In Mutts and Tigers or PVT TIM T HALL. Conditionally essential amino acids are only required for specific life stages. Examples include an increased need for glutamine in animals with sepsis, and increased need for arginine in individuals with liver or kidney disease, or in burn patients. Limiting amino acids are those essential amino acids in a diet that are present in low enough quantities that their concentration controls rate of protein synthesis. Complete proteins are those food sources that provide all essential amino acids and usually readily support ongoing protein synthesis. These usually are from animal sources. Plant proteins are more likely to be incomplete and/or limiting. A prominent example is lysine, which is limiting in corn. Complementary proteins are two protein sources that are themselves incomplete but that together provide all essential amino acids.

In ruminants, protein must pass through the rumen to be absorbed. Protein broken down in the rumen is available to microbes for synthesis of high-quality proteins and the remainder passes into the small intestine. Factors that affect the extent of protein breakdown in the rumen include the chemical structure and solubility of the protein, how long it is retained in the rumen, the particle size, the rumen pH, and the stage of plant growth. The breakdown in the rumen is vital; microbes in the rumen contribute up to 70% of the protein available for absorption in the small intestine. In some specific circumstances, which will be described later, ruminants are fed protein that will not be broken down in the rumen, called bypass protein, specifically to ensure that there is a large concentration of protein available for absorption from the small intestine.

In monogastric animals, proteins are broken down by pepsin and HCl into large polypeptides. In the small intestine, pancreatic enzymes (trypsin, chymotrypsin) break polypeptides down further into small peptides and amino acids. Absorption across the cell wall is sodium-dependent and requires energy (active transport).

Absorbed small peptides and amino acids are reassembled into new proteins in the liver and other tissues. Amino acids become tissue proteins (muscle, liver, etc.); enzymes, albumin, hormones, and other nitrogen-containing compounds; and are broken apart to provide energy. There is little storage of excess amino acids. Tissue proteins and serum albumin are a store of amino acids if necessary. When amino acids are deaminated, ammonia is produced. Ammonia and carbon dioxide combine to form urea, which is excreted.

Protein digestion is intertwined with energy use. If the cells are starved for energy, the amine group is removed and excreted and the rest of the molecule is broken down for energy. If the cells have a surplus of energy, the amine group is again excreted and rest of the molecule is converted to glucose and fat, and stored. It is valuable to think about energy needs when feeding protein because if the body cannot use the protein, it will be excreted or "wasted". Examples of circumstances where protein wasting occurs include lack of energy from other sources so the amino acids are used for energy only, if the diet supplies more protein than the body needs, if a single amino acid is provided in excess, or when the diet supplies low quality protein with too few essential amino acids. An example of a time when this information is valuable clinically is when weight loss is desired; an animal on an energy-restricted diet should get a generous amount of high-quality protein to help maintain lean body mass and ensure an appropriate intake of nitrogen intake to balance nitrogen use (= nitrogen balance).

- **Carbohydrates** – Carbohydrates are an important source of energy in all species and are the primary energy source in most plant products. At the molecular level, they are a "hydrate" of carbon, with C:H:O at a 1:2:1 ratio. Simple carbohydrates are monosaccharides (glucose, fructose), disaccharides, (sucrose, lactose), and oligosaccharides. Complex carbohydrates are polysaccharides (more than 9 CH2O units; cellulose) and fiber. Mono- and disaccharides are readily absorbed to provide energy. Examples of polysaccharides include glycogen (storage form of energy in the body), starch (storage form of energy in plants), and fiber (structure in plants). Polysaccharides are not digestible by mammals as they resist hydrolysis by digestive enzymes. Rumination (cattle, small ruminants) and hindgut fermentation (horses) are required for breakdown of these kinds of carbohydrates.

- In ruminants, dietary carbohydrates from forages like hay are primarily structural carbohydrates, such as cellulose, pectins, hemicellulose, and lignins. Some are non-structural carbohydrates, such as sugars and starches. Carbohydrates undergo microbial fermentation to form volatile fatty acids; this is described in detail later in these notes.
- In monogastric animals, there is limited digestion of carbohydrates in the mouth and stomach. Breakdown of carbohydrates is mediated by pancreatic alpha-amylase and brush border enzymes in the small intestine and by fermentation of undigested and unabsorbed carbohydrates in the large intestine. Fiber is not digestible in small animals but serves other purposes such as preventing constipation and normalizing intestinal motility. Cats handle carbohydrates uniquely; this is described in detail later in these notes.
- **Water-Soluble Vitamins and Minerals** – These compounds are needed in minute quantities. Water-soluble vitamins are the B-vitamins and vitamin C. They are organic micronutrients, required in small amounts but essential. They are not stored in the body so deficiency states can occur more quickly than with fat-soluble vitamins. If deficiency does occur, often more than one body system will be affected. Toxicity rarely occurs. Water-soluble vitamins often act as coenzymes.

Vitamin C can be synthesized in many species. Primates and guinea pigs are two species that require a dietary source of vitamin C.

Names of B Vitamins

B1	thiamine
B2	riboflavin
B3	niacin / niacinamide
B5	pantothenic acid
B6	pyridoxine hydrochloride
B7	biotin (sometimes called vitamin H)
B9	folic acid
B12	cobalamin

Minerals are inorganic elements in food. Macrominerals are those required in higher concentrations in the diet and include calcium, phosphorus, magnesium, potassium, and sodium. These are responsible for the structure of the bones and teeth, maintaining an action potential across cell membranes, fluid balance, acid-base balance, storage and transport of energy, and for acting as second messengers and co-factors. Microminerals often are associated with a specific enzyme, hormone, carrier protein, or vitamin, and include iron, copper, manganese, zinc, selenium, cobalt, and iodine. Other mineral compounds are classified as ultra-trace elements and are needed in very small amounts. Examples include molybdenum, fluorine, nickel, silicon, chromium, and vanadium.

LARGE ANIMAL NUTRITION BASICS

The Role of Nutrition in Large Animal Veterinary Practice

Some practitioners may choose not to include nutrition in the services they offer as a veterinarian. This is problematic because nutrition plays a key role in large animal veterinary care, especially in production medicine, and because avoiding nutrition issues removes your chance to help patients and clients, and is a loss+ of potential revenue. Feed is the largest input cost in animal production and what feed is provided varies with age, breed, production and gain needs, and pregnancy status of the animals, and season of the year, such that a given client may be responsible for a wide variety of different feeding regimens for the animals under their care. Feeding also is related to a significant number of large animal diseases, both directly (deficiencies and toxicities) and indirectly (through causing changes in metabolic and systemic disorders and in immune status and general health).

Animal Diseases Associated with Nutrition

SPECIES	DISORDERS / CONDITIONS ASSOCIATED WITH NUTRITION
Horses	Laminitis (founder) = inflammation of the hooves, associated with sudden change in diet or overfeeding of digestible carbohydrates Obesity, caused by overfeeding Feeding of mares during lactation Feeding foals and yearlings for growth Wobbler syndrome – a neurologic disorder Hyperkalemic periodic paralysis – a neurologic disorder associated with high potassium
Cattle (dairy and beef)	Rumenitis / acidosis = change in pH in the rumen and inflammation, secondary to increased carbohydrates in diet Liver abscess Milk fever = hypocalcemia = decreased calcium post-partum Ketosis = breakdown of fats and release into the metabolism post-partum Metritis = inflammation of the uterus post-partum Lameness and laminitis Displaced abomasum = twisted stomach Anestrus = delayed cycling due to inadequate nutrition

SPECIES	DISORDERS / CONDITIONS ASSOCIATED WITH NUTRITION
Sheep and Goats	Pregnancy toxemia = release of ketones secondary to a decline in nutrition and breakdown of fats in small ruminants carrying multiple offspring in late gestation
	Copper toxicity
	White muscle disease due to selenium deficiency
	Anestrus, low twinning rate, and general poor reproductive performance due to inadequate nutrition
Swine	Gastric ulcers in sows
	Anestrus and prolonged non-productive sow days (days the sow is not pregnant when she could be pregnant) – due to inadequate nutrition
	Dystocia = difficulty farrowing
	Poor lactation / baby pig mortality due to inadequate nutrition
	Poor growth rates in young pigs
	Poor disease resistance

Nutrition comes to the fore for large animal veterinarians because:

- Nutrition is often an option on your list for differentials for the cause of disease.
- Nutrition may be a limiting factor in production or performance.
- Inadequate nutrition may be a factor in development of disease.
- Improper nutrition is an unnecessary cost of ownership / management of animals.

Our role occurs at several levels, from as simple as advising on questions of feeding to troubleshooting production problems to diagnosing disease to formulating rations to acting as a nutrition program advisor (closely linked in production agriculture with records management and analysis). Other nutritional resources with whom we may work include owners / farmers, feed company personnel, independent nutritionists, feed product companies, extension personnel, university experts, and agronomy experts who study crops and their nutrient content. In practice, you will have an opportunity to apply your knowledge of nutrition every day.

Foods and Feeds

There is no hard definition that distinguishes "food" from "feed" but in general, food = what is actually eaten, mostly by people and non-farm animals (dogs, gerbils, birds, lizards, etc.) and feed = what may be mixed to produce animal food and/or what is fed to farm animals (cows, horses, chickens, sheep, etc.). Feeds may be characterized by origin or major type of the feed (plant, animal, mineral, vitamin) or by how the feed is processed (dried; ground = pulverized to decrease particle size; pelleted = extruded under high pressure and steam and therefore partially cooked; flaked = rolled and flattened; steamed; cooked; extruded; ensiled = anaerobically fermented).

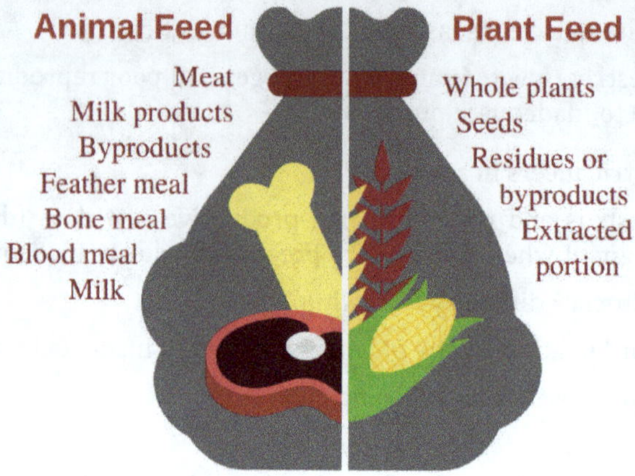

Animal Origin Feeds

- Meat
- Byproducts (protein sources from parts of the animal not used for human food)
- Meat and bone meal (cannot feed from ruminants because of concerns about bovine spongiform encephalopathy (BSE = mad cow disease))
- Blood meal (dried blood, great protein supplement)
- Feather meal (ground feathers, less digestible protein supplement)
- Milk and milk products (casein, whey, etc.)

Plant Origin Feeds

- Whole plants (corn, silage, alfalfa hay)
- Seeds (shell corn, wheat, oats, soybeans)
- Residues or byproducts (beet pulp = leftovers from sugar beet production, citrus pulp = leftovers from orange juice production, sweet corn stover, potato waste = leftovers from making French fries, almond hulls, cottonseed, distillers grains = leftovers from the bottom of the beer vat, brewers grains, straw)
- Extracted portion = soybean meal, corn starch, molasses, corn oil

How do we determine what is in a plant? A variety of extraction processes can be used. Ether extraction is used to identify the amount of fats / lipids. Nitrogen extraction is used as an estimate of crude protein – about 16% of protein is nitrogen. Ash is what is left after burning a plant and is the mineral content. Acid and detergent extractions are done to define the two forms of fiber, which are hemicellulose (neutral detergent fiber) and cellulose and lignin (acid detergent fiber). Subtracting these from total carbohydrates yields the non-fiber carbohydrates, which are sugars, starches, and pectins.

Types of Feed

Types of feed include dry forages (grass or legume hay), straw (plant parts remaining after grains are harvested), corn stover (parts of corn remaining after corn is harvested); wet forages such as green chop (undried grass and legume hays), and silage and haylage; byproducts = commodities; grains; protein concentrates; and lipid sources. Grazing animals also get fresh forage on pasture.

- **Silage and haylage** – The whole plant is harvested and chopped into small pieces, usually while in a vegetative state (before going to seed, more nutrient-dense). It is packed tightly to exclude air and is covered or sealed. Sugars in the plant feed bacteria that make acids in this anaerobic environment. As the pH drops, growth of microorganisms is inhibited, preserving the feed. This is also done with corn ("high moisture corn"). Silage and haylage are stored in upright silos (loaded from the top and so packs itself down, often cannot produce food quickly enough for large operations), silage piles (packed down by tractors), trench silos, or plastic bags (packed tightly by machines).
- **Dry feeds** – These include hay (grass or legumes (alfalfa or clover) that is cut, dried and then baled), grains, byproducts, minerals, and vitamins.
- **Hays** – Hays are best if cut early while in their vegetative, not reproductive, state (before they go to seed). If cut during the vegetative state, they have less cellulose and lignin and so are more digestible, and are higher in protein. Grasses include orchard, timothy, and fescue. Legumes include alfalfa and clover. If is stored dry, it will provide > 85-90% dry matter. If wet, it will mold and decay as it oxidizes and will lose nutritional value.
- **Straw** – Straw is the dried stems of crops that remain after those crops are harvested. "Straw should not be fed without supplementation because rarely does straw provide enough energy and protein to meet an animal's requirements. However, straw is a good alternative in rations for cows and sheep if properly supplemented with higher quality feedstuffs. Differences in feeding value do exist among the straws. Oat straw is the most palatable

and nutritious; barley straw is second and wheat straw has the lowest nutritional value of the main grains. Millet straw is more palatable and higher in energy and protein. Flax straw is lower in feed value than all the others because of its lower digestibility."

- **Grains** – Grains are the seeds of the plant. These include corn, wheat, oats, barley, sorghum, millet, and rice. They are usually high in energy and starch and are highly digestible. Grains are a major source of dietary energy for domestic animals and humans.
- **Protein concentrates** – These often are the seeds of plants as well, particularly legumes and oilseeds, including soybeans, cottonseed, rapeseed (= canola), and sunflower seeds. These often provide plant material after extraction of oils and often are a byproduct of some other process such as preparation of corn gluten meal or distilling. Others are animal byproducts such as meat and bone meal, blood meal, and feather meal.
- **Byproduct feeds** – These are leftovers from preparation of human foods and include beet pulp, citrus pulp, bakery waste, potato waste, brewer's grains, almond hulls, apple pomace, cannery waste, soy hulls, and wheat midds. Use of these as animal feed often solves what would otherwise be a major environmental problem.
- **Minerals** – These are ground and otherwise processed rock. Macrominerals include calcium, phosphorus, potassium, magnesium, sodium, sulfur, and chloride and often are provided as dicalcium phosphate, limestone, magnesium oxide, sodium chloride, potassium chloride, and sodium bicarbonate. Microminerals include selenium, copper, iron, zinc, manganese, cobalt, and molybdenum. There are important differences in biological availability, quality, and impact as fed to animals.
- **Vitamins** – Fat-soluble vitamins include A, D, and E. Vitamin K also is fat-soluble but rarely is added to large animal rations. Water-soluble vitamins added to feed are B vitamins such as thiamine, niacin, cyanocobalamin, and biotin. Vitamins usually are synthetic or fermentatively derived and are commonly added to rations without consideration for amount of those vitamins naturally occurring in other feed types.
- **Water** – Water is the single most important nutrient. It is cheap and is often ignored, for example by being limited in access or offered dirty. One must consider availability, cleanliness, flow, competition for water sources, and temperature.

There are a variety of ways nutrients in feed can be analyzed. You can find much information about nutrients in tables. For some feeds this is fine – salt is salt – but for others, the feed itself must be tested (for example, forages). Types of analysis include wet chemistry and near infrared analysis. Feed analysis is best used for directly measurable components (fiber, macronutrients, protein) and is poor for constituents with wide variation or error in measurement (microminerals). Energy and non-fiber carbohydrates can be assessed by calculation. Be cautious of feed tables that come pre-installed in computer programs.

Feed quality is dependent on the right feed component being used (be cautious of similar names), feed being collected at the proper stage of maturity and properly stored and processed, the bioavailability of the nutrients, and freedom from contamination, toxins, and micro-organisms. Feed delivery also can be a problem. Every single diet can be described as three diets – the one that is formulated on paper, the one that is delivered, and the one the animals eat. The goal is to make sure all three of these are the same for all animals intended to eat that diet.

FORMULATING RATIONS

Formulation is only one step and is not the end point. The key value is added by monitoring the implementation and the results of the feeding program. When in doubt, look at the animals! It is important to complete all 6 steps described below when formulating a ration.

- Describe the animal.
    - Species, breed, age, sex, production/rate of gain, stage of pregnancy/ lactation, exercise/activity, health status, environmental conditions – all of these factors play a role. For example, ruminants who have not been weaned (lambs and calves who are still milk-fed) are not functioning as ruminants.
- Describe the nutrient requirements.

This includes total food intake (usually best expressed on a dry matter basis [DMB]), energy (calories, essential fatty acids), protein (total and essential amino acids), fiber, macro- and microminerals, vitamins, and water. One must also consider how you feed animals in groups. If you feed the average animal in that group, you may be underfeeding high producing or fast growing individuals in the group. Diseased animals in that group (for example, those carrying parasites) also may require more nutrients. Feed intake is the limiting constraint to meeting nutrient needs in some animals because they cannot physically take in enough of a given ration to get all the nutrients available in that ration. This is particularly true of animals with high energy needs because of lactation, work, or life in harsh environmental conditions. This can be compensated for by adjusting animal comfort, access to feed (time, conditions, competition), physical forms of feeds, water content, palatability, and balance of feeds to enhance digestion.

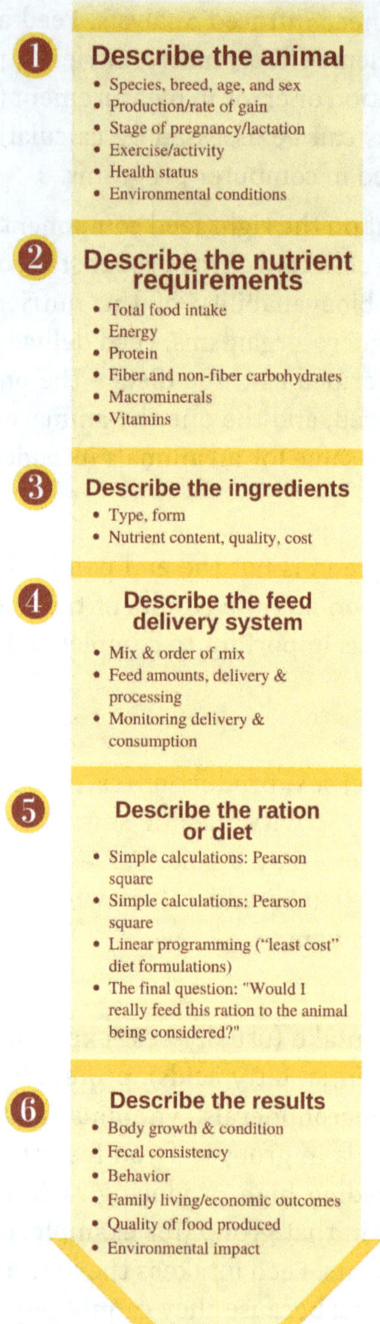

Energy

Energy cannot be measured directly in routine feed testing and is instead inferred from studies. In monogastric animals, energy may drive consumption; once the energy needs are met, the animal stops eating. If they do not, they become obese. If the diet is highly palatable, excess energy may be taken in. Energy density can be increased by using fats in the diet. Energy density can be decreased by increasing fiber, particularly in carnivores and omnivores.

Protein

Digestibility and types of protein present play a role. "Bypass protein" in ruminants is dietary protein that, either by some means of alteration or because of the type of protein, is not broken down by microbes in the rumen. Essential amino acids are those that must be in the diet; these vary by species. For example, taurine and carnitine are essential amino acids in cats. Corn is lysine deficient so soybeans may be added in rations to provide lysine. Protein sources are processed by heating, grinding, extrusion, and cooking to increase digestibility. Protein sources may be contaminated (for example, *Salmonella* sp, bovine spongiform encephalopathy).

Fiber and non-fiber carbohydrates

Concerns include digestibility, physical form, palatability, association with other nutrients (for example, nitrogen-containing nutrients to help break down carbohydrates). The more mature the plant, the less digestible the fiber. These include sugars, starches, pectin, hemicellulose, cellulose, and lignin.

Macrominerals

These are ground and processed rock and have variable bioavailability. They have reliably measured levels in feeds but levels present do not guarantee digestive availability. They typically are balanced for minimum needs and are adjusted for specific conditions.

Microminerals

These are unreliably measured in feeds and are typically added to satisfy complete requirements in food animal diets – this means a set amount is added regardless of how much may be in other components of the diet. They may interact with other microminerals (copper and molybdenum) or nutrients (selenium and vitamin E), or with macrominerals (most are divalent cations and so may alter each others' absorption).

Vitamins

Typically added to satisfy total needs – as above, vitamins are added without calculating vitamin content in all components of the diet. Need for water soluble vitamins varies with species and some have special needs – for example, guinea pigs, like humans, cannot synthesize vitamin C so it must be supplied in feed.

- Describe the feedstuffs.
    - Type, form, nutrient content, quality, cost

- Describe the feed delivery system.
    - Mix, order of mix, processing, feed delivery (amounts, timing delivery system), monitoring delivery and consumption
- Describe the ration or diet.
    - Doing the arithmetic. Computers do a lot of it. Work from an existing ration. Be careful about trusting the computer (Is the program up to date? Are the feed tables right? Are the nutrient requirements right?).
- Simple calculations: Pearson square
    - This is straightforward math and is easy to calculate but is rarely used when formulating a complex ration.

A = % desired nutrient in first type of feed

B = % desired nutrient in second type of feed

C = % desired nutrient in formulation

D, E and F are calculated

How to Use the Pearson Square

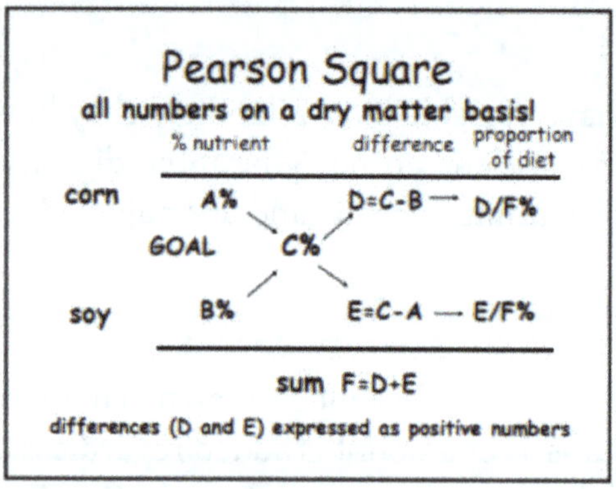

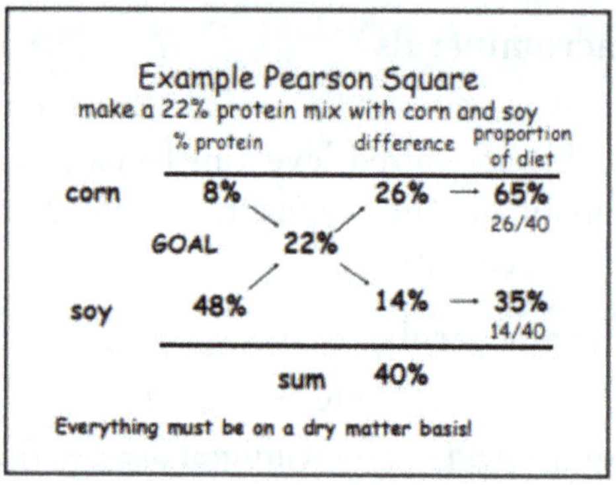

Cut and fit" formulation

Start by including some of the largest components (fiber in ruminants, protein in monogastrics). Add minerals and vitamins to meet needs. Fill remaining "intake space" with energy sources (carbohydrate, fats, fiber). Need to cut a little of something out of the ration to let something else fit in. Use trial and error until satisfied.

Linear programming

"Least cost" diet formulations – This is performed after a ration is formulated as a way of trying to optimize some particular aspect, for example, cost, while meeting the nutrient requirements and pre-set constraints. This commonly is used in food animal formulation. Results depend on accuracy of the definition of constraints and of nutrient content, and on the prices of feed used. Understand the approach and nutrition first, then use the tool. This can be a dangerous black box for the unsophisticated.

The final question

Would I really feed this ration to the animal being considered?

Describe the results.

Production – Growth – Body condition – Health – Fecal consistency – Behavior – Family living/economic outcomes – Family lifestyle; how hard is it to feed this diet? – Quality of food produced (wholesome, nutritious) – Environmental impact (for example, are we overfeeding something that will end up in the manure)

PET FOOD AND SMALL ANIMAL CLINICAL NUTRITION

What is the role of the veterinarian in small animal nutrition? The veterinarian provides nutrition counseling for healthy pets, for disease prevention, and for use of therapeutic diets. They are the link between the pet food manufacturer and the pet owner. You must also consider whether or not you will sell pet foods at your clinic and if so, how you will decide which you promote.

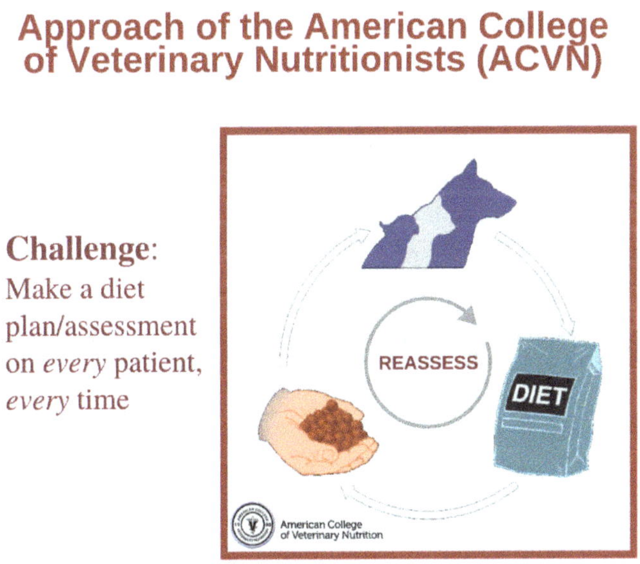

"The Circle of Nutrition," https://www.aaha.org/aaha-guidelines/nutritional-assessment-configuration/nutritional-assessment-introduction/

Clinical Goals

- To provide optimal nutrition

- To provide nutrition to support health and prevent disease
- To help clients select pet foods
- To address client misconceptions

Pet food industry in the United States – About 87% of dog and about 95% of cat owners in the United States feed at least 75% of their animal's diet as commercial pet food. There are fewer than 100 pet food manufacturers and are about 5000 different pet food labels in the US.

Percentages of Various Kinds of Foods Fed to Dogs and Cats

	CATS	DOGS
Canned	1	1
Mix of Canned and Dry	66	41
Dry	33	57

You should expect yourself to be able to physically examine pet food, calculate food dosage, and interpret pet food labels. You should always take a diet history which should include, at a minimum, what type of food(s) they're getting, how much they're being fed, and how often they're being fed.

Dogs and cats are fed a diet that is complete and balanced. Complete = all nutrients present and bioavailable. Balanced = feed to meet the pet's energy requirement and requirements for non-energy nutrients will automatically be met. This is very different from our approach as humans where we eat a variety of foods and hope for balance in our diet over time. Pet foods and pet food labeling are regulated by the American Association of Feed Control Officials (AAFCO). The front of the package will have a name for each product. The name tells you what likely percentage of a product is present.

Pet Food Package Labeling

INGREDIENT NAME	PRODUCT NAME	MINIMUM % OF INGREDIENT
Beef	All beef or 100% beef	95% beef
Beef and Chicken	Beef and chicken	95% beef and chicken with chicken at least 3%
Beef	Beef dinner	25% beef
Beef and Rice	Beef and rice formula	25% beef and rice with rice at least 3%
Beef	With beef	3%
Beef	Beef flavor	No minimum requirement

A new trend is unique game meats – for example, buffalo – 100% buffalo = buffalo meat with water sufficient for processing – This is not a complete and balanced diet and the label will reflect that.

Consumers read the brand name, then the guaranteed nutrient analysis, then the description of the food, and finally, the weight. About 1/3 of consumers in one study understood how nutritional adequacy was determined in pet foods and 2/3 did not. It is valuable for us to know how to read the labels so we can educate clients.

The label information panel must contain the following things: nutritional statement (adequacy claim), basis of nutrition claim, ingredient list, guaranteed analysis, manufacturer or distributor name and address, feeding directions, and universal product code.

Nutritional Statement

Nutrition in a diet may be determined either by the formulation method or by a feeding trial. If the formulation method is used, the label will have the following statement: "Diet X" formulated to meet nutritional levels established by AAFCO. Dog/cat nutrient profile for..." followed by which life stage is represented (maintenance, gestation, lactation, growth, all life stages). No animal studies are done. Nutritional statement by the formulation method is either calculated from known composition of ingredients in the diet or is determined by laboratory analysis of the food. Neither method considers digestibility or nutrient availability. Feeding trials are a superior way to determine nutritional adequacy. If a feeding trial is used, the label will have the following statement: "Animal feeding test using AAFCO procedures to substantiate that diet X provides complete and balanced nutrition for..." AAFCO feeding trials, for example for a maintenance food, must enroll 6-8 dogs, 1-6 years of age, with the food as the sole source of nutrition. The food is provided for a minimum time of 26 weeks, with a physical examination at beginning and end, body weight weekly, and labwork at the beginning, middle and end of the trial. All results must be normal for the food to "pass".

Two other options exist for the nutritional statement. "This product is intended for intermittent or supplemental feeding only" is on things like therapeutic diets, which are intended to be used short-term, under a veterinarian's supervision. No nutritional adequacy statement is needed on treats and other food products that are not intended to be fed as the sole diet.

Ingredient List

Ingredient versus nutrient – Nutrient = substance that must be consumed in the diet to provide a source of energy, substrate for growth or substance to regulate growth, metabolism, and energy production. Ingredient = the means to achieve nutritional and palatability goals – an ingredient may supply one nutrient, many nutrients, or none.

The ingredient list must show each ingredient, listed in descending order by weight and listed on "as is basis" (as it comes out of the bag or can).

Common Ingredients in Pet Foods to Provide Various Nutrients

	PROTEINS	CARBOHYDRATES	FATS
Dry Diets	Meat – Meat meal – Poultry meal – Poultry by-product meal – Fish meal – Corn gluten meal – Soybean meal	Corn – Rice – Barley – Sorghum – Potato	Animal fat – Fish oil – Vegetable oil
Canned Diets	Meat – Meat by-products – Poultry – Beef – Lamb – Fish	Corn – Rice – Barley – Sorghum – Potato	Animal fat – Fish oil – Vegetable oil
These ingredients provide...	Amino acids	Energy, some protein, some vitamins	Fats, essential fatty acids

Guaranteed Analysis = Proximate Analysis

Protein and fat are expressed as minimum amounts, and fiber and moisture are listed as maximum amounts. All are reported on an "as fed basis". Any other nutrient information is optional. Amounts will be close but not accurate.

Comparison of products requires evaluation on a dry matter basis (DMB). This allows you to compare foods with widely varying moisture content, knowing that you are not being misled by weight of moisture. As a rule of thumb, canned foods are 75% water and dry foods are about 10% water.

Dry matter (%) = 100 – moisture

DMB (%) = nutrient (%) divided by dry matter (%)

Example

A food is 12% moisture and 17% protein. What is percentage protein on a dry matter basis? Dry matter = 100-12 = 88. Percentage protein on a dry matter basis is 17 divided by 88 = 19.3%.

Dietary Protein Recommendations % Dry Matter Basis

	DOG	CAT
Minimum for adult (growth)	18% (22%)	26% (30%)
Minimum ideal	4%	8%
Recommended range	18-28%	30-45%
Common range	25-44%	35-52%

Dietary Fat Recommendations % Dry Matter Basis

	DOG	CAT
Minimum for adult (growth)	5% (8%)	9% (9%)
Recommended range	5-20%	9-30%
Common range	13-28%	11-16%

Feeding Guidelines

The general recommendation is to start at the low end of the recommended amount listed on the bag and to monitor body condition to ensure the animal is not being underfed or overfed.

Manufacturer or Distributor Name and Address

This permits the consumer / veterinarian to contact the company for accurate information that may not be readily accessed from the label and to bring forward concerns about the product.

Universal Product Code

This is a unique identifier of a batch of pet food and is valuable in face of a recall or other concern.

CHAPTER-11

HERBIVORES PROVIDE NUTRITION

Cattle, sheep, and goats are ruminants. Young that are still nursing do not function as ruminants as their rumen is still developing. Once weaned, all ruminants ferment food in the rumen and have unique nutritional needs.

Horses are not ruminants but still ferment food. They are hindgut fermenters, who ferment food in the cecum.

FEEDING DAIRY COWS

Cows, like all mammals, must give birth to make milk. They typically calve for the first time when 2 years old and have another calf every 13-14 months. Gestation length averages 280 days. They are not milked (dry) for 2 months at the end of pregnancy before the next calf is born. On average, cows have three calves before being replaced in the herd by their daughter (or the next cow's daughter). Cows are milked 2 or 3 times per day using milking machines that are cleaned and sanitized after each milking shift.

Cows are grazers. They are physiologically designed to consume large meals in a short amount of time. Meals are not chewed when consumed. Un-chewed feed is later regurgitated and chewed (the cud) so that particle size is reduced for further passage down the digestive tract.

The cow has four stomach chambers. The reticulum is a specialized pouch of the rumen located adjacent to the heart but separated from it by the diaphragm. It has a honeycomb appearance. It empties primarily into the rumen (large pieces of ingesta) but also empties in the omasum (small pieces of ingesta). It also collects abnormal objects eaten by the cow and so is sometimes called "the hardware stomach." The rumen lies on the left side of the abdomen. It is lined with papillae to create a huge absorptive surface. It contains muscular pillars. Basically, it is a huge fermentation vat filled primarily with anaerobic bacteria. It is not functional at birth. It serves to store feed for regurgitation, to soak feed, to physically mix and break down feed, and to ferment fibrous feeds, sugars, and starches into volatile fatty acids (VFAs), which are absorbed by the papillae. It also is a source of protein production (some of the rumen micro-organisms synthesize proteins and vitamins), and generates heat (great in the winter, a source of heat stress in the summer). The omasum absorbs water and breaks down the ingesta into small particles by passage through many closely connected layers ("plies"). None of the first three compartments secrete digestive enzymes. The abomasum is a "true stomach" that secretes enzymes; it is a glandular stomach as is seen in monogastric animals like the dog and cat. It secretes hydrochloric acid, mucin, pepsinogen, rennin (which clots casein, or milk proteins), and lipase (which breaks down fats).

Cows have a more complex digestive system than monogastrics. The food cows eat first passes into the rumen, then is regurgitated and re-chewed, and then passes again into the rumen and on through the three other chambers. In the rumen, bacteria and protozoa break down the food into nutrients the cow can absorb. This allows cows to digest food that humans (or chickens or pigs) cannot digest. Most feed, about 70%, is digested in the rumen by bacteria, protozoa and fungi. Micro-organisms are substrate-specific, breaking down either fiber or starch, for example. Micro-organisms produce VFAs from digested feed; this is the cow's primary energy source. Micro-organisms also provide a significant source of protein to the cow (microbial protein).

There is no oxygen in the rumen so when carbohydrates are broken down CO_2 and H_2O cannot be produced. The excess hydrogen is attached to carbon to make methane (CH_4), which is eructated (burped) or passed into manure. Fiber is broken down by rumen bacteria to create 2-carbon VFAs (acetate) and 4-carbon VFAs (butyrate) that are absorbed through the rumen wall. VFAs then go to the liver to be made into longer VFAs that contribute to milk fat. Starches and sugars are broken down to form 3-carbon VFAs (propionate) that are converted by the liver to glucose. Glucose plus galactose makes lactose – this is milk sugar and its production drives overall milk production.

Ruminant Digestion

The goals of feeding a milking cow are to maintain good cow health and reproduction, to support high milk production, to support good levels of milk components (3.7% fat, 3.2% protein in Holsteins) and to maintain adequate body condition. Cows are scored on a 1-5 scale with 1 being very thin and 5 being obese. Goals are a body condition score (BCS) of greater than 3 at calving, greater than 2.5 at peak lactation, and greater than 3.25 at dry off. After calving, it is 3-6 weeks until peak lactation. Prior to and at the peak, it is hard for a cow physically to eat enough to keep up with metabolic needs of milk production. She will meet energy needs by mobilizing fat and, to a smaller extent, protein. More protein is provided to cows in early lactation. After peak lactation, energy needs will gradually decrease until she is dried off two months before her next calf is due.

1 = rumen, 2 = reticulum, 3 = omasum, 4 = abomasum

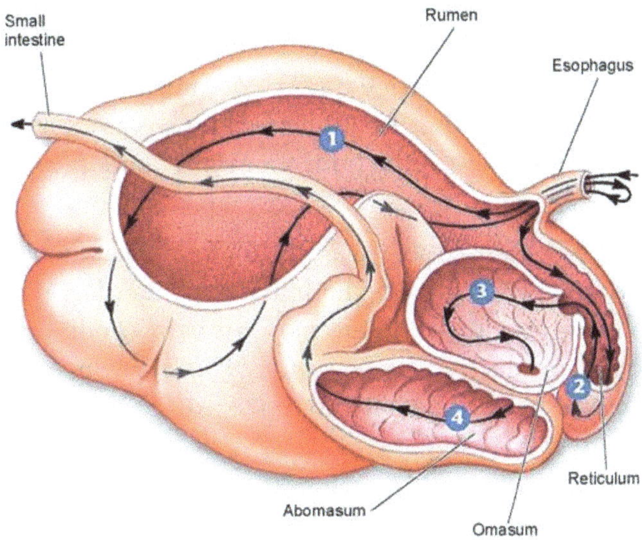

"Four-chambered stomach of a ruminant", https://schoolbag.info/biology/living/209.html

Overall Nutrient Needs

- Energy – Carbohydrates and VFAs from rumen and fats
- Protein – Supplied by diet and microbial protein. Cows also get bypass protein, which passes the rumen and is taken up in the small intestine intact. This is needed to support milk production.
- Fiber – Physically necessary in rumen and needed to support acetate production and subsequent creation of butterfat in the milk
- Fats
- Minerals
- Vitamins

Adult cows are fed differently depending on their stage of production. These may or may not be different diets and instead may be different amounts of the same diet. Stages are early lactation (7-70 days post-calving), peak lactation (71-140 days), mid and late lactation (140-305 days), dry cow (50-60 days before next calving), and transition from dry to lactation (3 weeks prior to calving and one week post-calving).

In early lactation there is a rapid increase in milk production. Cows cannot eat enough to take in sufficient energy to balance milk production. Dry matter intake is increased but is limiting as cows can only eat so much dry matter in a day. Protein needs are increased. A big concern in early lactation is rumen acidosis, a common condition where there is overproduction of lactic acid in the rumen with a decrease in production of the more valuable VFAs previously described. Causes of rumen acidosis include feeding of too much grain or concentrate and feeding of food in too small particles. Rumen acidosis is associated with lameness, low butterfat, weight loss, low production, poor reproduction, and eventual culling from the herd.

At peak milk production, intake again is limited by how much dry matter the cow can consume. The ration must be high in energy density, and high in protein; bypass protein often is provided. The cow may lose body condition due to inequality in energy out (milk production) versus energy in. Fiber must be provided and attention paid to size of particles introduced into the rumen to ensure normal rumen health.

At mid to late lactation, production gradually declines. Dry matter intake is associated with taking in enough nutrients to permit body condition to be restored. Cows are pregnant during this phase so the diet provided must support the developing fetus.

Cows are dried off (no longer milked) for about the last two months of gestation. The fetus is growing dramatically during this stage. Cows receive a very different ration during this stage than they had as milking cows, with an increase in forage to prepare the rumen for the next lactation and feeding of a ration with lower energy density. The ration generally is low in calcium and is acidifying; this keeps calcium metabolism pathways operational to reduce chances of post-partum hypocalcemia.

The transition period is the time spanning from 2-3 weeks before calving to about 1 week after calving. This is a stressful time in the cycle as there is a big metabolic shift. This is the most common time to see dairy cow disease – for example, one study demonstrated that cows that ate less dry matter prior to calving were more likely to suffer from uterine infection (metritis) after calving. During this stage, adequate high quality forage must be provided to maintain rumen fill and to stimulate rumination (regurgitation and re-chewing of the cud). The diet is gradually shifted to that of the milking cow to give the rumen microflora time to adapt.

Common feeds are as those described in the Nutrition-Basics section of the course. Other miscellaneous feeds that may be added include bypass protein (fish meal, blood meal, dried brewer's grains, soybean meal) and bypass fat (Megalac™).

A total mixed ration (TMR) is composed of (1) a base vitamin and mineral mix, (2) an on-farm dry ingredient premix made up of protein mix (protein and concentrate: grain mix), and corn and other grains and byproducts or commodities as described in the Nutrition-Basics section of the course, and (3) forages. Advantages of a TMR is that each mouthful is the same so there is better assurance of a balanced diet delivered to the rumen micro-organisms; there is less chance of a given cow selectively eating or avoiding a single type of feed; each individual cow can consume to her physical ability; and there is savings in labor and mechanization, especially in large operations. Delivery of the diet includes such factors as order of mixing of components, processing (grinding, heating, extrusion, drying, etc.), and how the feed is provided to the cattle (amount, timing, delivery system, and removal of feed that is not consumed).

Cows may be fed in stanchion barns with feed provided as separate components or as a TMR; fed in freestall barns with bunk feeding, primarily of a TMR; or fed in a variety of other ways including forage in bunks, racks or pasture; feeding of concentrate in the milking parlor; feeding of concentrates in "computer feeders" ,and feeding mineral free choice as loose minerals or salt blocks.

FEEDING DAIRY CALVES

Care of the newborn calf includes:

- Monitoring the calving process and assisting if needed
- Removing the calf from the dam ASAP and drying it – The goal is to remove the calf from the dam within 30-60 minutes of birth to decrease exposure to pathogens.
- Disinfecting the navel (for example, 7% iodine dip) to prevent umbilical infection
- Feeding colostrum with the first feeding within 1-2 hours of birth
- Placing in calf housing and feeding a milk diet until weaned at approximately 8 weeks of age

The Five Cs of Successful Calf Rearing

Colostrum – Calories (nutrition) – Comfort – Cleanliness – Consistency

Colostrum

Colostrum is the first milk produced after calving. It contains elevated concentrations of immunoglobulins (primarily IgG and some IgM and IgA), and of proteins and fats – see table below for a comparison between colostrum (first milking after calving), transition milk (second and third milkings after calving), and whole milk (subsequent milk produced).

Comparison of Milks After Calving

	COLOSTRUM	TRANSITION MILK	WHOLE MILK
Total Solids(%)	23.9	14.1	12.9
Protein (%)	14.0	5.1	3.1
Fat (%)	6.7	3.9	3.7
Total Minerals (%)	1.11	0.87	0.74
IgG (mg/mL)	48.0	15.0	0.6

Colostrum is important because cows have an epitheliochorial (6-layer) or a synepitheliochorial (5-layer) placenta. Immunoglobulins cannot cross this placenta to the fetus so calves are born without circulating protective antibodies. Passive transfer is absorption of antibodies by the newborn calf across the gut into the circulation (IgG, IgA, and IgM). Colostral immunoglobulins protect the calf against diseases for the first few months, until the calf can produce its own immune response. Failure of passive transfer (FPT) is defined as concentration of IgG in calf serum of less than 10 mg/mL when measured in blood drawn between 24 and 72 hours of age. In one study, 21% of United States dairy heifer calves had FPT. Benefits of having adequate passive transfer include reduced treatment and mortality rates in calves, improved growth rates and feed efficiency, decreased age at first calving, and increased first and second lactation milk production. Some of these parameters are not measured until cows are over 3 years of age so you can see that calf management has long-reaching effects.

The 5 Qs of a Successful Colostrum Management Program

Quality – Quantity – Quickness – sQueaky clean – Quantifying results

Quality

Quality of colostrum is defined by amount of IgG within that colostrum. Feeding of colostrum that contains at least 50 mg/mL of IgG is associated with achieving > 10 mg/mL IgG in the calf's serum, or successful passive transfer.

Factors that Affect Colostrum Quality

FACTORS NOT UNDER MANAGEMENT'S CONTROL	FACTORS UNDER MANAGEMENT'S CONTROL
Breed – Colostrum quality is higher in colored breeds than in Holsteins	Dry cow nutrition

Parity – Colostrum quality is higher in older cows than in first calf heifers	Stress during dry period (heat stress, overcrowding)
Pre-partum leaking	Vaccination during dry period – may be stressful but also important for increasing antibodies
	Clinical mastitis (infection of the mammary glands – this milk must be discarded)
	Time to first milking – Optimally harvest colostrum within 1-2 hours of calving; beyond 6 hours, quality significantly declines
	Dry period length – Colostrum quality suffers if the dry period is less than 3 weeks in length

Colostrum quality is measured using a colostrometer or Brix refractometer. A colostrometer measures specific gravity. Its sensitivity is 75% and specificity is 87%. It is inexpensive, rapid, and simple to do but the instrument is fragile and the test must be performed at room temperature. The Brix refractometer measures total solids. Its sensitivity is 90.5% and specificity is 85%. It is more expensive but is rapid and simple and the test is not temperature-dependent.

Quantity

Often we do not have a clear idea of how much IgG is in the colostrum. Most people hedge their bets by giving a large enough volume to ensure that calves are receiving enough IgG. To achieve IgG of greater than 10 mg/mL in serum, calves must consume more than 100 gm of IgG in colostrum. If calves are fed 4 quarts of colostrum, this goal will be met 87% of the time. The current recommendation is to feed 10% of body weight at first feeding – for the average Holstein calf, which weighs 43 kg (90 lbs), that would be 3.8 liters (4 quarts).

Quickness

Quickness refers to time to first feeding. Calves are born with an open gut that is able to absorb large protein molecules intact, such as IgG. Gut closure begins soon after birth with progressive loss of ability to absorb IgG. Closure is complete by 24 hours of life. The goal is to feed colostrum within 1-2 hours of birth and certainly before 6 hours of life. Colostrum can be fed using either a nippled bottle or an esophageal tube. Veterinarians can teach producers how to safely tube feed calves by teaching them proper technique and stressing sanitation and management of the equipment. Options for providing colostrum include:

- Milking the cow and feeding the calf within 1-2 hours – preferred
- Feeding the calf colostrum that was previously collected from a different cow and stored (refrigerated or frozen)

- Feeding a commercial colostrum replacer product
- The calf suckling the dam – This is NOT preferred as it is associated with high FPT rates and increases exposure of the calf to pathogens.

Queaky Clean

This refers to bacterial contamination. Colostrum is frequently an early source of microbial exposure. The goal is for colostrum to have a total plate count of fewer than 100,000 CFU/ml with total coliform count less than 10,000 CFU/ml. In one study, 82% of Wisconsin herds and 93% of Minnesota herds exceeded these amounts. If there are many bacteria in colostrum, this may prevent IgG absorption from the calf's GI tract and may directly cause disease. The three major sources of colostrum contamination are:

- Infection from the mammary gland or fecal contamination of skin on the teats
    - This is best avoided by discarding milk from known diseased cows, not letting the calf suckle the dam, cleaning and sanitizing the udder before milk collection, and not pooling raw colostrum to be sure that colostrum containing bacteria from one cow does not adulterate good colostrum from other cows.
- Contaminated collection or storage equipment
    - This is best avoided by scrupulously cleaning equipment.
- Bacterial proliferation in stored colostrum
    - This is avoided by feeding colostrum within 1-2 hours of collection, refrigerating it (use within 48 hours), or freezing it as soon as possible after collection.

Other techniques include feeding colostrum replacement products and heat-treating colostrum. Colostrum replacement products are powdered colostrum that is mixed with water. There is a minimum of 100 gm IgG per dose and cost is $25-30 / dose. It is a convenient, consistent source of IgG and controls disease transmission. One dose is equivalent to about 2 quarts of colostrum so most calves should receive at least two doses to try to avoid FPT. There is variation between products. Heat-treating is a relatively new technique. In one study, calves fed heat-treated colostrum were treated less and had less diarrhea (scours) than calves fed fresh colostrum.

Quantifying the Results

IgG in serum is not often measured. Total protein is more commonly measured; serum total protein of 5.0-5.2 gm/dL most accurately predicts serum IgG of 10 mg/mL. On-farm monitoring of passive transfer requires bleeding of about 12 clinically normal calves between 1 and 7 days old and measuring total protein with a refractometer. Goals are for 90% or more of the calves to have a total protein greater than 5.2 gm/dL. Higher is better!

Calories

Goals are for calves to double birth weight by 56 days of age (average daily gain (ADG) of 1.6-1.8 lb/day) and for calves to develop a functional rumen so the calf can be weaned off a milk diet and onto solid feed by 7-8 weeks of age.

Rumen Capacity as % of Total

The abomasum does not change in size as cows grow but the rumen changes dramatically in size and function.

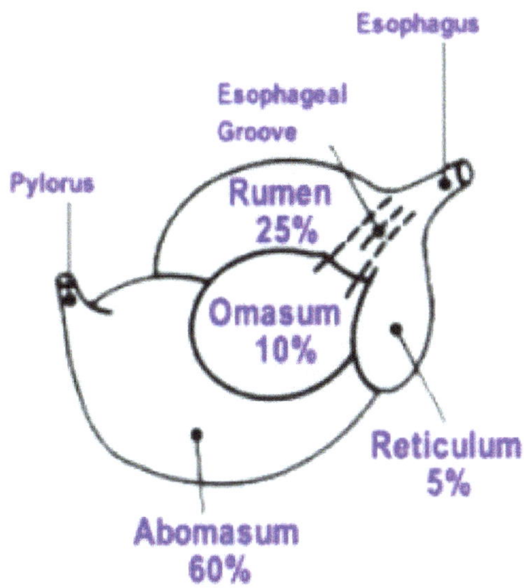

AGE	ABOMASUM CAPACITY	RUMEN CAPACITY
1 week	60%	25%
3-4 months	20%	65%
Maturity	7-8%	80%

Phases of Calf Development

There are three phases of calf development: Pre-ruminant phase (birth to 3-4 weeks) – Transition phase (3-4 weeks to weaning) – Ruminant phase (weaning to 225 lbs and beyond)

Pre-Ruminant Phase (birth to 3-4 weeks of age)

Baby calves do not have a functional rumen. They cannot digest solid feed and have limited rumen fermentation capacity. The rumen has no absorptive papillae and the rumen wall is thin. The abomasum is the main compartment involved in digestion. Calves are dependent on a liquid diet (milk) as their major source of nutrients. Their diet consists of high-quality milk replacer, calf starter (pelleted grain), and water. Calves are fed whole milk or milk replacer in a volume of 2-3 quarts twice daily in summer and 3-4 quarts twice daily in winter, when more energy is needed for cold stress; some producers feed three times on cold winter days. Offer free choice starter grain after 3 days of age and offer free choice water after 3 days of age. Some producers like to offer a small amount of dry hay but this does not contribute to rumen development prior to weaning. Milk generally bypasses the rumen via the esophageal groove and empties directly into the abomasum; reported stimuli for contracture of the esophageal groove include presence of milk solutes (proteins and other solids), the suckling of the calf, and the warm temperature of the fluid ingested. Esterase in the saliva begins fat digestion. Within the abomasum, milk clots within 10 minutes. Chymosin (rennin) acts on casein. The whey (liquid) fraction still includes many proteins, including antibodies. The milk clot is slowly digested by pepsin and HCl and is released to the intestines. Milk proteins but not vegetable proteins are best digested – look for this in milk replacers, as high-quality milk replacers will contain milk proteins, not soy or other vegetable-based proteins. In the small intestines, lactose is digested but starches and non-lactose disaccharides such as sucrose are essentially not digested during this phase. Pancreatic protein enzymes (trypsin and chymotrypsin) increase gradually.

Options for liquid feed for calves include milk replacer (generally 20% crude protein and 20% fat), whole milk, and pasteurized nonsaleable milk (for example, waste or discard milk). Considerations include desired nutrient intake to meet health and growth targets, disease control, complexity of managing the feeding program, and cost-benefit analysis.

Milk Replacer Programs

Nutrient Levels (e.g. 20 : 20 = Crude protein % : Fat)

- Crude protein: 18-30%
- Fat: 15-20% (up to 25% for Jerseys)

Protein Sources

- All milk – Whey protein: best mixing, highly digestible, most expensive
- Alternative proteins:
  - Soy protein concentrate
  - Soluble wheat gluten
  - Plasma

- Soy protein or modified soy flour isolate
- Egg protein

Fat Sources

- Lard – Probably the best and most economical
- Tallow – Can be less expensive at some times of the year
- Vegetable – Most expensive option today

Use of pasteurized non-saleable milk may be cost-effective. Pros include reduced pathogen transmission compared to raw milk, improved rate of gain compared to traditional milk replacer, improved calf health, improved economic efficiency, and use of a non-saleable product. Cons include cost of pasteurization and need for more intensive management and monitoring compared to conventional milk replacer programs.

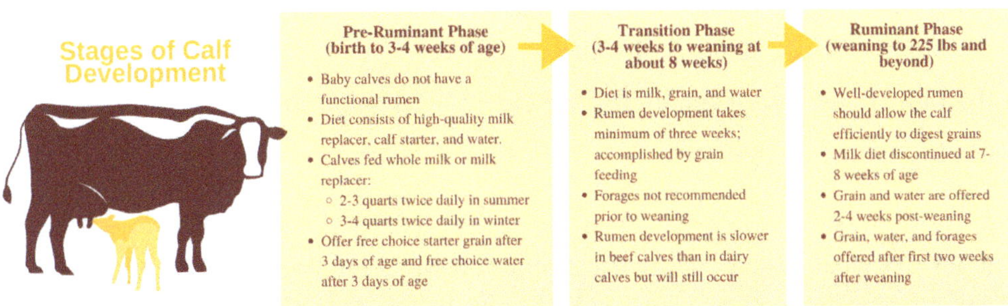

Transition Phase (3-4 weeks to weaning at about 8 weeks)

The diet is milk, grain, and water. During this phase, the calf begins to develop a functional rumen capable of digesting dry feed. Rumen development takes a minimum of three weeks. Rumen development is accomplished by grain feeding to promote butyric and propionic acid production, lowering pH and increasing growth of micro-organisms. This increases the size and muscularity of the rumen, and promotes development of papillae while the microflora is established. The rumen will not develop on a milk-only diet or on milk and forage. Grain feeding is required for development of the rumen in size and function. Forages are not recommended prior to weaning because microbes are not initially capable of fermenting forages, forage fermentation that may occur is associated with acetate production that does not stimulate rumen development, and forages fill the rumen and displace starter grains that would promote rumen development. Note that this is for dairy calves; beef calf management is described below.

Weaning Guidelines for Calves

Reduce stress by spreading out changes:

- Feed changes (weaning)
- Procedures: dehorning, vaccinations, tail docking
- Socialization/grouping, transport, environmental changes

Before weaning, calves should be:

- Eating starter for at least 3 weeks
- Consuming at least 2 lbs of starter per day for 3 consecutive days
- Receiving reduced milk diet by 50% in last 1-2 weeks to increase starter intake

Move to groups after weaning:

- Keep in individual pen on same grain > 7 days after weaning
- Move to small groups initially (6-8 calves)
- Continue on same grain for 1-2 weeks after grouping
- Introduce forages after 3-4 weeks post-weaning

Ruminant Phase (weaning to 225 lbs and beyond)

After 3-4 weeks in the transition phase, a well-developed rumen should allow the calf efficiently to digest grains. A milk (liquid) diet is discontinued at 7-8 weeks of age. For 1-2 weeks post-weaning, grain and water are offered. After that, grain, water, and forages (for example, hay) are offered.

General Considerations When Feeding Calves

Energy Status in Cold Weather

Strategies to improve energy status in cold weather include:

- Increase caloric intake:
  - Increase volume fed per feeding
  - Increase number of feedings per day
  - Add supplemental fat
  - Select liquid diet with increased energy density
- Decrease energy losses:
  - Keep calves dry
  - Prevent drafts
  - Use insulation: extra bedding (straw), calf jackets

- Use supplementary heat if needed
- Increase starter and water intake to promote rumen development
- Avoid illness by health management

Starter Management

You want to encourage starter intake to promote rumen development. This is needed before weaning to onto a cheaper diet of dry feed (no milk).

Calves prefer:

- Textured starters (pellets with corn/oats and molasses)
- Avoiding fines, dust
- Fresh (no mold), palatable, free choice

For best results:

- 21-23% crude protein (dry matter basis)
- Molasses content 5-8%
- Begin offering at 3 days and replace daily
- Provide free-choice fresh water
- Put in clean buckets
- Put in mouth after milk feeding

Free-Choice Water

Free-choice water promotes rumen development by providing an aqueous environment for microbes because milk bypasses the rumen by running through the esophageal groove but water deposits directly in the rumen. Water also promotes greater intake of dry feed. Water is essential to maintain hydration status, especially during periods of heat stress and illness (diarrhea = scours). Provide free-choice fresh water beginning at 3 days old and replace twice daily. Clean and disinfect buckets regularly. In winter, offer warm water for 1 hour after each milk feeding, then dump it before it freezes. In summer, check water at mid-day. Some calves are in an accelerated milk replacer program with high total solids – these calves absolutely must have free-choice water.

FEEDING BEEF CATTLE AND BEEF CALVES

What is fed to beef cattle varies widely. Beef cattle readily can use various rough feeds as are found on pasture and, in the United States, may be fed grain as well. As in other species and in dairy cattle, appropriate nutrition for beef cattle varies with life stage.

Breeding Cattle

Cows are bred to produce one calf per year. For the cows and bulls, grazed forage provides the bulk of the nutrition through the growing season. For the upper Midwest, this would typically be pasture from May through October, followed by grazing crop residue, primarily cornstalks, in November and December.

In addition to the grazed feed, beef cattle require supplemental vitamins and minerals for optimal health. These are delivered in the form of a loose mineral or a solid form. Solid products include a lick block, made from salt and minerals compressed into block form, or a lick tub, where vitamins and minerals are mixed with a protein source and molasses and cooked into a solid product that is delivered in a plastic or metal tub weighing 200 to 250 pounds. Supplemental vitamins and minerals are critical in grazing cattle to decrease the incidence of diseases such as pneumonia in the calves, as well as to prevent metabolic dysfunctions such as grass tetany (magnesium deficiency) in the cows.

Good pasture management is key to allowing maximum production of forage and maintain plant health. While not our primary role as veterinarians, as the most referenced source of advice on animal husbandry for producers it is critical to have a basic concept of how to manage grazing pastures, as poor grazing leads to unthrifty livestock and opens the door to parasitic infection.

For pastures in the upper Midwest and the Northern Plains, grass species are livestock's primary food source. In order to thrive, grasses need to have enough leaf to collect sunlight that the plant can then use to create energy. If the grass is grazed too tightly to the ground, the lack of a leaf inhibits sunlight capture.

To keep grass healthy, animals should only begin to graze a pasture once the grass has achieved twice its minimum required height. For the cool-season pastures common to Minnesota and the eastern Dakotas, this would be roughly 8-12″ tall. Once grass has been grazed to half its original height, it is time to move the animals to a new pasture. This gives the grass in the first pasture time to recuperate and regrow before being grazed again. Because of the need to move animals to new pasture throughout the grazing season, having multiple pastures, having a pasture cross-fenced into multiple paddocks, or having personnel to move the animals daily is a requirement for good grazing. This program of moving animals when they have grazed half the plant height is termed rotational grazing, as the animals "rotate" from one location to another. Due to the inconsistency of the weather, movements are not predicated on the calendar, but rather when grass height dictates moving. If done properly, the carrying capacity, meaning the number of animals the pasture can feed, will increase up to the level of doubling.

At the basic level, appropriate pasture management is critical to prevent malnutrition in livestock. Overgrazing early in the year can lead to a shortage later in the summer. Short pastures lead to poor body condition, lackluster reproductive performance and potentially weakened immune systems, allowing infectious disease to proliferate. Short pastures also open the door to increased parasite burdens, as was described in the chapter on parasite control. The life cycle of intestinal worms requires the larvae migrate up a blade of grass and be consumed livestock. This migration typically happens within the first 2″ of grass height. Therefore, if pastures are rotated as recommended at 4-6" of grass height, the members of the herd or flock consume fewer parasites, decreasing parasite burdens in the gut.

During the winter in the upper Midwest, cows and bulls often need to have feed delivered to them, as nothing will be growing and most crop residues are depleted. As ruminants, beef cattle have the ability to use an impressive variety of feedstuffs. This includes, but is not limited to, forages such as grass hay, alfalfa hay, corn, or other crop silage; grains such as corn, oats, or milo; and byproducts such as those left over from the production of ethanol, high-fructose corn syrup, or soybean oil. Because of this variety, testing each type of feed to determine the quality and quantity of macro and micro nutrients is a necessity. These test results can be used by a ruminant nutritionist to provide a balanced ration to keep cows in good condition through the cold of the winter.

Feeding Beef Calves

Most calves are born in the early spring. This is done to match the most economical forage, grazed pasture, to the time when cows are at peak lactation, the first 6-8 weeks after the calf is born. As lactation requires much energy, aligning calving so peak lactation occurs in late spring when grasses are most nutrient-dense is a common strategy. Calving may occur at other times of the year for a variety of reasons. The most common is labor-related, as calving can be a labor-intensive process for the rancher. If spring is occupied by other endeavors, such as planting crops, calving may occur in the winter or in the early fall, when it doesn't overlap with farming.

Just like the dairy calf, the beef calf is born as a pre-ruminant. However, beef cattle are permitted to nurse from their dam, and unlike the managed process of rumen development that occurs with dairy calves, beef calves' rumens develop on their own, as they remain with the cow for several months. Beef calves develop their rumen through eating forages out of curiosity, taking small nibbles at a few weeks of age, and progressing to grazing more as they age. While cows' milk makes up the entirety of the calves' diet for the first few weeks after birth, it is gradually outpaced after that by grazed forage. Weaning typically occurs in beef cattle around 6-7 months of age, usually in September, October or November. The reason for timing is once again cow-nutrition based—the process of nursing a calf takes energy from the cow and if she does not recover her body condition prior to winter, she will have difficulty during cold weather. By weaning a few months before winter, cows can store up body condition to have extra insulation for the incoming cold weather.

At weaning, calf diets start off forage-based, but must quickly progress to a supplement/forage blend. The reason for this transition is because calves' nutritional requirements are higher for protein and energy than simple grass hay can provide. Supplements, such as grains, fill that gap, but if the conversion happens too quickly, the rumen pH can drop rapidly and lead to acidosis. Alternatively, if the change happens too slowly, calves robbed of necessary nutrition are more susceptible to health issues, predominantly pneumonia. At this critical juncture, it is essential for calf diets to be formulated by a nutritionist.

Once calves are comfortable eating their initial diet, the subsequent diet will be one that matches the ultimate destiny for each particular group of cattle. For calves destined for the breeding herd, the diet remains forage-based, with grains and/or byproducts supplemented at a low level to meet the calves' energy requirements. The goal is for both heifers and bulls to be sexually mature at or before 15 months of age, to allow for them to successfully produce calves when they are two years old.

For cattle destined for slaughter in the Midwest or the Great Plains, the diet is transitioned to a grain-predominant diet, or so called "grain-fed beef". It is important to not confuse grain-fed as grain-exclusive diets, as all cattle require some forage to keep their rumen functioning. For grain-fed cattle in the upper Midwest, approximately 10% of their diet is rough forage, such as grass hay, ground corn stalks or chopped straw. The rest of the diet typically consists of ground corn, corn silage and ethanol by-products. This is done for three reasons. First, grain-fed cattle are ready for slaughter much sooner than those fed forages alone. A grain-fed animal reaches the 1300-1500 lbs slaughter weight at 14-16 months of age, as compared to 20-24 months for forage-fed cattle. Second, in order to keep a steady supply of fresh beef coming to market, some cattle will need to be fattened during the winter. Stored forages do not have the energy necessary to fatten cattle and without grain, the harsh winters of the central United States would inhibit cattle from fattening for a few months. This is why warmer climates, like Brazil or New Zealand, can provide fat, forage-fed beef year around. Lastly, the flavor profile of grain-fed cattle is preferred by many customers of beef both in the United States and abroad. This creates a lucrative market for grain-fed beef, causing the high-value cuts of US and Canadian beef to command a premium world-wide.

FEEDING SHEEP AND GOATS

Sheep are bred in the fall and lamb in the spring after a 147 day gestation. Important times to consider changes in nutrition are one month prior to breeding, in the first month after bred, in the last month of gestation, and in the first 45 days of lactation. Lambs are weaned at 60-120 days of age and go to market at about 5 months of age.

The production cycle of goats is similar. The typical dairy goat is bred in the fall while still lactating from her previous pregnancy. Gestation is 150 days. She is dried off for the last 60 days of her pregnancy and kids in the spring. Lactation is 305 days.

The information below refers to goats but is applicable to sheep as well; the complete document from which this is drawn is in the External Resources folder for this section.

The greatest asset of goats is the ability and tendency to use woody plants and weeds not typically consumed by other species of animals (cattle and sheep), converting them into a saleable product. Therefore, these plant species can be inexpensive sources of nutrients and make for a very profitable goat enterprise. Goats typically consume a number of different plant species in any one day and can use some poisonous plants because they do not consume enough to be toxic. Similarly, goats are believed to have a relatively high ability to detoxify absorbed anti-nutritional factors. Goats are more resistant to bloating than other ruminants, and after a brief adaptation may graze alfalfa without bloating.

Body Condition Scoring

The adequacy of a nutritional program can be assessed by observing changes in body weight and condition of the animal. If animals lose weight, body condition will be reduced (animal is thinner), alerting an observant manager to a problem. Body condition is particularly responsive to energy and protein adequacy. Body condition scoring is a system of assigning a numerical score based on physical characteristics indicative of fatness. These include the amount of muscle and fat covering the spine in the loin area and ribs and fat pad at the sternum. Body condition scores range from 1 (very thin) to 5 (obese) in one-half score increments. Animals should achieve a certain body condition during specific periods of the production cycle. For example, animals should have a body condition of at least 2.5 but no more than 4.0 at the beginning of the breeding season. Prior to entering the winter a minimum score of 3.0 is desirable. Also, if body condition score is 4.5 or greater, pregnancy toxemia prior to kidding is likely, as also is the case with a score of 2.0 or less.

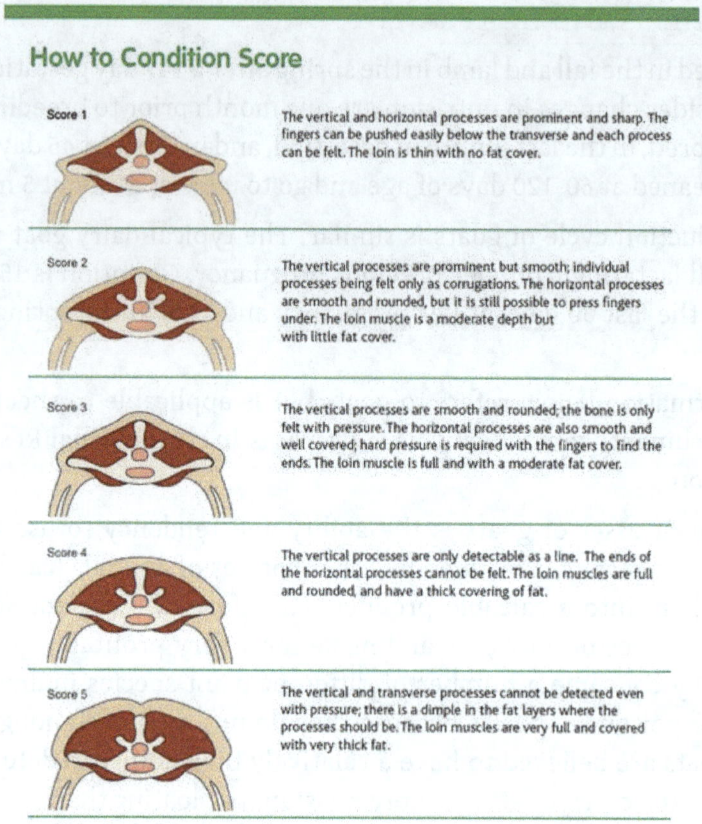

"Condition scoring of ewes", https://www.farmhealthonline.com/wp-content/uploads/2015/12/AHDB-Ewe-Condition-Handout-2015.pdf

Nutrients must be provided using feedstuffs such as pasture, hay, concentrate, and minerals. For most goats throughout much of the year, nutrient requirements can be met by available pasture, a mineral supplement, and water. During times of limited forage availability or quality such as winter, or feeding poor quality hay or stockpiled forage, a supplement will be needed to supply deficient nutrients. The level of supplemental feeding should be adjusted with changes in animal requirements, such as increased needs of late pregnancy. Sometimes it may be preferable to put an animal in a lot and feed a complete diet or one high in concentrate such as with dairy goats.

There may be periods when nutrient requirements cannot be met, resulting in loss of body weight. This is acceptable at certain times in the production cycle if body condition is sufficient for the animal to draw upon body reserves and maintain the desired production level. An example would be weight loss during early lactation because sufficient nutrients cannot be consumed. However if the doe is in poor body condition, is a growing yearling, or has severe weight loss during this time, milk production will be depressed. During a drought, it may be acceptable for open or early pregnant animals that are not lactating to lose weight. During late pregnancy, inadequate nutrition can have adverse effects on pregnancy outcome and subsequent lactation. Severe undernutrition can cause abortion, reduced livability of the kid(s), and reduced milk production, and can adversely affect maternal behavior.

Feeding Different Classes of Goats

Feeding Bucks

Mature bucks can obtain most of their nutrients from pasture. However, yearling and 2 year old bucks have greater nutrient requirements since they are still growing. Bucks need to be in good body condition (BCS greater than 3) before the breeding season because feed intake may be relatively low during that time, with loss of body weight. Thus, body condition should be evaluated 3 months before the breeding season. Decisions can then be made on the supplemental nutrition needed for the buck to achieve the desired BCS. Whenever bucks cannot meet nutritional needs from pasture, supplementation is necessary. Under most conditions, whole shelled corn or sweet feed at 0.25 to 0.5% of body weight will be adequate (0.5 to 1 lb of feed for a 200 lb buck). Feeding bucks high levels of grain (greater than 1.5% of body weight) for a long period of time makes them prone to urinary calculi. The levels of grain recommended above are safe for bucks. When pasture is scarce, bucks can be fed medium quality hay free-choice.

Feeding Does Throughout their Life Cycle

The four production periods of does are dry nonpregnant, pregnant, late gestation, and lactating. Does that are open (nonpregnant) or in the early stage of pregnancy (< 95 days) have fairly low nutrient requirements. For open does, the goal is to gain a little weight to be in good condition for breeding. A medium quality pasture, such as in late summer, or a medium quality hay is sufficient to prepare for breeding and the early stage of pregnancy. However, adequate quantities of feed are necessary. Flushing refers to the practice of providing extra nutrition to does approximately 2 weeks prior to breeding and for a variable portion of the breeding period (e.g., 1-2 weeks) to increase the number of ovulations and have a greater proportion of twins and triplets. This is widely advocated with sheep producers and Angora goat producers. Producers have extrapolated the practice to meat goats. However, several controlled studies with Spanish goats in reasonable body condition (BCS 2.5 – 3.5) have shown no response in kidding or conception rate of meat goats to flushing with extra protein, energy, or both. The practice may have utility for meat goats in poor body condition, but there does not appear to be justification for flushing does in acceptable body condition.

- Medium quality pasture or medium quality hay is sufficient
- Adequate quantities of feed are necessary

Pregnant

- Early to mid-winter
- Goal is to maintain body condition & keep them warm
- Feed forage and supplement components
- Forage can consist of hay, stockpiled forage, or cheap byproduct roughage
- Supplement usually contains energy, protein, and vitamins and minerals

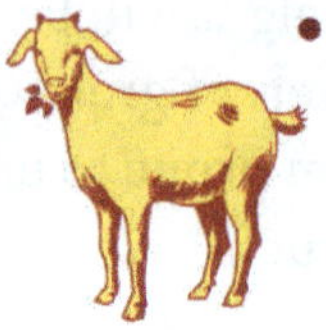

- Supplements include whole shelled corn, range cubes, sweet feed, protein & molasses blocks or tubs, & liquid feed

Late Gestation

- Energy requirements increase
- Feed intake may be reduced in the last 4 to 6 weeks of gestation
- Will need a more nutrient dense diet & exercise

Lactating

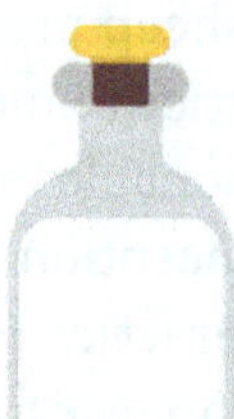

- Doe has very high nutrient requirements
- Nutrient requirements decline as stage of lactation

Winter Feeding of Does

Early to mid-winter is a time when does should be in early pregnancy. The goal of a wintering program is to economically provide the necessary nutrients to maintain a reasonable body condition, lose no weight, and keep them warm. In general, most wintering programs consist of both forage and supplement components. The forage component can consist of hay, stockpiled forage, or a cheap byproduct roughage feed. The supplement usually contains energy, protein, and often vitamins and minerals, although these may be provided separately as a mineral mix. Commonly used supplements include whole shelled corn (inexpensive source of energy), range cubes (inexpensive source of energy and protein), sweet feed, protein blocks, molasses blocks or tubs, and liquid feed. Stockpiled forage is forage that is grown during the summer or fall upon which animals are not allowed to graze, reserving it for the winter months. In drier areas, the forage is well preserved, but in a more humid climate quality declines rapidly, making the practice less satisfactory. Stockpiled forage is a very inexpensive forage source since it does not have to be mechanically harvested (baling forage doubles the cost of forage). Animals harvest stockpiled forage by grazing, which also decreases cost. Animals make much more efficient use of stockpiled forage when strip grazed (using temporary electric fence to limit animal access to an area containing a 1 to 3 day supply of forage) to minimize trampling. Fescue is used in many temperate regions for stockpiling and retains its quality well into late winter even in humid areas. Most recommendations for stockpiling fescue include late summer fertilization, clipping, and deferred grazing. Warm season grasses such as native range and Bermuda grass can be stockpiled. The amount of deterioration is dependent on grass species and rain.

Feeding Does in Late Gestation

Energy requirements increase dramatically in late pregnancy. Doelings require more supplementation than mature does, as the doelings are still growing. Feed intake may be reduced in the last 4 to 6 weeks of gestation by the growing kids that reduce available abdominal space. Pregnancy toxemia is a metabolic disease usually caused by animals being too fat (body condition score greater than 4) prior to kidding, although very thin animals (body condition score less than 2) are subject to the disease also. It is caused by a high demand for nutrients by the growing fetus in late pregnancy that is not being met (excess fat in the body and the growing fetus limit room in the stomach for food, reducing intake of the diet). This unmet nutrient demand causes a rapid breakdown of fat reserves, forming ketone bodies at high levels which are toxic. Treatments include administration of propylene glycol, large doses of B vitamins, glucose given intravenously, and possibly C-section. Prevention of the disease is far easier and more effective than treatment. Simply monitor animal body condition and adjust nutrition, especially energy, to manipulate body condition. Do NOT sharply reduce feed in late gestation as this may cause pregnancy toxemia. Also, pregnant goats in the last third of pregnancy will need a more nutrient dense diet (higher quality) due to fetal growth and reduced intake because of reduced stomach capacity. Exercise will help. Does can be encouraged to exercise by separating hay, feed and water at a substantial distance, forcing them to walk more.

Feeding the Lactating Doe

The lactating doe has very high nutrient requirements. During lactation, the doe can consume nearly enough nutrients if an abundant supply of high quality pasture is available, such as in spring or early summer. However, does will likely lose some bodyweight due to the high demands of peak lactation (weeks 3 to 8 of lactation) and an inability to consume an adequate quantity of feed. Kidding should take place when there is an adequate supply of high quality pasture. If there is not adequate pasture, supplemental feed will be required. Inadequate nutrition will decrease body condition, reduce milk production, reduce kid weaning weight, and increase kid mortality. When feeding high levels of grain, the animal should go through an adjustment period of two to three weeks during which time the grain portion of the diet is gradually increased to prevent digestion and other problems from occurring. Feeding a dairy ration and hay to a doe during late gestation and the lactating period will cost approximately $30 per animal. Utilizing available pasture as a feed source is a much cheaper alternative. Kids are usually weaned at about 12 weeks of age. Milk production of the doe begins to decrease after the 6th week of lactation and is quite low by the 12th week. Nutrient requirements decline as stage of lactation advances, enabling the doe to maintain body condition or even increase it on pasture alone. Kids may be creep fed while nursing to increase growth rate of the kids and reduce nutrient demands on the doe for milk production.

Creep Feeding

Creep feeding is a method of providing feed for the kids only. This is accomplished by fencing around a feeder and using a creep gate that has holes about 5 inch wide by 1 ft high. These holes are small enough so that kids can enter the feeder, but adults are excluded because they are too big to go through the hole. Creep feeding will provide extra growth for the kids and train them to eat feed, facilitating weaning. A commercial creep feed with at least 16% crude protein that is medicated with a coccidiostat should be used. It requires about 6 lbs of feed to produce 1 lb of animal gain. The more rapid growth from creep feeding may be beneficial for producing show prospects. An alternative to grain-based creep feeds that is used in the beef cattle industry is to creep graze calves, using a creep gate that allows calves access to ungrazed high quality pasture. This may have application for goats using high quality pastures (crabgrass or sudangrass that is planted for the kids). In rotational grazing of cattle, the calves are often allowed to creep graze the next pasture before cows so that they have relatively high nutrient intake. Those pastures often have less parasites and disease organisms because of the time since last grazing.

Effect of Kidding Season on Nutrient Requirements

Nutrient requirements of does change dramatically with stage of production. Requirements increase dramatically the last 6 weeks of gestation due to increasing fetal growth and remain high in early lactation. During the month prior to kidding and for the following 3 months (assuming weaning at 12 weeks of age), the doe will consume nearly as much nutrients as in the remaining 8 months of the production cycle. Thus, during that time it makes sense to supply nutrients from an inexpensive source, typically pasture. The cost of providing the same nutrients as hay is more than twice that of pasture, and supplying through purchased feeds may be four to five times greater than for pasture. Kidding should be planned for a time when pasture is rapidly growing. This period corresponds to late spring for pastures comprised of warm season forages such as Bermuda grass or native range, browse, and forbs, but could be either fall or early spring for cool season grasses such as ryegrass, wheat, orchard grass, and fescue. Cool season grasses usually produce less forage per acre than warm season forages, but generally are higher in energy and protein. Rapidly growing pasture is high in protein and energy. A major consideration in determining the date to kid is level of forage production at that time. However, there are other considerations in selecting kidding date, such as parasites and market opportunities. Some markets provide a substantial price premium from kidding at a specific time of the year, such as producing prospect show wethers or registered animals. However, it may take a considerable market premium to cover the cost of purchased feed, so general reliance on pastures and forages is best.

Artificial Raising of Kids

Sometimes it is necessary to bottle feed young kids due to death of the mother or the mother refusing to take them. It may be avoided by crossfostering kids onto another doe. If a bottle-raised kid is with other kids and does, they may learn to 'steal' sufficient milk to raise themselves. Kids can be raised on cow milk replacer, goat milk replacer (expensive) or, if none is available, cow milk from the store may be used. It is very important that kids receive colostrum within 12 hours of birth. After 12 hours, antibodies absorption decreases. Colostrum may be milked from another doe that recently kidded. Colostrum contains antibodies that strengthen the immune system for the first months of life. A kid should be fed one ounce of colostrum per lb of weight (average birthweight 7 lbs, therefore, 7 ounces of colostrum) at each of three feedings in the first 24 hours. If the kid is too weak to nurse, it is appropriate to provide the colostrum via stomach tube. This does take some practice, but obtaining colostrum is critically important to kid survival. Initially kids can be fed using a baby bottle or a nipple such as the Pritchard teat which fits on a plastic soda bottle. Kids can be bottle fed twice a day, although three times a day the first 4 to 6 weeks of life may increase growth rate. Kids are very susceptible to bloating and other gastrointestinal problems from milk replacers that contain a high level of lactose due to use of dried whey in their formulation. Reduced lactose milk replacers will reduce bloating problems. A calf starter feed (with a coccidiostat such as Rumensin or Deccox, sometimes called medicated) and high quality hay should be made available the second week of life. Deccox can be used in the milk from week 2-6 to prevent coccidiosis. After 4 weeks of life, kids can be limit fed milk at one pint in the morning and also in the afternoon. This will stimulate consumption of starter feed and facilitate weaning. Kids can be weaned after 8 weeks of age if they are consuming 2 ounces of starter per day and weigh two and a half times their birth weight (about 18 lbs). Weaning shock can be reduced by going to once daily milk feeding for several days to encourage consumption of the starter.

Note: *Remember that any time you're talking about medicated feed, under new legislation, a Veterinary Feed Directive is required – see the Drug Management chapter to learn more about veterinary feed directives.*

Considerations in Ration Formulation

Rations should be balanced not only for protein and energy, but calcium and phosphorus contents should be calculated, macrominerals supplemented, and a trace mineralized salt used to provide microminerals. A vitamin premix should be used to provide at least vitamin A and E. If the diet is being fed at high levels to bucks or wethers, there is risk of urinary calculi. To prevent urinary calculi, the ration should be formulated with a minimum of phosphorus, over twice as much calcium as phosphorus, and a urine acidifier such as ammonium chloride at 0.5-1.0% of the diet. Salt can also be included in the diet, such as at 1%, to reduce incidence of urinary calculi. If the ration is being fed at high levels, sufficient fiber should be included in the diet to prevent acidosis. Dried brewers yeast and probiotics are often used in rations fed to animals at high levels to help prevent them from going off feed. Feeds may have a coccidiostat included in the formulation to prevent coccidiosis. There are a number of coccidiostats, but Food and Drug Administration approved drugs commonly used include Deccox and Rumensin. Since goats are very susceptible to coccidiosis when stressed, such as at weaning or shipping, many starters and show feeds contain coccidiostats and have the term 'medicated' on the feed tag. Management considerations to reduce coccidiosis incidence include sanitation, cleanliness, and dry housing.

Feeding Systems

There are many methods of feeding goats. Feeds should be offered in such a way to minimize mold growth or fecal contamination that reduces intake. Mineral mixes must remain dry and should be replenished at 2 week intervals to avoid caking. Feed troughs should be designed to facilitate removal of feces and leftover feed. Troughs generally require a bar running above the length of the trough to keep goats from defecating in them. Self feeders can be used for feeds containing sufficient roughage for use as a complete feed or for feed that has a built-in intake limiter. For large range operations, feeds such as whole shelled corn or range pellets or cubes are often fed on the ground. The feeding area is moved each day to have clean ground upon which to feed. Round hay bales should be fed in a rack off the ground. Feeding round hay bales on the ground results in hay wastage and leaves a mess that is difficult to clean. Hay can be fed in a manger or hay feeder with keyhole slots, but horns may cause problems preventing access to feed. For large operations, unrolling round bales on the ground works well.

FEEDING HORSES

Horses are social animals with an established hierarchy. Wild horses are nomadic, following the food, and don't defend a set territory. They are herbivores with a forage-based diet. They are grazers or trickle feeders, designed to eat numerous small meals throughout the day. They tend to feed more heavily at dawn and dusk.

Horse Anatomy

Horses have hypsodont teeth that erupt over the life of the horse. Horses prehend with their tongue and incisors, moving the bolus to the back of the mouth where it is ground by the cheek teeth (premolars and molars). Side-to-side chewing motion maximizes grinding. Differences in tooth wear are noted between forage and concentrate-based diets. Intense mastication by the cheek teeth leads to reduction in particle size and stimulates production of saliva, which is 99% water and serves primarily as a lubricant. There are virtually no digestive enzymes in equine saliva but it does provide buffering of gastric contents. Saliva secretion increases with increased dry matter (DM) intake (i.e. forage requires more chewing than concentrates and is associated with larger volume of saliva). Careful chewers will reduce particle size of ingested feeds to 1-2 mm, which allows for more complete exposure of feeds to enzymatic digestion in the small intestine.

The esophagus is 1.2-1.5 meters (4-5 ft) long from the pharynx to the cardia of the stomach with upper and lower esophageal sphincters. It is lined with stratified squamous epithelium and has no secretory function. The sequence of motility follows – food enters pharynx, upper esophageal sphincter relaxes, peristalsis, distal movement of bolus, lower esophageal sphincter relaxes, bolus enters stomach – total transit time is 4-10 seconds.

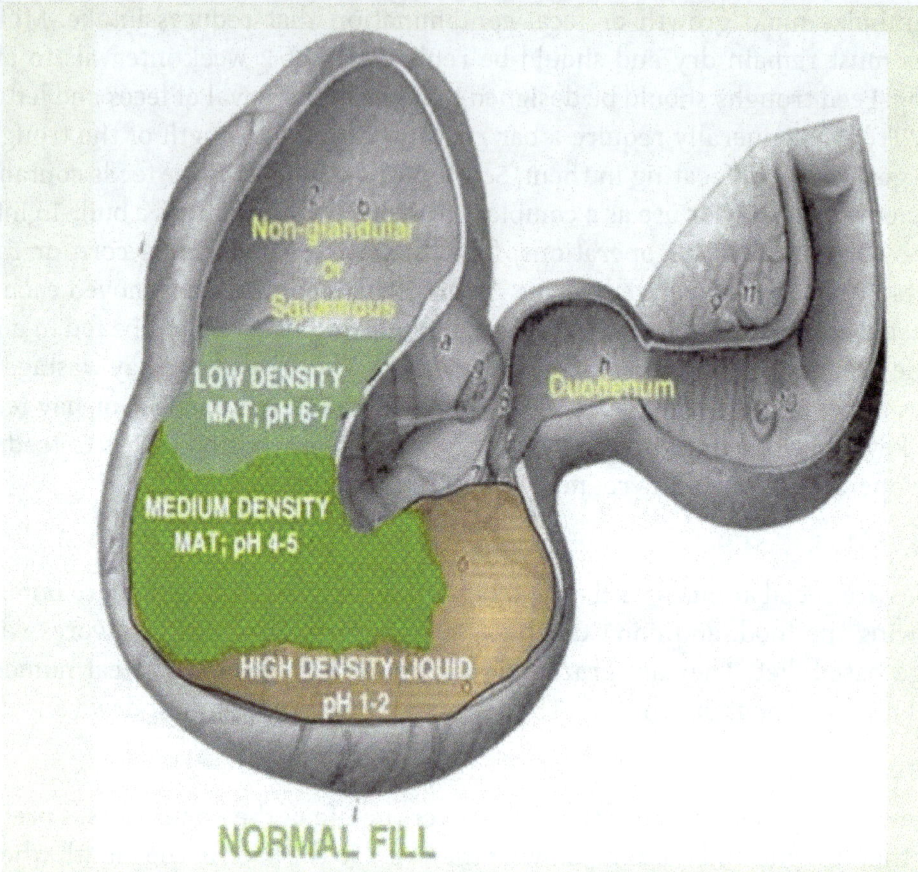

"Horse digestive tract", https://slideplayer.com/slide/6123276/

Stomach volume is 8-15 L (about 8% of the total GI tract). The proximal half is non-glandular, and the distal half is glandular. The fundic mucosa produces HCl (continuous, highly influenced by type of feed), and the pyloric mucosa produces gastrin. The gastric bacterial population contributes to digestion of non-structural carbohydrates – this population is pH dependent and produces lactic acid and VFAs. Gastric emptying time for water is 30-90 minutes, for high-fiber / low-starch diets about 90 minutes, and for low-fiber / high-starch diets 2-4 hours; meal size also affects rate of gastric emptying. Little absorption of nutrients occurs here.

The small intestine is 25 meters (82 ft) long – passage of foodstuffs occurs at a rate of 6-90 cm/min. This is the major site of enzymatic digestion and absorption of nutrients such as glucose, amino acids, fatty acids, fat-soluble vitamins, calcium, phosphorus, magnesium, and water. The small intestine is the only site of calcium absorption in the equine GI tract.

The hindgut is made up of the cecum, large (ascending) colon, small colon, and the rectum. This is the major site of microbial fermentation and fluid absorption – horses are hindgut fermenters. The hindgut processes plant components that do not get broken down in the small intestine. A huge resident microbial population is responsible for digestion of fibrous matter and includes bacteria, fungi, and protozoa. VFAs, fructans (complex sugars), nitrogen, sodium, chloride, and water are absorbed. Simple sugars (glucose, fructose), amino acids, fatty acids, and fat soluble vitamins are not absorbed in the hindgut. The small colon is responsible for desiccation and formation of fecal balls.

Nutrient Requirements of Horses

- **Water** – Requirement is 30-60 ml/kg/day in adults (4-8 gallons or 15-30 L). Requirements fluctuate with ambient temperature, exercise, pregnancy, lactation, etc. Water may be consumed with diet when on pasture (40-60% water). A goal is to maximize water consumption. Horses can be very finicky about temperature of water, bucket, location, etc.
- **Energy** – Horses eat to meet their energy needs. Need is heavily influenced by life stage, body condition, and ambient temperature. The most useful term for practical purposes is digestible energy (DE) = gross energy minus energy lost in feces – Maintenance DE (Mcal/day) = 1.4 + (0.03 x BW in kg) for horses 600 kg or less (1 Mcal = 1000 kcal).
- **Carbohydrates** – The principle source of energy in equine diets and come from forages and grains. Some are hydrolyzed to simple sugars in the small intestine, leading to absorption of glucose into the bloodstream, and some undergo bacterial fermentation in the hindgut. More energy is derived from those broken down in the small intestine than from those metabolized in the hindgut. There are no established maximum or minimum requirements for carbohydrates.
- **Protein** – A source of energy and is the major component of most tissues in the body. It is obtained from feed and is digested and absorbed primarily in the small intestine. Quality of the protein affects its digestibility and therefore the amount that must be fed. Digestion of protein is initiated in the stomach through the actions of HCl and pepsinogen and is completed in the small intestine. Undigested protein is absorbed as nitrogen in the cecum. Essential (also called indispensable) amino acids cannot be synthesized and must be obtained in the diet. Dispensable amino acids can be synthesized. For conditionally indispensable amino acids, pathways exist but at times the body cannot make them in sufficient quantities. The essential amino acids in horses are lysine, methionine, threonine, isoleucine, leucine, valine, phenylalanine, tryptophan, histidine, arginine – Lysine is the first

limiting amino acid in equine diets (first one to be used up and therefore prevent further protein synthesis), followed by threonine and methionine.

- **Lipids** – A source of energy absorbed in the small intestine as fatty acids; fats are highly digestible and are required for absorption of fat-soluble vitamins (A, D, E, K). Essential fatty acids (FAs) must be supplied in the diet and include linoleic (0.5% of DM) and alpha-linoleic acids. Omega FAs – omega 6 = linoleic, gamma-linoleic and arachidonic acids – these are potent inflammatory mediators from soy, corn, sunflower, and safflower oils. Omega 3 = alpha-linoleic, eicosapentaenoic acid (EPA), and docosahexaenoic acid (DHA) – these are less potent inflammatory mediators from flaxseed oil or fish oil. Forage diets (fresh forage and hay) are naturally higher in omega 3 FAs. Cereal grains, soybean meal, rice bran, and vegetable oils are higher in omega 6 FAs. Dietary recommendations for horses are still under investigation. Supplementation is aimed at inflammation and immune function – flaxseed and fish oil often are used. Benefits of fat supplementation are increased energy density for weight gain and replacing carbohydrates as sources of calories. Palatability is the major factor in how much fat you can supplement. Fats must be added gradually to the diet. Oxidation also is an issue. Vitamin E supplementation is suggested when adding fat to the diet.

- **Vitamins and Minerals** – Vitamin requirements are set based on daily DM intake. For fat-soluble vitamins, toxicities are rare and deficiencies are more common. There are high concentrations in fresh forage. In dried forage (hay), vitamin A, D, and E levels decrease rapidly. Supplementation is recommended for horses not on pasture. Water-soluble ("natural") vitamin E is more bioavailable than are synthetic forms. Water-soluble vitamins are thiamin and riboflavin. Macrominerals that are required in the diet include calcium, phosphorus, sodium, chloride, magnesium, and potassium. Calcium absorption is estimated at 50% and is variable depending on the source. Vitamin D plays a smaller role in Ca:P homeostasis in horses than in other species. Phosphorus absorption varies widely, averaging 33%. Ca:P ratio more important than absolute numbers; ideal is a ratio of 1.5:1 to 2:1. High calcium can negatively impact phosphorus absorption and vice versa. Microminerals that are required in the diet include copper, zinc, iron, selenium, manganese, cobalt, and iodine. Dietary toxicity can be seen if microminerals are fed in excess. Selenium should be a maximum of 0.5 mg/kg DM intake. Selenium deficient soils exist in different parts of the United States, so having an understanding of local growing conditions (and/or a hay analysis) is key to making good decisions about supplementation. The maximum tolerable concentration is 2 mg/kg DM; selenium toxicity is a clinical concern.

Types of Horse Feed

Forage

The stems, leaves and stalks of plants – pasture = fresh forage, hay = dried forage. Horses should consume at least 70% of their diets (ideally 80-100%) in forage. No forage is 100% complete so some vitamins/mineral supplementation will be required. Minimum requirement = 1% of BW in forage daily (ideally 1.5-2%). Type of forage available varies with region and time of year. Cool season grasses = orchard grass, Kentucky bluegrass, timothy, ryegrass, bromegrass, tall fescue. Warm season grasses = Bermuda grass, teff. Legumes = alfalfa and clover.

Concentrates

Cereal grains such as corn, oats, barley, wheat, rye, and millet. These are highly digestible with a high concentration of soluble carbohydrates. They are usually processed by cracking, grinding, steaming, and flaking. Many have an inverted Ca:P ratio. Grain should be limited to less than 30% of the overall diet. Concentrates can be used to supplement calories, vitamins, and minerals lacking in forage.

Supplemental Feeds

These may be added to forage. These may be pelleted, and may be cereal grains, and supplemental protein or vitamins/minerals, for example Purina Ultium. Ration balancers are very concentrated sources of vitamins and minerals designed to be fed with either grass forage or alfalfa forage, for example Nutrena Empower Grass Balancer. Complete feeds are designed to be fed as the sole source of nutrition in the absence of forage. These are forage-based and often are pelleted and softened by the addition of water, for example, Purina Equine Senior.

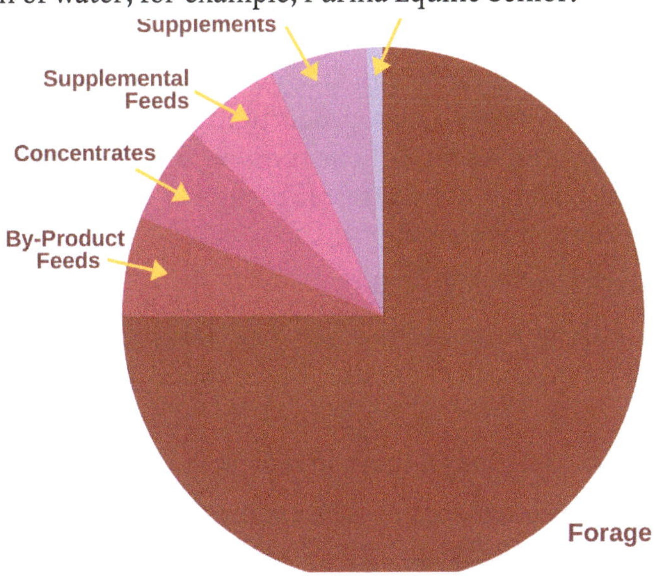

By-Product Feeds

These are as in other species and include beet pulp, wheat bran, and rice bran.

Macronutrient Supplements

Protein may be added to improve quality of forage and to aid in building muscle, hair and hooves. Owners can use as a protein supplement, a complete feed, or alfalfa (forage or pellets). Don't use human supplements; equine-specific supplements often are soy or whey-based. Other examples are soybean meal, fish meal, meat and bone meal, cottonseed, and linseed. Fats may be plant or animal based. Examples are rice bran, fish oils, and flax. Fat supplements have variable palatability and digestibility. Essential fatty acids vary between oils – omega 3 flax>soy> canola>sunflower> corn. Flax oil has an omega 3:omega 6 ratio of 4.2. Corn oil has an omega 3:omega 6 ratio of 0.2. Feed supplemental vitamin E when feeding > ½ c oil/day (1000-2000 IU vitamin E/cup of oil). Limit flax to ½ cup oil or 1 pound of flaxseed per day.

Salt and Trace Minerals

Salt should be provided free choice. Salt blocks may contain iodine. Loose salt may be added to the bucket to encourage water consumption (1-3 tsp BID). Trace mineral blocks are okay if only one horse has access but it is hard to guarantee adequate consumption. Trace mineral blocks are not necessary if the diet is complete. Many vitamin and mineral mixes are available and again are not necessary if the diet is complete.

Ideal Feeding Practices

Feed horses like horses – Horses are designed to eat for up to 18 hours per day. Their cycle is eat – drink – sleep – repeat. Horses selectively graze areas where they have not defecated and remove the tops of plants that are actively growing. Continuous grazing maximizes saliva production, and decreases risk of gastric ulcers, colic, and vices. Horses on 24 hour turn-out will consume about 2 to 2.5% of their body weight /day in dry matter. If pasture is limited, they will actually consume more per hour. It is ideal to:

- Monitor the horse's body weight
    - When estimating, consistency is key. Have the same person do the measurements each time, use consistent landmarks, and take digital photos.
- Monitor the horse's Body Condition Scoring (BCS)
    - Monitor as in other species. A BCS of 5 on 9-point scale is ideal. Evaluate the horse from all angles and do a hands-on evaluation as well. Key areas to evaluate are the neck, shoulder, barrel (ribs), and tailhead. A

horse with BCS less than 4 needs more calories and a horse with BCS greater than 6 needs fewer calories.

Humans may mess up horses' body weight and condition by:

- Limiting access to feed – Horses will eat 2-3% of their body weight daily. Forage must be available. 80-100% of their diet should be forage. Horses should go no more than 2-3 hours without forage intake. Forage can be fresh or dried.
- Overfeeding – Not all horses will self-regulate, especially when turnout is restricted. Compensating for decreased turnout with free choice hay may work but must be monitored.
- Overfeeding concentrates, supplements, treats – Cereal grains are very high in non-structural carbohydrates, are not tolerated by all horses, and are not needed by all horses, leading to disease (obesity, equine metabolic syndrome, and laminitis).
- Underfeeding supplemental feeds – Feeding a concentrate at less than label recommendations can lead to nutrient deficiencies. If forage is fed solely in the form of hay, vitamins A and E will need to be supplemented.

Consequences of poor feeding practices include obesity, poor performance, starvation, insulin resistance, colic, gastric ulcers, and laminitis.

EXTRA RESOURCES

Monitoring the horse's body weight: https://www.youtube.com/watch?v=IVVQcTgynDc

Monitoring the horse's body condition scoring (BCS): https://ker.com/wp-content/uploads/body-condition-score-chart.pdf

Goat nutrition: https://pressbooks.umn.edu/app/uploads/sites/7/2019/08/Goat-nutrition-for-health.pdf

CHAPTER-W12

NUTRITION: CARNIVORES AND OMNIVORES

Swine and dogs are omnivores. Cats are true carnivores.

FEEDING SWINE

Pig Terminology Used In This Chapter

Boar	Intact male pig
Barrow	Castrated male pig
Gilt	Young female pig not having produced her first litter
Sow	Older female pig having produced at least one litter
Pig	Younger swine (less than about 120 lbs)
Hog	Older swine (more than 120 lbs)
Weaner	Young pig (18-60 days of age)
Early-Weaned Pig	Pig weaned at less than 21 days of age
Litter	Multiple pigs born from same pregnancy
Gestation	115 days of pregnancy
Lactation	18-25 days after birth where sows nurse baby pigs
Grow-Finish	Production phase from 60-260 lbs body weight
Wean-to-Finish	Production phase from 10-260 lbs body weight
Nursery	Production phase from weaning to 60 lbs body weight
Feeder Pigs	40-60 lb pigs sold for feeding to market weight
Market Hogs	Hogs weighing 240-280 lbs, ready for slaughter

Production Phases of the Breeding Herd

Male Reproduction – Boar

Female Reproduction – Gilt development / pre-breeding to breeding to gestation to farrowing / lactation to weaning to rebreeding to gestation, etc.

Growing Pigs to Market – Nursing pigs (nursing off the sow, eating creep feed) with three phases (phase I 12-15 lb body weight, II 15-25, III 25-50) to grow-finish in four phases (phase I 5-100, II 10-150, III 150-200, IV 200-250) to market

Pork Production Measures for Growing Pigs

ADFI	Average daily feed intake
ADG	Average daily gain = average amount of weight gained daily
F/G or G/F	Feed conversion = feed efficiency
% carcass lean	Ratio of lean:fat
Lbs lean gain/day	Lbs of lean body weight gained daily
Lean gain efficiency	Lbs feed per lbs lean body weight gained

Pork Production Measures for Breeding Herd

NPD = non-productive sow days	Time that sows are not pregnant or lactating – goal is fewer than 50 NPD/female/year
Litter size	Number of piglets in the litter
Litter weaning weights	Weights of piglets at weaning – this is a reflection of milking ability of the sow
Wean-estrus interval	Days from weaning to re-breeding – goal is 4-7 days
Farrowing rate	Percentage of females mated that farrow – goal is 85+%
Litters / sow / year	Goal is greater than 2.2

PHASE FEEDING

Pigs are commonly phase fed. This is a system of separating pigs by weight and feeding specific diets to those groups of pigs. The value of this is demonstrated in the graph below. The curved line shows daily lysine requirement. The stepped lines show either a 6-phase feeding program or a 2-phase feeding program. Note how pigs in these groups (or phases) are occasionally underfed and occasionally overfed as they grow. The goal of phase feeding is to minimize the amount of over- and underfeeding. There is increasing economic advantage in increasing number of phases (and therefore, number of group of pigs and number of diets provided) in pig production.

Phase Feeding Swine

"Swine nutrient recommendations and feeding management", http://porkgateway.org/resource/growing-finishing-swine-nutrient-recommendations-and-feeding-management/

Feed Budgets

It is essential to get the right feed to the right pig for the right amount of time. An example is shown below, demonstrating how amount of food provided varies with phase (grower phases I-III and finisher I-III) and with body weight of those pigs.

Feed Budgets by Phase

PHASE	G1	G2	G3	F1	F2	F3
BW (LBS)	60-80	80-110	110-140	140-180	180-220	220-250
AMT OF FEED (LBS)	46	76	84	123	137	193

Split-Sex Feeding

Sometimes specific diets must be provided by sex. As an example, gilts have higher amino acid requirements and have a 5% greater lean growth potential than barrows. Gilts consume less than barrows so different diets must be provided for gilts and barrows when they reach about 80 lbs body weight. Another example is the change in diet required of sows as they go through their reproductive cycle. Assessment of body condition score (see image below) allows one to watch how sow weight varies and to feed to try to keep as consistent a body weight as possible. Generally, the sow is heavy until the time of farrowing and lactation, when she loses a lot of weight from giving birth and from milk production. It is difficult for sows to eat enough during lactation to gain weight and it is wise to keep a record of how much they eat (average daily feed intake) to plan for future pregnancies. Sows regain body condition after they wean piglets and generally are at a higher weight at the time of the next pregnancy, and then the cycle starts again.

Swine Body Condition Score Assessment

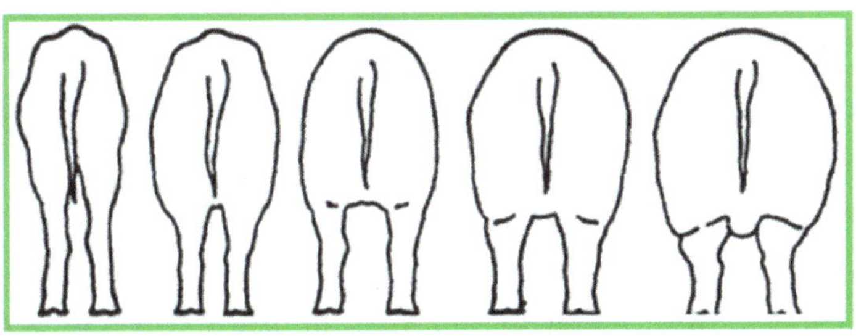

SCORE	LAST RIB BACK FAT DEPTH	CONDITION	BODY SHAPE
1	<15	Emaciated	Hips, spine prominent to the eye
2	15-18	Thin	Hips, spine easily felt without pressure
3	18-20	Ideal	Hips, spine felt only with firm pressure
4	20-23	Fat	Hips, spine cannot be felt
5	>23	Overweight	Hips, spine heavily covered

—"Swine nutrition guide",https://prairieswine.com/rsc/swine-nutrition-guide-2/

Nutrition Goals

Nutrition goals in commercial pork production include the following: Maximizing net profit / pig space by minimizing cost of inputs (feed is 65% of the total cost of production; providing good nutrition to improve productivity, which reduces facility and labor costs/cwt* pork produced); supporting and maintaining high health; minimizing nutrient excretion and odor emissions; and ensuring pre-harvest food safety. * = *hundredweight*

Factors affecting feed cost/cwt pork produced are:

- Factors altering cost/ton of complete feed (cost of feed manufacturing and quality control, cost of service for commercial products, cost of feed delivery, profit margin of manufacturer)
- Factors affecting the rate of gain of body weight per lb of feed (diet digestibility, diet nutrient levels relative to requirements, feed wastage). Attention to proper nutrition and proper feeding of a correct diet supports pig health and economics for the producer.

Understanding Nutrient Requirements

Animals require amounts of nutrients per day, not % of nutrients in the diet. A key concept is that feed intake times nutrient concentration equals the amount of nutrient consumed per day. For example, let's say a lactating sow is consuming 4.5 kg (which is 4500 gm) of feed per day and that the feed she is consuming contains 1.0% lysine. Her daily lysine requirement is 50 gm lysine/day. Is this diet adequate to meet her needs? Using the calculation above, feed intake (4500 gm/day) times nutrient concentration (0.01) yields a total consumption per day of 4.5 gm. This is deficient. This could be corrected by giving her more to eat of her current diet or by offering a diet that is higher in lysine.

Nutrient requirements vary with production phase due to genetics, gender, health, and housing conditions.

- Energy – Generally provided as starch (carbohydrates) and fat.
- Amino Acids – The ten essential amino acids (required in the diet) are lysine (first limiting), methionine (2nd limiting), threonine (3rd limiting), tryptophan (4th limiting), histidine, arginine, leucine, isoleucine, valine, and phenylalanine. "Limiting" refers to the composition in feed ingredients – lysine is the first amino acid to be inadequate in a corn-based diet, because there is limited lysine in corn.
- Macrominerals – Those supplemented are calcium, phosphorus, sodium, and chloride. Trace minerals supplemented are iron, copper, zinc, iodine, manganese, and selenium. Vitamins supplemented are the fat-soluble

vitamins (A, D, E, K) and some water-soluble vitamins (riboflavin, niacin, pantothenic acid, choline, folic acid, biotin, B12).

- Water – Attention must be paid to water quality, quantity, and availability – Water is used for metabolism and to regulate body temperature, and it is a constituent of body tissues.

Feed Ingredients = Nutrient Sources

Most swine diets in the United States are comprised of corn (primary energy source), soybean meal (primary amino acid source), monocalcium phosphate (primary P source), limestone (primary Ca source), and a vitamin and trace mineral premix. Depending on cost and availability, other ingredients are partial substitutes for corn and soybean meal. Corn substitutes are barley, wheat, sorghum, and dried distillers grains with solubles (a mix of corn, rice and other grains that is a byproduct of distilling for brewing or creation of ethanol). Soybean meal substitutes are meat and bone meal, dried distillers grains with solubles, and synthetic amino acids. Nursery diets include lactose, dried whey, spray dried porcine plasma, fish meal, spray dried blood meal, and supranutritional levels of copper and zinc.

Feed Manufacturing

Grain is ground using a roller mill or hammermill – reduced particle size = increased nutrient digestibility. Average particle size should be 700-800 microns. Ingredients are mixed to ensure uniform dispersion in a complete feed. Most diets are fed in meal form. Nursery diets are fed in pellet or crumble form – these are complex diets with multiple ingredients.

Life-Cycle Feeding for Swine

Pigs are provided ad libitum access to feed (all they can eat, feed available continuously) in all phases except pre-breeding, breeding, and gestation. Sows are fed limited amounts (4-8 lbs/day) to control body weight gain and body condition.

Typical Ranges in Daily Feed Consumption Levels for Swine

STAGE	AMOUNT (LBS/DAY)
Pre-Breeding	4-8
Breeding	4-6
Gestation	4-6
Lactation	8-20
Weaning-Rebreeding	4-8
Nursery Phase I (12-15 lbs BW)	0 – 0.5
Nursery Phase II (15-25 lbs BW)	0.5-1.5
Nursery Phase III (25-50 lbs BW)	1.5-2.5

Grow-Finish Phase I (50-100 lbs BW)	2.5-3.5
Grow-Finish Phase II (100-150 lbs BW)	3.5-4.5
Grow-Finish Phase III (150-200 lbs BW)	4.5-5.5
Grow-Finish Phase IV (200-250 lbs BW)	5.5-.65

Feeder Design and Feeder Management

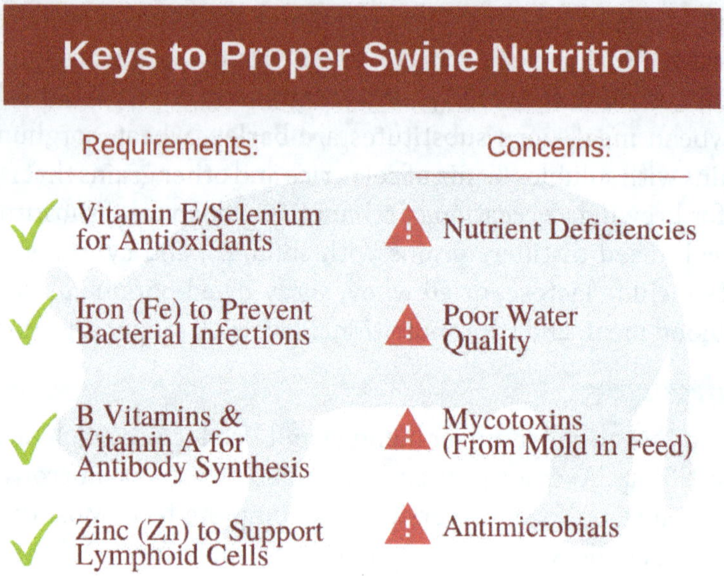

Feeder space and design is important to minimize chances of pigs fouling the feed with feces and to minimize feed wastage. Feed wastage can be as high as 20% due to inadequate design and/or management. In a study of grow-finish pigs, 5% feed wastage increased feed cost / pig by more than $2 and 20% wastage increased it by more than $8.

Nutrition and Health Conditions

Proper nutrition supports the immune system (Vit E / selenium are anti-oxidants, Vit A – antibody synthesis, Fe (too high or too low) – increased susceptibility to bacterial infections, Zn – role in lymphoid cells, B vitamins – deficiency reduces antibody synthesis). Concerns include nutrient deficiencies and toxicities – water quality – mycotoxins (toxins due to molds in feed = aflatoxin, doexynivalenol [DON], zearalenone, fumonisin), and antimicrobials (antibiotics, growth promoting levels of Cu and Zn).

DOGS

Feeding and Hunting

Dogs must be fed by life stage. Dietary goals include good quality of life, maximum longevity, optimization of performance, and disease prevention. For example, obesity is the number 1 nutritional disease in dogs and cats and is present in 12-40% of animals. It is associated with health risks (musculoskeletal disease, cardiovascular disease, cancer, diabetes mellitus, reduced immunocompetence), and with decreased life span. Other conditions associated with nutrition in dogs are dental disease and urolithiasis.

Wild dogs live in hierarchical groups. They hunt in packs and the dominant dog(s) eat first. They consume large meals (up to 16% of their body weight in a single meal). Dogs retain the "social value" of food. Their behavior is influenced by breeding, selection, and interaction with humans.

Nutrients

A nutrient is any food constituent that helps support life. Essential (also called indispensable) nutrients are those that the body cannot synthesize and that are needed at all life stages. Conditionally essential (conditionally indispensable) nutrients are those that are required only during certain physiologic or pathologic conditions. Nonessential (dispensable) nutrients are those that can be synthesized by the body.

Canine Feeding Behavior

Dogs are omnivores. They eat 1-3 meals/day and feed during daylight. They are glutton feeders (built to eat large volumes of food infrequently) and recognize the social value of food (food is a resource to guard).

Free Choice Feeding = ad libitum or ad lib

- Advantages: less labor and knowledge required, better share for non-dominant dogs
- Disadvantages: increased risk for obesity, skeletal disease, less knowledge about intake by each animal, for dry/semi-moist foods only

Food Restricted or Meal Feeding

- Advantages: best control and knowledge of intake, best control of body weight, reduced risk of obesity and skeletal disease, facilitates house training
- Disadvantages: labor-intensive, need to calculate food

Determination of food dosage is the basis for nutritional management and is a basic skill in nutritional therapy. We must calculate food dosage recognizing that dogs may be fed a complete and balanced diet, supplements, and treats.

Energy Requirements

Resting energy requirement (RER) is the energy used by an adult at rest in a thermoneutral environment. This level does not support activity, growth, or reproduction and is a function of metabolic body size. RER (kcal/day) = 70(BW in kg)$^{0.75}$ or 30(BW in kg)+70 – use latter if body weight is between 2 and 46 kg. Canine maintenance energy requirement (MER) = 1-1.8 x RER and varies by intact status and life stage. These are averages; needs for specific individuals may be considerably higher or lower.

Canine Maintenance Energy Requirement

TYPE OF DOG	MER (value x RER)
Intact adult	1.8
Neutered healthy adult	1.6
Adult prone to obesity	1.4
Geriatric animal	1.4
Adult needing to lose weight	1.0 (note that this would be RER at ideal weight)

Daily energy requirement (DER) is affected by breed, neuter status, age, activity, environment and so may be higher than MER – for example, daily energy requirement for dogs doing light work equals 2 x RER, for those doing moderate work equals 3 x RER, and for those doing heavy work equals 4-8 x RER. Animals that are late in pregnancy and are lactating have increased nutrient requirements. Animals that have been spayed or castrated have decreased energy requirements.

Food Dosage Determination

Calorie content is not required on pet food labels so to determine number of calories per cup, you may need to check the website or call the pet food company.

- Estimate RER as described as above
- Factor RER if necessary to get estimated maintenance energy requirement (MER) or daily energy requirement (DER)
- Select specific food, determine energy density
- Energy requirement divided by energy density = food dosage

Because individual animal needs vary, body condition scoring is important to determine if the amount of food calculated is ideal for a given animal. New ideal

BCS = 4-5 on a 9-point scale – see chart below. This was defined by the Purina lifespan study – 48 Labrador retriever puppies were paired by weight and sex, with one member of the pair fed 25% less than the other. Dietary restriction resulted in lower prevalence and severity of osteoarthritis. The age when 50% of dogs were first treated for chronic conditions was 2.1 years later in restricted-fed dogs and the restricted-fed dogs had a 15% longer median lifespan and were considerably healthier than their free-fed littermates.

As an example of food dosage calculation and nutritional assessment, Ms. Gray owns a 5-year-old spayed female Beagle. The dog weighs 26 pounds and has a body condition score of 5/9. You collect a diet history and find that Ms. Gray is feeding 1.5 cups of food/day of a food that has 350 kcal/cup. No other food or treats are given. She wants to know if this is enough food. – First, calculate RER. Body weight is 26 pounds (11.8 kg). RER = 30(BW in kg)+70 = (30)(11.8)+70 = 424 kcal/day. She is a neutered healthy adult so her MER = 1.6 x RER = 678 kcal/day. She currently is eating 525 kcal/day (1.5 cups x 350 kcal/cup). Her body condition score is fine so this appears to be a good amount of food for her for right now. The owner should watch body condition and if the dog appears to be getting thin, she certainly could be getting more food, up to about 2 cups per day (678 / 350 = 1.9).

DOGS - BODY CONDITION SCORING

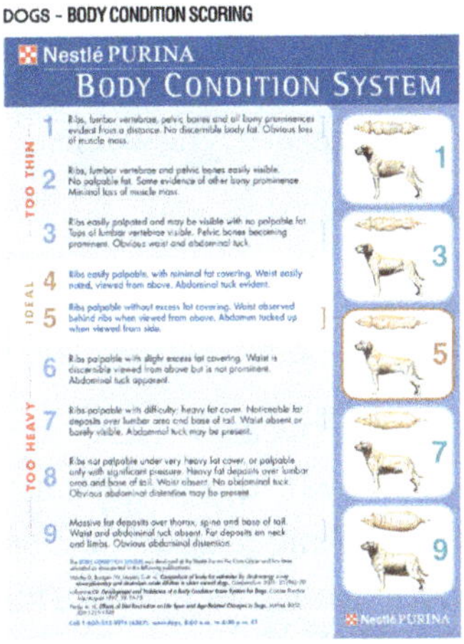

https://www.morrisanimalfoundation.org/sites/default/files/filesync/Purina-Body-Condition-System.pdf

Specific Versus All-Purpose Diets

Specific purpose diets are produced to feed dogs for specific life stages or specific activities. Examples include diets for growth, lactation, adults at maintenance, athletes / performance, and geriatric animals. Breed-specific diets exist. Veterinarians can prescribe diets to specifically treat disease, for example, highly digestible diets for intestinal disorders and diets with unique proteins for dogs that are allergic to common pet food ingredients.

Feeding Specific Types of Dogs

Gestation and Lactation

For the first 6 weeks of gestation, MER = 1.8 x RER and for the last 3 weeks of gestation, MER = 3 x RER. During lactation (the equivalent of heavy work), MER = 4-8 x RER with ad lib feeding. During lactation, carbohydrate is conditionally essential so the recommended diet has 20% of calories as carbohydrate. In the latter part of pregnancy, the bitch needs an increase in calories. She either can be fed more of her regular food or can be fed a growth or performance food.

Nursing Pups

Puppies that are nursing should gain 2-4 g/kg adult weight/day. Offer solid food (growth / lactation diet) at 3-4 weeks of age and wean off the dam at 6-7 weeks. Feed growing pups to have a slim figure (ideal BCS of 4-5) to promote normal hip development. Overconsumption of food after weaning (excess energy and calcium) is associated with development skeletal diseases such as hip dysplasia, osteochondrosis, panosteitis, angular limb defects, and other bone and cartilage dysplasias. Genetics and environmental factors also increase risk. Feeding recommendation for growth at < 4 months of age = 3 x RER, from 4-12 months of age = 2 x RER, and at greater than 12 months of age = 1.6 x RER. Feed the right diet (protein 25-35% DMB, calcium 0.9-1.5% DMB, energy 3.4-4.2 ME/g/DMB – feed the diet right – calculate starting point – evaluate every 2 weeks – adjust to maintain lean body condition.

TRENDS IN CANINE NUTRITION

Home-Prepared Diets

Owners may wish to prepare diets at home because they equate nutrition with nurturing their pets, they want control over quality of ingredients (natural, preservative-free, color-free, organic), or to meet specific health goals for their pet. In 2020, survey data from over 3600 pet owners in the United States, Canada, Australia, New Zealand, and the United Kingdom described about 2/3 of dogs and 1/2 of cats receiving some homemade food at least some of the time, with more than half of dogs and at least half of cats sometimes getting raw diets.

Raw Diets

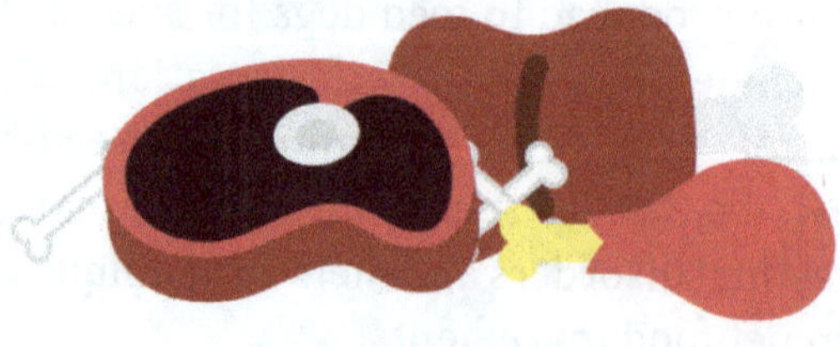

Three common names in the raw diet conversation for dogs are Billinghurst BARF, Schultz, and Volhard. All claim that no extra knowledge is required by owners to feed this diet. They all are based on raw meat, bones, and some vegetables and are intended not to be complete and balanced but to achieve nutritional balance over time. An increasing number of commercial raw preparations are available. Some are formulated to meet AAFCO nutrient profiles and may be complete and balanced in each meal. They are usually very highly digestible, with high quality ingredients, high water content that helps with satiety and weight control, and provide a sense of nurturing. However, there is no scientific evidence that raw diets provide superior nutrition, they may have nutritional excesses or deficits, vitamin A and D have the potential to be excessive if offal is used as an ingredient, and calcium is a nutrient of concern especially in growing large breed puppies. Other concerns include the possibility of bones in the diet fracturing teeth and perforating intestines. Nutritional problems take years to manifest into clinical disease and people who choose to create a raw food diet or any homemade diet are encouraged to work with a veterinary nutritionist. Raw diets also pose safety concerns for the very young and very old (animals and humans) due to concerns about bacterial and parasitic contamination; studies suggest that 3-50% of adult dogs fed raw food diets may be asymptomatic shedders of Salmonella into the environment. In one study of dog owners feeding raw food diets, confirmed transmission of Salmonella from the pets to the people was 0.2%, with very young, very old, pregnant, and immunosuppressed people at greatest risk. Finally, it is valuable to help clients understand that some things they provide for their pets are uncooked and pose a risk of bacterial spread. This includes rawhides and pig ears provided as treats.

Grain-free diets

Grain-free diets contain a high proportion of peas, lentils, other legumes, and other ingredients including potatoes. The rationale is that dogs would not eat a significant amount of grain in the wild. In 2018, the FDA warned pet owners of a possible link between eating foods labeled as grain-free and development of a heart condition called dilated cardiomyopathy. Cause-and-effect of this association has not been defined.

CATS

Feeding and Hunting Behavior

Cats are obligate carnivores. Their molars are vertically oriented and they have almost no lateral jaw motion. Their molars are not intended for grinding, as in omnivores and herbivores. They lack salivary amylase, and have a simple stomach and short intestinal tract.

Five traits of a cat are nocturnal (crepuscular), predators, territorial, solitary, and maternal.

Cats are exceptional hunters. In cats, hunting behavior is independent from feeding behavior, and they are solitary hunters and eaters, with no concept of the social value of food. Cats are constantly attuned to hunting, with hearing very acute when hunting at night and vision (motion) very acute when hunting during the day. Cats prefer to eat 10-20 small meals/day and in the wild, would spend 6-8 hours daily stalking prey. The average rat carcass provides about 5.7 kcal/gm of energy. How much cats eat is dependent on how much energy they get from it, not on the bulk of food eaten. Cats have specific preferences for temperature, odor, and physical form of food. Wild cats maintain body weight and fitness. House cats lose the ability to regulate energy intake due to readily available food and lack of physical activity. Best tips for cat owners are to feed smaller, more frequent meals throughout the day; provide food puzzles or other feeders that foster hunting behavior, feed individual cats separately in multi-cat households, and feed from an elevated location that is away from noise and visual threats.

Food Selection

Food selection is highly variable in dogs and cats and is based on senses (odor, temperature, mouth feel) and on past experience. Neophobia (disliking new things) is important in veterinary patients, who may choose not to try a new food. Milk composition is affected by maternal diet so pups and kittens may develop preferences at a very early age. Aversion to new foods is greater in cats than in dogs.

Nutrition and Energy Requirements

- Water – the most important nutrient. Age affects thirst, total body water, and water balance (intake versus loss). Domestic cat breeds are descendants of wild desert cats and so will concentrate urine significantly before they drink more water. They are not driven by thirst. In the wild they will get some water from their prey (1.5 – 2 mL / gm of prey eaten).
- Energy – In general, their daily energy requirement (DER) = 1.2 x RER
- Protein – Cats are missing some key enzymes and other enzymes are not adaptive (that is, they do not upregulate or downregulate relative to the presence of substrate). This contributes to their high protein requirement. For example, they require arginine to synthesize ornithine and citruline in the gastrointestinal tract as part of the urea cycle. A single meal devoid of arginine will lead to excess ammonia in the blood stream (hyperammonemia). Another example is taurine. Taurine is present in most animal tissues and can be synthesized from cysteine and methionine.

Cats lack the enzymes necessary to consistently synthesize taurine and lose it through the gastrointestinal tract as it binds bile acids. In general, cats require protein as %19 of the diet – food animal tissue should be listed within the first two ingredients on a dry food and within the first three ingredients for a canned food.

Feeding adult cats – Atkins-type diet for cats = high protein and fat, low carbohydrate – The natural feline diet is %7 carbohydrate (DMB) so this kind of diet is well suited for cats.

- Lipids – Consume up to about %65 of the diet without negative effects. Cats require linoleic acid (like dogs) but also require arachidonic acid.
- Low Carbohydrates – Cats lack sucrose taste buds, their small intestine has low sucrase and lactase activity, they have non-adaptive sugar transporters that do not upregulate with a high carbohydrate diet, they lack salivary amylase, and their pancreatic amylase concentration is only %5 that of dogs. Carbohydrates can be up to %30 of the diet.
- Vitamins and Minerals– Cats have some unique vitamin requirements – Key vitamins required in high amounts or preformed are vitamins A and D, and niacin. Vitamin K may be required in the diet during long-term antibiotic therapy. Mineral requirements are similar to that in dogs. Calcium and phosphorus deficiency is the most common deficiency reported, especially in those cats who are on all meat diets. The sodium requirement in cats is three times that in dogs.

FEEDING SPECIFIC TYPES OF CATS

Gestation and Early Lactation

Queens have an increased requirement for energy, protein, fat, calcium and phosphorus, soluble carbohydrates, taurine and copper. Unlike in bitches, who need a change in diet to one with increased energy at mid-gestation, queens should gain weight gradually throughout pregnancy and so should be changed to a growth / lactation diet as soon as it is known that they are pregnant. At the end of lactation, when kittens are weaning, the queen should have a gradual reduction in energy provided as follows: the day prior = little / no food, weaning day ¼ DER, next day ½ DER, next day ¾ DER, 3rd day full DER.

Kittens

See chart below as a reference. Kittens should gain 50-100 g/wk. Feed a growth/ lactation diet beginning at 3 weeks of age, wean kittens at 8-10 weeks of age, and then free choice or meal feed three times daily.

Key Nutritional Factors in Finding the Ideal Kitten Diet

Energy	4.0-5.0 Kcal/g
Protein	35-50% DM
Fat	18-35% DM
Carbohydrate	10% DM
Crude Fiber	<5% DM
Calcium	0.8-1.6% DM
Ca:P ratio	(1.1-1.5):1
Potassium	0.6-1.2% DM
Magnesium	0.08-0.15% DM

Neutered Adult Cats

Cats that have been spayed or castrated have decreased RER associated with a 25% reduction in DER, increased food intake, and decreased insulin sensitivity. Because cats naturally eat many small meals, it can be difficult to decrease calories and maintain body condition without exercising cats. Options for ways to increase exercise in cats can be found through the Indoor Pet Initiative and Purrfect Fence.

Current Trends

Raw Diets

Concerns are as in the dog. Feeding "human grade" tuna is a concern because that tuna is high in polyunsaturated fatty acids and is associated with vitamin E deficiency, steatitis (fatty inflammation), vitamin K antagonism, loss of B vitamins when the fish is cooked, excess in minerals (for example magnesium), and possible fixation on specific foods.

Vegetarian Diets

In cats, feeding of vegetarian diets is associated with inadequate protein / amino acids (taurine, arginine) and arachidonic acid, and alterations in other nutrients (vitamin A, B12, niacin, calcium, iron, zinc, copper).

Homemade Diets

Feeding of homemade diets may be associated with problems especially if they contain all meat or very high protein, deficient calcium, excess phosphorus, excesses of vitamins A and D toxic to the liver, and deficient microminerals. Thiamin may be deficient in raw fish diets. Homemade diets can be made safely and be complete and balanced but involve cost and effort. Consultation with a veterinary nutritionist is recommended.

CATS - BODY CONDITION SCORING

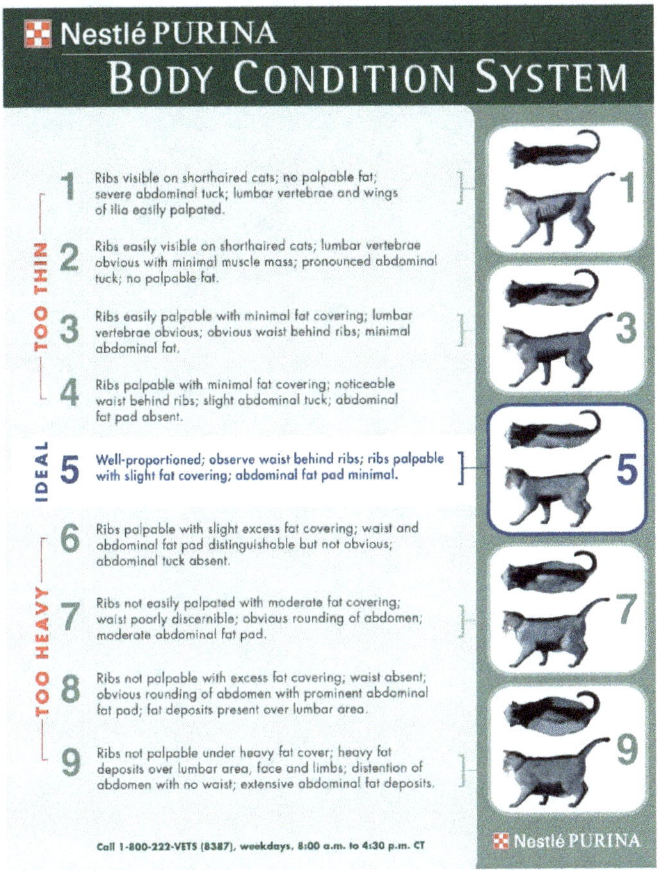

https://www.in.gov/boah/files/Cat-BCS-from-Purina.pdf

CHAPTER-13

BIOSECURITY: AN OVERVIEW

BIOEXCLUSION AND BIOCONTAINMENT

Biosecurity is split out by some into bioexclusion, also called external biosecurity (preventing disease from entering a facility) and biocontainment, also called internal biosecurity (managing a disease once it is on the premises). Biosecurity in general is a concern for populations of animals and the facilities where they are housed. If the disease of concern is a zoonotic disease, precautions to protect those who work in those facilities or otherwise interact with those animals also are in order.

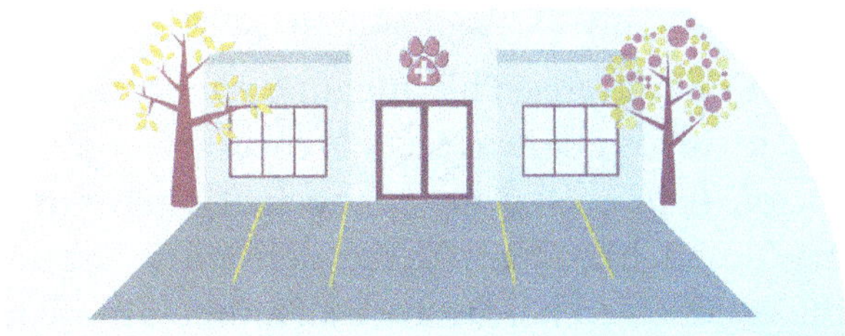

Bioexclusion
(keeping disease out in the first place)

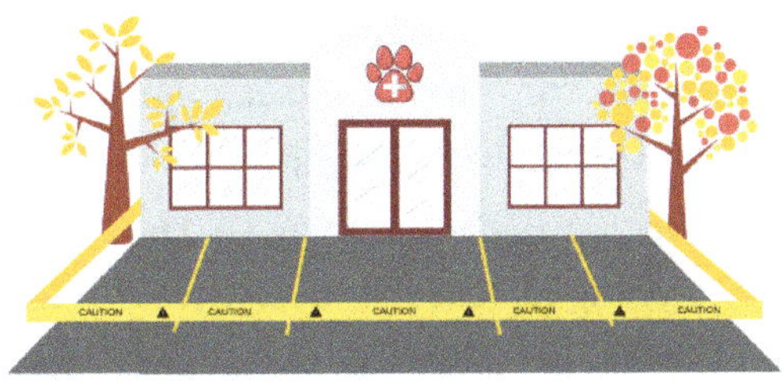

The concepts of biosecurity are presented here to help you see the continuum of infection control in veterinary medicine. We often concentrate on infection control in the hospital (wearing gloves or other personal protective equipment, using foot baths in the large animal hospital to prevent spread of disease by traffic through the facility, properly using isolation facilities). For many veterinarians, that is the full scope of their responsibility in addressing biosecurity. For others, including everyone who works with groups of animals, whether that be a herd of cattle or a group of cats in a rescue facility, knowledge of principles of biosecurity can prevent disease from being introduced or spreading in a facility and is a cornerstone of preventive care for those animals.

Concepts of biosecurity are of concern for any disease-causing organism. Some organisms and diseases rise to a higher level of concern and oversight. These reportable diseases are those that we are required by law to report to the state Board of Animal Health so appropriate biosecurity measures may be enforced to prevent widespread disease with subsequent economic consequences and the potential for loss of human and animal life. The list of reportable diseases in Minnesota, the timing of reporting, and the type of testing to be performed are updated constantly.

FOOD ANIMAL FACILITIES

Much of the information in this section is from the following website: http://www.omafra.gov.on.ca/english/livestock/vet/facts/04-003.htm

Biosecurity at the farm level can be defined as the management practices enabling producers to prevent the movement of disease-causing agents onto and off of agricultural operations. This includes environmental contamination. Biosecurity therefore involves many aspects of farm management, such as disease control and prevention (e.g. closed herd, vaccinations), nutrient management, and visitor control. Closed herds are those defined as having no new animal introduction into the established herd; either all animals move as a cohort, leaving the facilities empty for a while (all in-all out), and/or all replacement animals are born on the farm (a process called internal multiplication). Keeping the herd closed is extremely difficult for a producer, so most choose to introduce new animals into the herd after they undergo testing and quarantine before introduction. Although controlling and limiting the movement of livestock is recognized as the most important biosecurity measure for most diseases, many important hazards can be carried on contaminated clothing, boots, equipment, and vehicles.

Biosecurity has become a major concern to the agriculture industry as a result of foreign and emerging disease issues, the globalization of agriculture, and increasing public concerns over food safety. Individual farms are less isolated and inputs are entering the farms of today from further away, often from other countries. Issues such as bovine spongiform encephalopathy, foot and mouth disease, avian influenza, and Newcastle disease have brought world concerns closer to the local farm level.

Practices do not have to be cumbersome, confusing or expensive, but a small investment in time and money can yield big benefits for the farmer, the industry, and for the consumer through improved food quality and safety.

Disease Spread Risks

What are the chances of introducing disease? The single biggest risk factor in disease is purely mathematical in that the higher number of animals in any facility or on any one site, the greater the chances of disease spread. Other risk factors include:

- Direct contact between animals on the farm and newly purchased animals
- Mechanical spread by animal transporters
- Mechanical spread on contaminated farm equipment, boots, clothing, and contractors cables and tools
- Movement of birds, mice, rats, flies, dogs, cats, and wildlife
- Airborne spread in aerosols or dust / dirt, affected by the herd location, wind, animal density, and neighbors
- Contamination of feed, water, and bedding
- Contamination of the environment on farm – moving animals from diseased pen or hospital leads to dirty passages and yards
- Biting insects

Mechanical Transmission

Infection present in feces, saliva, nasal secretions, blood, milk, or semen may be mechanically transmitted between animals on a variety of inanimate objects (fomites). The body fluid is not the fomite. If you sneeze on your cell phone, the cell phone is the fomite. The time that these fomites remain infectious depends on the resistance of the organism, the temperature, amount of sunlight, dryness, and level of disinfection.

Guidelines for Buying Breeding Stock and Minimizing Risks

If you have any doubts about the health of breeding stock, don't buy those animals! Health is worth far more than genetics. Producers should work with veterinarians to make sure the veterinarian completes all necessary health assessments and testing. The buyer should only work with sellers who are completely open about the health status of the animals. Isolate incoming animals for at least 3-4 weeks and if possible limit the number of intakes of live animals. Guidelines for buying breeding stock include:

- Know the disease status of both the recipient and source herds.

- Consider the location of both herds and the surrounding disease risks.
- Recognize the limitations of recipient herd biosecurity.
- Select an appropriate single source for replacements.
- Check and test disease status including history and past and present customers.

Biosecurity Checklist

Facility Guidelines

- [x] Vehicle parking must be off-site and easily cleaned and disinfected
- [x] Farm boundary must be clearly defined with a wildlife-proof perimeter fence
- [x] Feed bins should be sited on perimeter with own blow pipes
- [x] Good facilities for slurry collection and disposal

Animal Housing & Purchase Guidelines

- [x] Long loading race to outside perimeter of animal unit
  - Should go through the perimeter and have assembly yards at each end
  - Outer yard should be washable and drain away
  - Truck drivers should remain on the ramp and farmer should remain in the yard
- [x] On-site isolation facilities for purchased animals
- [x] Animal housing and buildings should be inaccessible to dogs, cats, and vermin
- [x] Completely separate off-site bay for carcass collection

Facility Worker & Visitor Guidelines

- [x] Farm facilities workers must have access to:
  - Changing / showering facilities with separate clean and dirty areas
  - Hand washing stations
  - Regularly cleaned toilets
  - Dedicated farm equipment
  - Protective clothing, boots and vehicles
- [x] All visitors need to understand the possible risk they present when entering a farm, what a farmer expects from them, and what precautions need to be taken between farms
- [x] Foot baths should be strategically placed, well maintained, and regularly disinfected
  - Boots and foot baths are the biggest biosecurity weak point
  - Must be clean and an effective disinfectant used that is regularly replaced

Guidelines for Isolation Units

No matter how reliable the health status of the herd of origin is, it is important that incoming animals undergo a period of isolation for at least 3-4 weeks. The biosecurity of the quarantine unit ideally should be better than that of the home unit, and the isolation unit should preferably be on another site, managed by different staff or at least with dedicated boots, clothing, and equipment used. There should be no slurry or drainage crossovers and an all in-all out policy should be in place with thorough cleaning and disinfection between batches. Regular clinical and veterinary inspections / tests should be carried out with all diseases and deaths being investigated.

Checklist of Physical Biosecurity Measures

- Strategically placed, well maintained disinfectant footbaths
- Off-site vehicle parking, easily cleaned and disinfected
- Defined farm boundary and wildlife-proof perimeter fence
- Changing / showering facilities with separate clean and dirty areas
- Hand washing and regularly cleaned toilets
- Dedicated farm equipment, for example, protective clothing, boots and vehicles
- Long loading ramp to outside perimeter of animal unit
- Completely separate off-site bay for carcass collection
- On-site isolation facilities for purchased animals
- Feed bins sited on perimeter with own blow pipes
- Bird and vermin proof buildings
- Good facilities for slurry collection and disposal

Livestock Loading and Unloading

Animal loading areas are always a weakness. The ramp is often not long enough, or far enough away from the buildings. It should go through the perimeter and have an assembly yard at each end with the outer yard washable and draining away from the unit. Truck drivers should not come into the unit, they should remain on the ramp and likewise, the farmer should not go onto the truck.

Disinfection and Disinfectants

Disinfection is targeted at reducing disease spread from contaminated boots, buildings, yards, equipment and vehicles. Disinfection will not work without proper cleaning and removal of all organic matter. It is vital to dry and rest buildings before final disinfection and equally vital that all surfaces are saturated. The drying and resting of buildings for 3-4 days before final disinfection improves efficacy to over 99%. The sequence for cleaning a building looks like this – (1) soak all surfaces with water – (2) powerwash to remove the bulk of the organic matter – (3) use detergent to break down what's left – (4) powerwash again – (5) let the building dry – (6) apply disinfectant.

In any operation, boots and foot baths are the biggest weaknesses! Clean boots are vital and every farm should have them for staff and visitors alike. Remind everyone to be biosecurity conscious and to reduce transmission between buildings, hospital pens, and birthing pens. Foot baths must be clean and an effective disinfectant used that is regularly replaced. Remember that the boots must also be cleaned of organic matter; use of footbaths alone will not disinfect boots adequately. The ideal disinfectant has the following characteristics:

- Proven broad spectrum activity and efficacy
- Fast acting to rapidly kill very infectious agents
- Active in the presence of organic matter
- Stable after dilution, especially in footbaths
- Safe for environment, animals and people
- Non-corrosive and suitable for a range of surfaces, for example, porous and other applications
- Easy to store, move and dispose of
- Cost effective – do not judge by smell

Truck Wash and Disinfection

As mentioned earlier, trucks can and do bring infection onto a farm. They are often washed at the factory or rendering plant and contaminated equipment, hoses, and boots are put onto the truck. Wheels and wheel arches are a big risk. Ideally an off-site washing stand is required at the truck driver's home base.

Vermin Control

Animal housing should be inaccessible to dogs, cats, and vermin. Control of birds and insects is vital to prevent spread of disease.

Biosecurity for Workers and Visitors

Staff training and their vigilant attitude is the best defense. How often do they have explained to them the importance of changing clothes and boots and doing the biosecurity disciplines? Do you have standard operating procedures (SOPs), which are agreed ways of doing each task? Simply written, these should improve staff members' understanding of why certain procedures are in place.

All visitors need to understand the possible risk they present when entering a farm, what a farmer expects from them, and what precautions need to be taken between farms that are visited. This applies to anyone entering or leaving the premises who may be visiting other livestock operations, and not just those of the same species or commodity type. The list includes:

- neighbors and friends;
- agribusiness and service representatives;
- veterinarians;
- municipal/regulatory personnel, inspectors;
- dead stock collectors / renderers;
- custom manure/biosolids haulers and applicators.

Visitors can unknowingly bring harmful agents onto a farm via contaminated clothing and footwear, equipment, or vehicles. Equipment used to repair buildings and machinery, to treat or handle animals, and to carry out testing or procedures are all potential sources of contamination. The risk is increased with visitors who regularly go from farm to farm as part of their employment or routine. Such individuals, businesses, and organizations are encouraged to develop and follow a biosecurity plan. All visitors, farm owners, and their employees have a shared responsibility in biosecurity. Visitors need to be aware of that farm's level of biosecurity and need to follow their recommendations. Visitors must be prepared to accept all reasonable directives from the farmer when visiting his or her operation. In many swine operations, for example, showering in and out of facilities is a requirement.

Farmers and their employees also have a responsibility to prevent hazards from leaving the premises. Wear clean clothing and footwear when leaving the farm, particularly if visiting other farms, feed supply agencies, veterinary facilities, or auction markets.

All visitors should make an appointment so that both parties can make best use of their time. The visitor should ask the farm operator about his or her biosecurity protocol and any special measures that must be taken.

Assessing Visitor Risk and Controlling Access

Risk assessment is a method of determining the likelihood and severity of the risk posed by a visitor. By identifying key risk factors, appropriate procedures and protocols can be determined.

Guidelines for Visitor Risk Assessment

	LOW RISK	MODERATE RISK	HIGH RISK
Number of farm visits per day	No other farm contact	One or occasionally more than one farm per day	Routinely visits many farms or auctions
Protective Clothing	Wears sanitized shoes or boots. One pair of clean coveralls per site	Wears sanitized shoes or boots – If clean, may not change coveralls	Does not wear clean or protective clothing
Animal Ownership	Does not own and/or care for livestock	Owns and/or cares for a different species	Owns and/or cares for a similar species and production type
Contact with animals	No animal contact	Minimal or no direct contact – exposure to housing facilities	Regular direct contact with animals
Biosecurity knowledge	Understands and promotes biosecurity for industry	Aware of basic biosecurity principles but is not an advocate	Little appreciation or understanding of biosecurity principles
Foreign travel	Does not travel out of the country	Limited travel outside of the country without animal contact	Travel to foreign countries with animal contact in those countries

- Biosecurity Guidelines for Visitor Control
- Provide a farm gate sign indicating biosecurity levels in effect on the farm. Place restricted entry notices on the doors to animal facilities.
- Keep service vehicles as far away from the animal facilities as is feasible. Designate a parking area for vehicles entering the farm, away from traffic areas used by farm vehicles and away from feed and manure. Visitors' vehicles should be visibly clean of manure and organic matter.
- Establish one area of the farm for visitors to enter if required. All visitors should go directly to the entry point. Consider installing a bell or alarm system for visitors to indicate their arrival.
- Keep a visitor log or record of the names, dates, and vehicles that visit.
- Determine if, when and what types of farms have been visited prior to your farm. As a precaution, 48 hours may be required between visits (1 week for foreign visitors).

- Restrict access to animal facilities to essential visitors only. Keep visitors out of animal pens and feed alleys, and do not allow direct contact with animals if not essential.
- Insist on clean clothing and/or supply clean boots and clothing at your farm.
- Do not allow foods of animal origin to be brought onto the premises.
- Provide a container or plastic bag for collecting dirty clothing or disposable items used by visitors.
- Ask visitors to wash their hands prior to leaving the premises, especially if in contact with animals. If hosting tours, provide hand washing facilities or disinfectant hand gel. If food is to be served, do this away from the animal facilities and after hand washing.
- Provide a footbath and a container of an appropriate disinfectant solution with a scrub brush at the entrance to each facility. Maintain these with daily cleaning, remove accumulated organic matter, and replenish disinfectant regularly. Footbaths alone are not an effective means of disinfecting footwear.
- Ensure all equipment used by visitors has been thoroughly cleaned and disinfected and stored appropriately before being used on your premises. Also clean and disinfect all borrowed equipment and tools prior to use on your farm and before returning them.

Proper use of disinfectants is a critical component of biosecurity. Use all disinfectants according to product recommendations.

Some facilities use ultraviolet (UV) germicidal chambers to decrease number of pathogens on objects that could introduce disease into farms. Recent work by Dr. Torremorrel and Summer Scholar Katelyn Rieland from the University of Minnesota College of Veterinary Medicine has verified that use of these products reduces risk of introducing pathogens but does not guarantee it. Guidelines that should be followed when using products such as these include frequently cleaning the chambers and replacing the UV bulbs, and rotating objects for optimal exposure to UV light.

Manure and its Concerns

Many important diseases can be transmitted by manure, either directly or indirectly, via contaminated clothing and equipment. The pathogens responsible can be classified into four major types:

- bacterial (e.g., *Salmonella*, *E. coli*, Johne's disease, tuberculosis);

- viral (e.g., hog cholera, foot and mouth disease, bovine viral diarrhea);
- protozoal (e.g., coccidiosis, cryptosporidiosis);
- parasitic (e.g., ascariasis, sarcocystosis).

Fungal diseases, such as aspergillosis, are less likely to be shed in manure, but may be present in contaminated bedding and litter. As production costs increase, more producers are contracting professional manure handlers and haulers. However, there is a risk of disease being introduced by hiring custom labor. Improper sanitation procedures between farms can potentially spread a number of diseases. Ensure manure management equipment is properly maintained and cleaned, especially if being used at several farm sites. Wash all exterior surfaces of manure handling equipment; check that they are visibly free of organic matter before arriving on a farm.

Summary for Food Animal Facilities

Biosecurity is an essential component of many on-farm food safety programs and provides:

- greater consumer acceptability of the quality and safety of the food supply;
- healthy animals that are more productive;
- improved animal welfare and well-being;
- improved efficiency and profitability for the farmer.

Whether it is the relatively controlled environment of a poultry production facility, or the more open pasture of a beef or dairy operation, biosecurity is critical. Over the past decade, food safety, public health and animal health have gained greater importance throughout the world. Quality assurance and HACCP (Hazard Analysis Critical Control Points) programs originate at the primary production level – the farm – with biosecurity planning a key role for the entire food production chain.

Because hazards and risks vary among species and types of operations, what works for one farm may not be appropriate or effective for another. Each farm needs to develop a specific, documented biosecurity plan in consultation with their veterinarian. Visitor control as presented in this information is just one component of the complete biosecurity plan.

The fundamentals of developing a biosecurity plan are:

- Identify possible risk factors.
- Identify critical control points for your operation.
- Set limits or standards for your farm.

- Set up a monitoring schedule and procedures.
- Keep effective records.

COMPANION ANIMAL FACILITIES

Horses

General principles of biosecurity apply although facilities that house horses often are less stringent than facilities that house food animals unless a disease outbreak has occurred. This is a good thing for us to watch for when we visit equine facilities as we can help them improve biosecurity and prevent disease outbreaks. Attention should be paid to likelihood of new animals introducing disease into an established group of horses. Some vaccinations also are more likely to be recommended for horses that have greater exposure to groups of horses, for example at shows or sales barns. In any horse facility that has animals that are not healthy, it is wise to always care for the healthy animals first, including young animals, and then care for those that are ill, so there is less risk of the person who provides daily care transmitting disease through fomites. Foot baths are a good measure to try to minimize disease movement within and between buildings.

Most medical facilities for horses will have a dedicated area for isolation of horses with potentially contagious disease. This is not true at all locations that board or otherwise house horses and it is valuable to help owners recognize when there is a serious risk to biosecurity. General guidelines for immediate admission of horses to an isolation unit as they enter a medical facility include:

- Any 2 of the following 3 signs – diarrhea, fever, neutropenia (low white blood cell number)
- A primary complaint of diarrhea that is not obviously physiologic
- A positive diagnosis of a known contagious / zoonotic disease
- Fever greater than 102°F accompanied by any 2 of the following signs – cough, nasal discharge, lymphopenia (low number of lymphocytes)
- Clinical signs suspicious of equine herpesvirus 1 (neurologic signs)

Clients should be made well aware of the list above, so they know to contact their veterinarian immediately if any of these signs occur, both for the sake of the affected animals and for other animals in the facility.

Dogs and Cats

As with equine facilities, often facilities that house large numbers of dogs and cats do not have stringent biosecurity protocols unless a disease outbreak occurs. Boarding kennels usually require some sort of verification of health of animals before they are allowed to enter but these often are superficial and not based in science. For example, most boarding facilities require that dogs and cats be vaccinated for specific diseases before entry, but will permit those vaccinations to have been given the day before, such that animals are brought to the facility well before any immune response could have been generated.

Most biosecurity protocols that are published for animals are for humane societies and small animal clinics, where there is great likelihood of mixing of healthy and diseased animal populations. Policies to minimize introduction and spread of disease in these facilities, as generated by the American Animal Hospital Association, include:

- Having separate entrances for animals with possible infectious disease and having signs to direct people to those entrances appropriately
- Requiring staff to wear appropriate personal protective equipment
- Posting and following very specific cleaning and disinfecting measures
- Using specific examination rooms or housing areas for animals with infectious disease, perhaps even disease-specific (a set of runs only used for dogs with suspected parvovirus, for example)
- Having dedicated staff for infectious disease patients who do not interact with healthy animals in the facility
- Training all staff and faculty in biosecurity protocols
- Developing a surveillance program to ensure that breaks in protocols are identified and that disease outbreaks are caught early

CHAPTER-14

CHICKENS IN THE BACKYARD, CAGED BIRDS, FISH, REPTILES, AND AMPHIBIANS

Information in this and the next two sections (Mammals I and Mammals II / Marsupials) is not inclusive of all disease conditions or common concerns in these species and instead will focus on relevant aspects of housing, vaccination / diseases, parasite control, behavior, dentistry, biosecurity, and nutrition. The information about poultry is about backyard chicken flocks and not all of this information is appropriate for large-scale poultry production operations.

BACKYARD POULTRY

Unique Anatomy – External

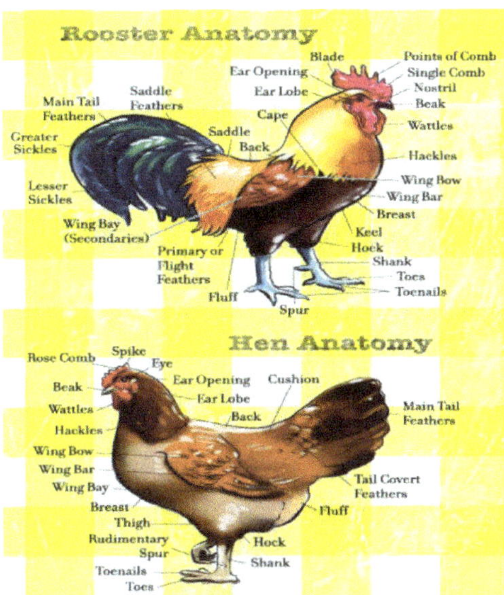

"Rooster and hen external anatomy", https://mrandmrscoletti.wordpress.com/category/uncategorized/

Unique Anatomy – Internal

The respiratory tract of birds is dissimilar to that of mammals in that they have no diaphragm. Air is pulled in and forced out by movement of the rib cage and keel. Chickens have a trachea that bifurcates into two lungs. The syrinx (voice box) is located at the bifurcation. From the lungs, air moves into large air sacs.

The gastrointestinal tract begins at the beak. The tongue has barbs that help direct food into the esophagus. Birds do not swallow; movement of the tongue forces food into the upper esophagus. The crop lies midway along the esophagus. It is a place where food can be stored and moistened; no digestion takes place in the crop. The crop serves the same purpose in prey birds as rumination does in cattle, in that it permits the bird to ingest a large amount quickly and then to digest it later, in a safer location. From the lower esophagus, food moves through the proventriculus (glandular stomach) into the ventriculus or gizzard (muscular stomach) where it is physically broken down. Food then moves into the small intestine where enzymatic digestion takes place and nutrients are absorbed. Paired ceca lie at the junction of the small and large intestines. Not all ingesta pass into the ceca, which primarily function to break down dietary fiber. The short large intestine is attached to the cloaca, which is a common chamber for the gastrointestinal, excretory, and reproductive tracts.

The excretory tract consists of paired, trilobed kidneys that lie posterior to the lungs and bilateral ureters that empty directly into the cloaca. There is no urinary bladder. Metabolic wastes (urates) are deposited onto the feces before being expelled.

The reproductive tract in chickens is unilateral. The left ovary and oviduct are functional and the right ovary and oviduct regress. The left oviduct is made up of the infundibulum, which catches the yolk as it released from the ovary; the magnum, which secretes albumen; the isthmus, which secretes the inner shell membranes; the shell gland, which secretes the calcium carbonate shell; and the vagina, which secretes the outer cuticle of the shell and any pigments, and directs the egg for laying (oviposition). Birds begin laying eggs at about 6 months of age and lay until about 3 years of age. It takes 23-26 hours for an egg to form and be layed. Chickens will lay a clutch of 3-8 eggs and then take a day or so off before beginning laying of another clutch. Roosters need not be present for hens to lay eggs.

Housing

Local ordinances determine whether or not people can keep chickens, especially in urban areas, and may place restrictions on gender of birds (no roosters, for example) or total number of birds. It is the client's responsibility to investigate and follow these ordinances.

Most backyard chicken flocks are small. Single chickens are lonely and if you have only two chickens, they are likely to fight. For that reason, a minimum of three chickens works well for most people.

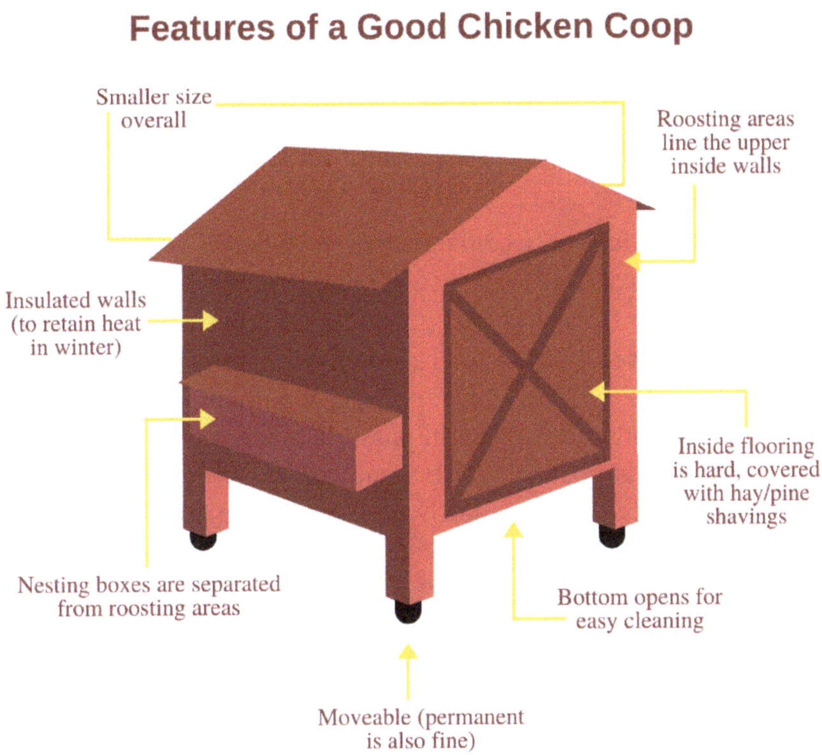

You do not want the coop to be too palatial; a smaller, insulated space will retain heat better in the winter. You should provide about 2-5 square feet per bird in the coop and 8-10 square feet per bird for outside enclosures. Chickens should be provided with indoor housing where they can nest and roost. The chicken coop should contain nesting boxes that are separate from roosting areas and are not directly below roosting areas, so they do not become soiled with droppings. You should have at least one nest box for every 3-4 birds. Birds will roost at the highest point available to them. Coops can be permanent, on a concrete or wood base, or can be movable and placed on grass or pasture. Hard flooring should be covered with clean, dry straw or pine shavings. Protection from predators includes protection from owls and hawks; a covered, fenced area is recommended for birds given access to the outside. The coop should be well ventilated to permit enough air flow to decrease moisture and thereby minimize odor of ammonia from droppings. Keeping bedding clean and dry also will help control insects. Keeping feed securely stored, ideally in closed containers, will help control rodents.

Chickens are sensitive to daylength. Chickens require about 12-14 hours of light daily to continue laying; with decreasing daylength, they layer fewer eggs and eventually molt, which will stop egg laying temporarily. Nest boxes should be checked for eggs 1-2 times daily.

Droppings must be regularly cleaned out of the coop. Disposal or management of waste is dependent on local ordinances. Uncomposted chicken droppings cannot be used directly as fertilizer as the high nitrogen content will burn plants.

Fresh water must be available at all times and in winter, care must be taken that water does not freeze.

Clients who keep chickens in cold environments may wish to insulate the coop; a student from the class of 2019 informed me that chickens in Minnesota can freeze off their combs if it gets too cold in the coop. Combs and wattles are needed by the birds to help regulate their body temperature. A student from the class of 2022 tells me that freezing can be minimized by applying petroleum jelly to the wattles and comb but be aware that freezing is still possible if the temperature is well below freezing and the coop is not insulated. Some owners provide heat lamps. Use of electricity in a coop may be controlled by local municipalities.

Vaccinations and Disease Control

Many diseases in chickens can be controlled by vaccination of breeding hens to produce disease-free chicks or by vaccination of chicks themselves. It is always best to get chicks from a breeder or hatchery that is part of the National Poultry Improvement Plan. Any drug therapy must be evaluated for its use in laying hens as it may affect use of eggs layed by treated hens or ability of the owner to use those hens for meat. Indiscriminate use of antibiotics will not consistently prevent or control disease in flocks.

Overall, to prevent disease in backyard poultry, the following steps should be taken:

- Purchase birds from breeders or hatcheries that follow the National Poultry Improvement Plan.
- Thoroughly clean the coop to remove organic materials before disinfecting; cleaning and disinfection of the coop and tools (feeding scoops, rakes, etc.) should be performed daily.
- Restrict human traffic in and out of the area where the birds roam.
- Protect the chickens from exposure to wild birds including waterfowl.
- Properly dispose of dead birds (follow local ordinances).

Diseases Of Concern Include

- Infectious bronchitis
- Newcastle disease
- Laryngotracheitis
- Fowl pox
- Infectious coryza
- Mycoplasma
- Fowl cholera
- Marek's disease
- Avian influenza

Infectious Bronchitis

This is probably the most common respiratory disease of chickens. It is caused by a coronavirus with variable antigenicity; new serotypes arise regularly. Signs and severity of disease vary with the specific coronavirus, age of the bird, and presence of any secondary infections. The virus is highly contagious and spreads readily between birds by direct contact, aerosol spread, or via fomites (inanimate objects). Spread of the disease through a flock is worsened by poor ventilation and overstocking of birds. Clinical signs include depression, loss of appetite, coughing, gasping, and diarrhea. This disease is best controlled by vaccination.

Newcastle Disease

This is a highly contagious disease caused by paramyxovirus-1. This is a high morbidity disease with depression, loss of appetite, respiratory signs, twisted neck (stargazing), and leg paralysis. The disease is transmitted between and within species of birds, via aerosols, and by fomites including visitors to the facility. This disease is best controlled by vaccination.

Laryngotracheitis

Infectious laryngotracheitis is caused by a herpesvirus with variable pathogenicity. Spread between birds is slow but the disease can be spread between farms by fomites or aerosol spread. Signs include gasping, coughing up of mucous and blood, and ocular and nasal discharge. The hallmark clinical sign for this disease is "pump handle respiration", which is where the bird is trying to breathe in such a way that its head goes up and down, looking like an old well pump handle. Control is through vaccination if the disease is enzootic (regularly present in a population) or epizootic (a sudden widespread outbreak) in an area. Sick birds that recover and vaccinated birds should be housed separately from susceptible birds. Infectious laryngotracheitis is a reportable disease in Minnesota.

Fowl Pox

Fowl pox is a pox virus that manifests as skin lesions and pharyngeal plaques. Fowl pox can have both dry and wet forms. Respiratory signs are evident only with the wet form. The wet form of this disease can present very similarly to infectious laryngotracheitis. Spread through a flock is slow. Transmission is through skin abrasions or by the aerosol route; birds, mosquitoes, and fomites may transmit the virus. The disease is more common in male chickens because of their greater tendency to fight and suffer skin wounds, and in areas where there are biting insects. Birds will be sick for about 2 weeks and there is no effective treatment. This disease is best controlled by vaccination.

Infectious Coryza

This is a chronic, highly infectious disease of chickens caused by *Avibacterium* (formerly *Haemophilus*) *paragallinarum*. This disorder is more common in the southern United States and in California than in the upper Midwest. There is rapid transmission through direct contact between birds in a given flock. Signs include swelling of the face and wattles, purulent ocular and nasal discharge, sneezing, and dyspnea. Various antibiotics may be used for treatment but the disease is best controlled by stocking birds only from known disease-free breeders or hatcheries. Vaccinations may be used in areas of high incidence.

Mycoplasma

Chronic respiratory disease due to Mycoplasma gallisepticum or Mycoplasma synoviae may be seen in chickens. The organism can be spread through aerosols, airborne dust or feathers, or by direct contact. Recovered birds remain infected for life and may express disease when stressed. Birds show respiratory signs as described above and also may show arthritis. Treatment with some antibiotics is possible; secondary disease conditions must be addressed and the environment cleaned. The disease is best controlled by stocking birds only from known disease-free breeders or hatcheries.

Fowl Cholera

Pasteurella multocida is the bacterial cause of this highly contagious, high mortality disease in chickens. Transmission is through direct contact with nasal exudate or feces of infected birds, or via fomites including contaminated soil, equipment, and workers. Clinical signs include loss of appetite, ruffled feathers, coughing, ocular and nasal discharge, swollen face and wattles, arthritis, and diarrhea. Risk of disease is worsened if concurrent infections are present or if birds are overstocked. Treatment with antibiotics is possible but disease may redevelop after medication is stopped. The disease is best controlled by vaccination.

Marek's Disease

Marek's disease is caused by a herpesvirus that has several manifestations. Neurological disease may be evidenced as paralysis of the legs and wings. The visceral form is evidenced as growth of tumors in the cardiac and skeletal muscle, lungs, and reproductive tissues. The cutaneous form is evidenced as tumors in the feather follicles. Peripheral nerve enlargement and "Marek's eye" also may be seen. Mortality in affected chickens is 100%. The route of infection is through the respiratory tract and transmission may occur through exposure to affected feather dander or via fomites. There is no treatment. The disease is best controlled through vaccination of chicks. A combination of vaccines commonly is used to ensure broad immunity is induced. Genetic resistance exists and breeders may select for stock with increased frequency of the gene that confers this protection. Again, chicks should be purchased through breeders or hatcheries that provide vaccinated birds.

Avian influenza

Avian influenza is caused by an influenza type A virus and can infect domestic and wild poultry and waterfowl. Low pathogenicity avian influenza is commonly carried by migratory waterfowl. It can infect domestic poultry but rarely causes illness. Highly pathogenic avian influenza (HPAI) is extremely infectious, spreading rapidly between flocks, and causes serious illness or death. Clinical signs of chickens infected with HPAI include depression; difficulty breathing; swelling or purple discoloration of the head, comb, and wattle; decreased egg production; and sudden death. Avian influenza is a reportable disease in Minnesota. Owners of backyard flocks are recommended to protect their flock from HPAI by avoiding attracting wild birds, especially waterfowl by enclosing feed and reducing standing water, limiting movement of chickens to and from the property (for example, to attend shows or sales), and limiting visitors to the property that interact with the birds. Good information is available from the University of Minnesota Extension Service and the USDA.

External Parasite Control

External parasites found in birds include:

- Biting lice
- Feather and leg mites
- Red mites and northern fowl mites

Biting Lice

Lice are spread by direct contact between birds and from infested litter. Life cycle of the parasites is about 3 weeks. Rapidly moving insects will be visible at the base of the feathers on the abdomen or around the vent. Clumps of eggs (nits) may also be visible at the base of the feathers. Various powders and sprays are approved for application on birds including malathion and pyrethroids. Treatment may need to be repeated as not all life stages of the parasite are killed by these drugs. Prevention involves inhibiting exposure of chickens to wild birds and regular removal of infested litter.

Feather and Leg Mites

These parasites cause chickens to pull out feathers and cause thickening of the scales on the legs. Mites are visible on scrapings but not with the naked eye. Conditions may be treated by dipping the affected part in a parasiticide or by applying mineral or vegetable oil. Prevention involves inhibiting exposure of chickens to wild birds. In small flocks with ongoing problems, culling of affected birds might be considered.

Red Mites and Northern Fowl Mites

These are blood-sucking mites that may transmit diseases including fowl cholera. The grey or red mites may be visible to the naked eye. Affected birds are restless and may have pale combs and wattles. Young birds may die from anemia. Control of mites in the environment and on the birds is vital for treatment and control. Pyrethroids, organophosphates, and carbamates may be used, and other treatments include use of citrus extracts, mineral oil, and vegetable oil, or hanging cotton bags of sulfur dust in areas where the birds will rub against them. The environment must be thoroughly cleaned and fumigated. Cracks in the environment should be filled in and the birds and environment regularly monitored so disease can be controlled before birds are severely affected.

Internal Parasite Control

Internal parasites found in birds include:

- Coccidia
- Gapeworm
- Roundworms
- Cecal worm
- Tapeworm
- Hairworms or capillary worms
- Coccidia

Coccidia are protozoan parasites. Various species of coccidia infect different regions of the intestinal tract. Affected chickens are depressed, and have ruffled feathers and poor appetite. They may have diarrhea and show depigmentation.

Chickens commonly are provided with coccidiostatic drugs, such as sulphonamides or amprolium, in their feed or water.

Gapeworm

Syngamus trachea is a nematode parasite that infects the trachea of chickens. Infection is via the oral route by ingestion of earthworms, slugs or snails, or by direct ingestion of gapeworm eggs. The condition is more common in birds maintained on soil or kept on pasture. The birds stand with their mouths agape and show dyspnea and loss of appetite. The condition is treated and prevented by administration of drugs such as flubendazole in feed.

Roundworms

Roundworms are nematodes of the *Ascaridia* species. Infection is via ingestion of roundworm eggs. Affected birds may be asymptomatic or may show poor growth, depression, and diarrhea. Treatment with various anthelmintics is curative. Prevention involves keeping feeders and waterers clean of droppings and rotating on which pastures birds are housed.

Cecal Worm

Heterakis gallinarum is a nematode that infests the ceca of chickens that feed off the ground. The worm itself is not that pathogenic but it may carry a protozoan parasite, *Histomonas meleagridis*, that causes blackhead disease. Transmission of cecal worms may be by direct ingestion of worm eggs or by ingestion of earthworms that have ingested the eggs. Treatment is possible using various anthelmintic drugs. Chickens may be housed on hard surfaces or hardware cloth placed over soil to prevent ingestion of earthworms.

Tapeworm

Tapeworms are regularly transmitted through invertebrate hosts such as earthworms or beetles and are therefore more common in birds housed on soil. Most birds show no clinical signs of disease but may show lack of weight gain or unthriftiness. Treatment with various drugs is possible but care must be taken to evaluate withdrawal times.

Hairworms or Capillary Worms

Hairworms are nematodes of *Capillaria* species that may infest the esophagus or crop. Infection is via ingestion of eggs; transmission through ingestion of earthworms also is possible. Most birds show no clinical signs but birds may show unthriftiness or die acutely. Treatment is with anthelmintic drugs. Prevention is through control of exposure to earthworms and thorough cleaning of the environment.

Behavior

Aggression, including pecking out the feathers or pecking at the vent of another bird, are not uncommon behavior problems in flocks of chickens. Any underlying causes of stress including overcrowding, unsanitary conditions, and presence of disease, should be identified and addressed. Observation of the flock may identify one individual that is particularly aggressive; that individual may need to be removed. Beak trimming may prevent the problem but does not address underlying stresses and is considered unethical in some countries.

Backyard birds value enrichment. Chickens will spend up to 80% of their time foraging and if they are not given ways to forage and exercise, behavioral problems will develop. Physical forms of enrichment include changes in the environment (for example, creating areas for birds to perch or fly to such as arrangements of logs and branches) and dust baths (shallow pans of sand / soil birds roll around in as a way to clean their feathers and control parasites). Nutritional forms of enrichment include anything that makes them work for their food, such as pushing a stick through an apple and sticking it into the ground for them to peck at, making a hole through a cabbage and hanging it up for them to peck at, freezing fruits and vegetables in water in a pan and then turning it out – this is a particularly good form of enrichment on hot summer days – or dropping a pumpkin from a height and letting the birds find all of the seeds and broken bits.

Biosecurity

Diseases of concern that can be passed from chickens to people include bacterial diseases such as salmonellosis, psittacosis, and tuberculosis; viral diseases such as influenza; fungal diseases such as histoplasmosis; and parasitic diseases such as giardiasis. Humans can decrease likelihood of contracting disease from chickens by wearing dedicated clothing to clean, feed, or handle the chickens; always washing hands after handling birds or equipment used with the birds; never eating or drinking in the area where the birds roam and never allowing birds into areas where human food and drink is prepared or consumed; and minimizing contact of live birds with the very old, the very young, and any immunocompromised people. The CDC has recognized a series of Salmonella outbreaks in backyard chickens since 2015. They reported the following in 2019 regarding these outbreaks:

- There have been 1003 ill people reported from 49 states; 175 of these people have been hospitalized. Two deaths have been reported, one in Ohio and one in Texas. Most people infected with *Salmonella* develop diarrhea, fever, and stomach cramps, are ill for 7-4 days, and recover without treatment.
- An increase in *Salmonella* infection linked to live poultry usually is seen in the spring and summer, when more people are purchasing chicks. People

who got sick in the 2019 outbreak reported getting chicks from places such as agricultural stores, websites, and hatcheries.

- People can get sick from *Salmonella* after touching poultry or the places where they live and roam. Birds carrying the bacteria may appear healthy and clean.

The following are their recommendations for backyard flocks and their owners:

- Do not snuggle with or kiss birds or touch them anywhere near your mouth.
- Do not permit poultry into the house.
- Remember that backyard poultry are not like family dogs, no matter how much you love them.

Some clients may ask whether or not they can slaughter their chickens when they are no longer laying. Live slaughter is not permitted at a residence anywhere in the Twin Cities. There are processors to which you can refer these clients, for example, Long Cheng – Hmong Livestock and Meat Processing plant in South Saint Paul.

Nutrition

It is recommended to feed a commercial ration to ensure proper nutrient balance. Make sure that young birds are fed a starter or grower ration and not a layer ration, which is much higher in calcium and could cause improper bone growth or renal failure if fed to young birds. Laying hens must be fed a layer ration and can also be provided with supplemental calcium. Birds can be provided with scratch grains (cracked, rolled or whole corn, oats, barley, or wheat) but this should be less than 10% of the total food provided daily. Grains may be soaked to make them easier to digest. Grit also may be provided if scratch grains are offered, to help birds break down these grains. Birds on grass or pasture also may eat grass and insects. Other sources of food for chickens include greens (fruits and vegetables) and mats of oats or wheat grass. Chickens will also eat mice (they can be good mousers in a farm setting) and frogs.

All feed must be maintained in containers that are airtight and watertight and that cannot be accessed by rodents.

Fresh water must be available at all times and in winter, care must be taken that water does not freeze.

CAGED BIRDS

Unique Anatomy – External

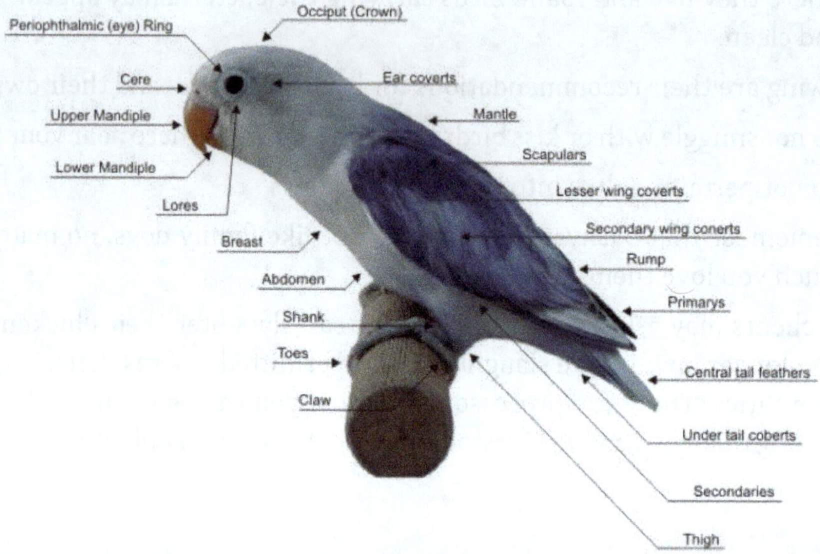

"Standard bird body parts of a psittacine (parrot-like) bird", http://www.sciencepartners.info/module-6-birds/bird-anatomy-bones-muscles/bird-anatomy-from-the-outside-in/

Many caged birds are parrot-like, but you also may work with finches, doves, and other types of caged birds.

Two specific parts of the head we talk about in caged birds are the lores and the cere. The lores are the spaces between the top of the beak and the eye. The cere is a fleshy mass at the top of the beak within which the nostrils are located. All birds have lores and a cere but the cere is especially prominent in psittacines. Species of birds show differences in size and structure of the beak dependent on their primary diet.

Unique Anatomy – Internal

Internal anatomy of caged birds is generally very similar to that of chickens with the exception of the reproductive tract. Depending on the species, it may be unilateral (as in chickens) or bilateral. In most species of caged birds, females have a unilateral reproductive tract on the left side. Knowledge of specifics of the reproductive tract is valuable as direct observation of the gonad of a bird by laparoscopy (surgical sexing) is one method of determining sex of birds from species that are not sexually dimorphic.

Specifics of anatomy and other information about caged birds can be found in the Manual of Exotic Pet Practice, pp 250-298.

Housing

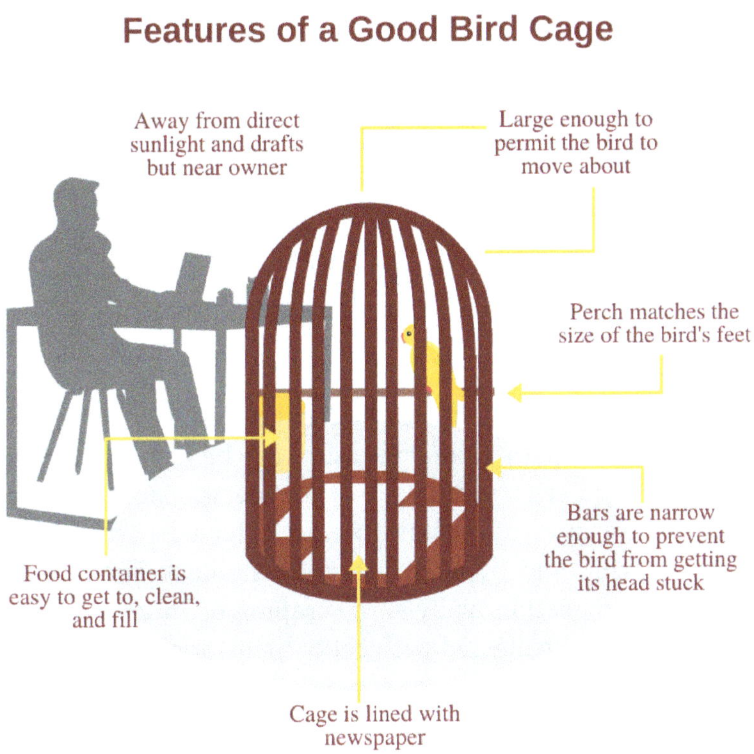

Most companion birds will be caged for the majority of the day. The cage should be placed away from direct sunlight and drafts. Exposure to natural light is important in some species of birds as it may alter molting, egg-laying, and singing behaviors. Many birds appreciate placement of the cage where they can see and interact with their owners. Cages generally should not be put in a kitchen or in any area of the house where chemicals or any other products that give off strong vapors are used or stored. Cages must be large enough to permit the bird to move about and spread its wings. The bars of the cage may be made of a variety of metals and may or may not be painted / powder-coated. Birds often chew at their enclosures so only non-toxic and durable products should be used. Bars of the cage should be narrow enough to prevent the bird from sticking its head through and getting caught. The cage should be easy to clean completely, with water and food containers that can easily be filled and an easy way for the owner to clean the floor of the cage. Cages often are lined with some sort of disposable material, such as newspaper, to facilitate removal of feces; this should be changed at least every 2-3 days. Any spilled seed or seed hulls should also be cleaned from the cage every 2-3 days to prevent insect infestation. Perches should be appropriate for the size of the bird's feet and should be cleanable. Any toys or other enrichment should be appropriate for the size of the bird. For example, toys for budgerigars should be not given to large parrots, who may chew them apart and ingest small pieces.

Vaccinations and Disease Control

While there are a variety of viral diseases that can infect caged birds, the only one for which a vaccine is available is polyomavirus. This disease causes death in birds ≤ 4 months of age. Prevalence of the virus in adult birds, who are asymptomatic, is considered to be high so there may be little use in vaccinating birds other than those used for breeding or in facilities with a known problem.

Parasite Control

Caged birds rarely can be infected with internal parasites including roundworms, tapeworms, and *Giardia* sp. Intestinal parasites can be identified by fecal flotation or direct inspection and are treated as in other species. More commonly in birds, parasite concerns are due to infestation with external parasites, usually mites causing feather picking and hyperkeratosis of the beak and legs. Mites can be identified by direct inspection or by skin scraping or by microscopic evaluation of skin and feather debris collected with cellophane tape. Mites are treated on the bird and in its environment with sprays or other direct formulations.

Behavior

See Behavior chapter.

Biosecurity

There are very few zoonotic diseases of concern. Psittacosis (*Chlamydia [Chlamydophila] psittaci*) is the most common, with fewer than 100 cases reported in the United States annually. Affected birds generally are not clinically ill.

Nutrition

All birds require a source of clean water at all times. Nutrition varies with the species of birds, as some require primarily a seed-based diet (for example, canaries) and others do better with a pelleted diet and fresh fruits and vegetables (for example, budgerigars). Fruit should be offered no more than 2-3 times weekly. Dark green, red, and orange vegetables can be offered daily. Fresh fruits and vegetables should be offered in a separate dish from pelleted food; pelleted food can be available at all times but the fruits and vegetables should be offered for only 30-60 minutes and then removed to prevent spoiling. Birds should never be given avocadoes, onions, garlic, fruit pits or seeds, high-sugar or high-fat foods, or chocolate. Seeds or pellets should be purchased as fresh as possible to minimize loss of nutrients in storage and should be stored to prevent infiltration of insects, especially seed moths. Most caged birds do not require a calcium supplement unless they chronically lay eggs, but calcium supplementation in the form of cuttlebone is inexpensive and also provides enrichment.

FISH

Unique Anatomy and Classification

There are over 20,000 species of fish and over 1000 have been kept in captivity. Fish can be separated into fresh water, brackish water, and salt water species. Among the freshwater fish, there are temperate and tropical species. Temperate species are sport or game fish, such as sturgeon, pike, walleye, bass, trout, sunfish, and eels. These generally are not kept as pets. In Minnesota, game fish can be kept in a tank legally if they are purchased from a dealer that is licensed by the Department of Natural Resources. The fish maintained in the tank count toward the state angling possession limit for that species.

Freshwater tropical fish are those most commonly maintained in home fish tanks.

FAMILY	COMMON EXAMPLES
Characins	Tetras
Cyprinids	Goldfish, carp (koi are an ornamental mutation of carp)
Catfish	Catfish
Killifish	—
Rainbowfishes	—
Gouramies	Bettas
Livebearers	Mollies, Guppies
Cichlids	Angelfish

Bony fishes are covered with scales and an overlying mucous coat. These serve to protect the fish from trauma and from invasion of pathogens. The scales also provide camouflage or are used for signaling behavior within or between species. When handling fish, it is good to minimize loss of scales or mucous.

Fish have paired pectoral and pelvic fins, and single dorsal, anal, and caudal fins. The dorsal fin is made of two parts in some species. Fins are used for steering, balancing, and braking.

The primary respiratory organs are the gills. The gills are covered by the bony operculum. The gills absorb oxygen, excrete ammonia and carbon dioxide, and regulate absorption and excretion of ions and water. Fish have a simple 2-chambered heart. The lateral line is a mechanosensory structure that permits the fish to sense changes in sound waves and water pressure. There is great variation in the gastrointestinal tract of fish by species. Carnivorous species have a much shorter GI tract than do herbivorous species. Not all species have a stomach. Some species have pyloric cecae that secrete digestive enzymes. Fish have a large liver and a single large kidney with anterior and posterior segments. Another abdominal organ is the swim bladder or air bladder; this is a gas-filled single or double sac that enables fish to maintain depth without expending energy by swimming.

Housing

The environment provided for fish is a miniature ecosystem within which the fish, the water, the substrate, and anything else added to the tank all play a part. Tanks are preferred to bowls for fish as it is easier to create a stable environment for the fish in a larger volume of water. In general, larger tanks are better for the fish than are smaller tanks. Required temperature in the tank varies with the species of fish. Some require very warm water but that is not true of all tropical fish. Fish can tolerate a variation in temperature of about 10°F. Type of light required again varies by species but in general, full spectrum fairly bright light with a 12-hour dark:light cycle is appropriate. Filtration of the water to remove wastes is required. The filter often also contains a system for aeration of water to ensure oxygenation. The substrate in the tank is part of the overall ecosystem. Gravel is easy to clean. Development of a healthy bacterial community within the tank is important and can be managed either with artificial introduction of bacteria (often through a filtering mechanism) or by permitting development of a fine sediment component to the substrate. Addition of artificial plants, tiny deep-sea divers, treasure chests and other inert objects provide places for fish to hide. Make sure they are approved for use in fish tanks so no unexpected compounds are added to the water and do not add so many that it overcrowds the tank. Live plants are more work to establish in the tank but provide shelter and security for the fish, add oxygen to the water, and compete with algae for nutrients, keeping down the development of algae within the tank. Algae also can be controlled by adding an algae-eating species of fish or snail to the tank.

High water quality is vital for health of the fish. Some pet stores provide free water quality testing. At-home kits can be purchased and commercial laboratories also provide water testing. Components of concern are concentration of waste products (ammonia, nitrites, nitrates), pH, and oxygenation. New tanks should be tested daily until the system stabilizes. Fish should be added very gradually to new tanks and stabilization permitted before new introductions. If a tank is set up with a large number of fish at once, acute mortality of all fish may result. In established tanks, 10-20% of the water should be replaced every 1-3 weeks and water quality should be evaluated intermittently.

Nutrition

Fish may be herbivores, omnivores, or carnivores. Most fish require a high percentage of protein in their diet and need dietary fat as a source of energy. Fish digest carbohydrates poorly and require very little carbohydrate in their diet. Fish must be fed food that is appropriate for their species.

Vaccinations and disease control

Vaccinations are not commonly used to control disease in hobby fish tanks; vaccines are used in some commercial fish farming operations. Discussion of fish farming is beyond the scope of this course.

Parasite control

Preventive diagnosis and treatment of parasites is rarely done in hobby fish tanks except at the time of introduction to the tank (see Biosecurity).

Behavior

Fish may hide, dart around quickly, or spend time on the bottom of the tank as normal behaviors. Fish may fight and some fish naturally eat other fish. Attention must be paid to which species will not readily co-exist in a tank. Fish acting listless, swimming erratically, or gasping at the surface may be suffering from poor water quality or illness.

Biosecurity

New fish should be quarantined before being added to the tank. Length of quarantine varies with where the fish were purchased or captured; wild-caught fish are more likely to harbor parasites or infectious diseases. Fish should be checked for external parasites and other signs of disease and potentially treated for internal parasites before being added to a tank.

REPTILES

Many states prohibit ownership of venomous reptiles and large constricting snakes.

Many of the concerns we see as veterinarians are because reptiles are not fed and housed properly. A colleague from the class of 2022 offers the following suggestions to pass along to clients who tell you they are interested in getting a reptile as a pet:

- It is widely reported that the majority of pet reptiles (75-90%) die within the first year after purchase due to poor husbandry. Thoroughly research your reptile of interest before bringing them home and have their habitat ready to go before you purchase your new pet.

- Find a veterinarian who will see your reptile before purchase. In many rural areas, there are few to no veterinarians readily available with training and equipment or interest in caring for pet reptiles. Reptiles, like all pets, benefit from regular visits to a veterinarian.
- The majority of the reptile cases seen by veterinarians have problems due to inadequate husbandry. When you take your reptile to a veterinarian, be prepared to answer questions about the ambient temperature, lighting sources, humidity level, and feeding protocol you use.
- It was once widely believed that reptiles could be euthanized at home by putting them in the freezer. It has been found that this is actually a very painful process for the reptile and is not considered an appropriate form of euthanasia due to animal welfare concerns. If you believe your reptile needs to be euthanized, that should be done by a veterinarian.

Unique Anatomy and Classification

The reptiles are a diverse group of animals. There are four orders of reptiles. The order Testudines includes turtles and tortoises. The order Squamata includes the suborders Serpentes (snakes) and Lacertilia (lizards). The order Crocodilia includes crocodiles, alligators, caimans, and gavials. The order Rhynchocephalia contains one or two species of tuatara from New Zealand. Most pet reptiles are from the orders Testudines and Squamata and that information will be the focus of this chapter.

Reptiles have an opening caudal to the tongue called the glottis that only opens when they are breathing. Snakes can extend their glottis laterally to permit them to breathe while eating. They have a trachea that bifurcates into two lungs. Reptiles do not have a diaphragm but do have ribs and breathing is controlled by the intercostal muscles with assistance from the muscles of the trunk and abdomen and smooth muscle in the lungs. There are significant variations in the cardiorespiratory tracts of underwater species.

Reptiles are ectothermic (cold-blooded; depending on external heat sources to regulate body temperature). Like amphibians, reptiles have a preferred optimal body temperature that alters cardiac and respiratory function. This in turn will alter the absorption, metabolism, distribution, and excretion of drugs. Squamates (lizards) and chelonians (turtles and tortoises) have a three-chambered heart with a single ventricle; this ventricle does contain an incomplete septum that can permit the heart to function as if it has four chambers. Functionally they have a dual system that always has a potential of mixing oxygenated and deoxygenated blood. Crocodilia have a 4-chambered heart.

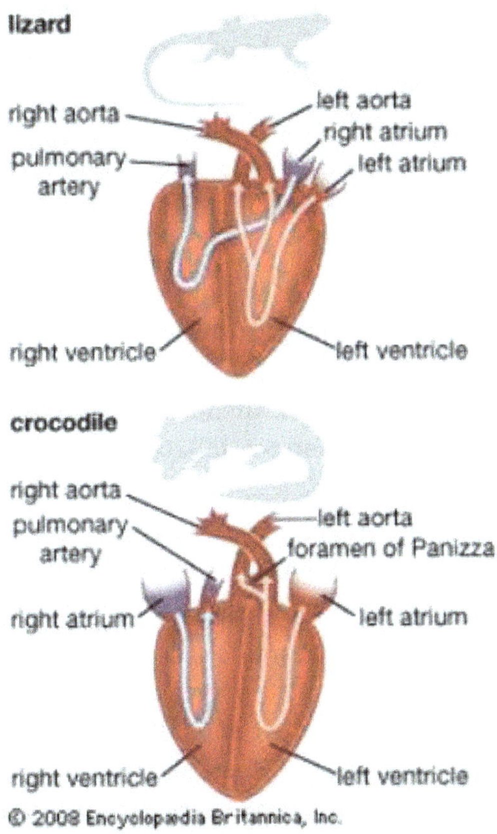

"Types of reptilian hearts", https://www.britannica.com/animal/reptile/Circulatory-system

Reptiles also have a renal portal system where blood from the caudal half of the animal (dorsal body wall, hind limbs, tail, urinary bladder, cloaca and reproductive organs) passes through the kidneys prior to returning to circulation. This allows for tubular excretion of nitrogenous waste during dehydration. This is of clinical significance when administering drugs.

All reptiles naturally are covered with scales. Some reptiles also have a specialized feature called osteoderms, which are bony deposits located within their scales or skin. This is of special consideration during imaging, surgery, and injections. Some reptiles have been selectively bred to be scaleless, and extra care is required for these animals as they are more sensitive to dehydration and temperature fluctuations. With reptiles and amphibians, different color variations have been selectively bred and are referred to as morphs in the hobby. The care for these animals is often the same, but there can be genetic diseases that are strongly linked to certain morphs.

Snakes and lizards have teeth and may have more than one row of teeth on the maxilla and mandible. Tortoises and turtles do not have teeth and instead have a hard beak used for pulling apart their food; an appropriate diet is important to prevent beak overgrowth. Reptiles generally do not chew their food. Species that swallow their food whole have a highly distensible esophagus. Reptiles do have ureters and a urinary bladder and do produce liquid waste. Liquid and solid waste both are passed through the cloaca.

Reptiles may or may not have eyelids. In general, turtles and lizards have eyelids but some geckos do not. Snake eyes are protected with a transparent scale, called a spectacle, which is replaced when snakes shed. The tongue-flicking behavior of snakes and lizards reflects the use of the tongue to capture chemical cues from the environment that are then applied to the animal's vomeronasal (Jacobson's) organ to permit them to identify prey and dangers.

Snakes shed their scales in a normal process called ecdysis. Snakes have small overlapping scales on the dorsum and sides and have ladder-like short, wide scales on their ventrum, called scutes. New scales form over the entire animal under the old scales. Lymphatic fluid accumulates between the new and old scales, dulling the appearance of the skin and markings, and making the spectacles (the scales over the eyes) opaque. The skin clears about 3-4 days before shedding begins. The snake will rub to start the shed and generally will shed the whole skin in one piece.

Specifics of anatomy and other information about all orders of reptiles can be found in the Manual of Exotic Pet Practice, pp 112-249.

Housing

Reptiles are solitary animals and prefer to be alone. A majority will fight or resource guard if another animal is present, especially if it is of the same sex. Sometimes this fighting will result in death or serious injury. Having more than one animal in the same enclosure causes undue stress on both, but especially on the less dominant animal. For these reasons, reptiles should be individually housed.

Nearly all reptiles need to be kept in enclosures with tight-fitting lids, with either weights or a lock to prevent escape. A screened lid is often used to permit ventilation, and can be partially covered to aide in proper humidity. Glass tanks work well for smaller animals. Larger animals, however, may require specially built structures. Many commercial reptile cages are made of plastic or glass making them easy to clean and sanitize. Cages need to be cleaned frequently to avoid buildup of waste and bacteria. Chlorine bleach solutions can be used for disinfection, however, cages need to be thoroughly rinsed and dried before the animals are returned to the environment. The size and shape of the habitat is dependent on the species, number of animals, activity requirements, and necessary enrichments.

For example, a tree-dwelling (arboreal) snake requires a higher enclosure than a burrowing (fossorial) snake.

The best guide for reptile habitat is to create one that closely mirrors its natural environment, including considerations of appropriate temperature and humidity. There are three types of habitats that meet the needs of most reptiles and amphibians. Aquatic habitats are appropriate for animals that are wholly aquatic. Semi-aquatic habitats are appropriate for animals that live on land and in water. They may be swimming species that come up on land for food or to sun themselves. Terrestrial habitats are appropriate for species that spend their lives on land.

Aquatic Habitats

Very few reptiles are fully aquatic, but many amphibians are fully aquatic during their larval stage of life. A typical setup includes a filtration and aeration system. This is especially important for tadpoles that cannot breathe air at the water surface. Mudpuppies prefer well-aerated tanks in which they can remain on the bottom and use their gills. Filtration is important because amphibians, like fish, generate ammonia as a waste product. Turtles are especially dirty, and require double the filtration power. Aquariums without filtration systems will need water changes every 2-3 days to prevent buildup of excrement and loss of oxygen. Substrate that cannot be ingested is ideal for the bottom of the tank. Large river stones or slate slabs are much better than sand or gravel, as there is no risk of impaction. Tap water must be treated before adding it to the tank as it often contains heavy metals in addition to chlorine. Chemicals used to treat the water for fish will work for reptiles and amphibians if the directions are followed. Allowing the water to sit in open containers for 48 hours to allow the chlorine to evaporate will get rid of the chlorine, but not the heavy metals. Plants, rocks, and tree branches provide hiding places and mimic the natural habitat.

Semi-aquatic Habitat

All animals kept in a semi-aquatic habitat need to have access to an area that allows them to leave the water completely and dry off if they so desire. Many turtles do well in a tank that is aquatic but has spots that allow them to exit the water completely and dry off. Depending on the species, you may wish to create a split tank. You can create a split tank by dividing an aquarium with a plexiglass wall, using silicon caulking to make each section water tight. In the dry area, create a terrestrial habitat, ensuring that you use substrate that the animal cannot ingest. Add leaves, bark, branches, and plants to make it more like a natural habitat. Ensure that the animal can easily go between the water and the terrestrial side. The water side should be similar to the aquatic habitat. The water side will need a strong filter with a guard, as the animals often drag substrate into the water.

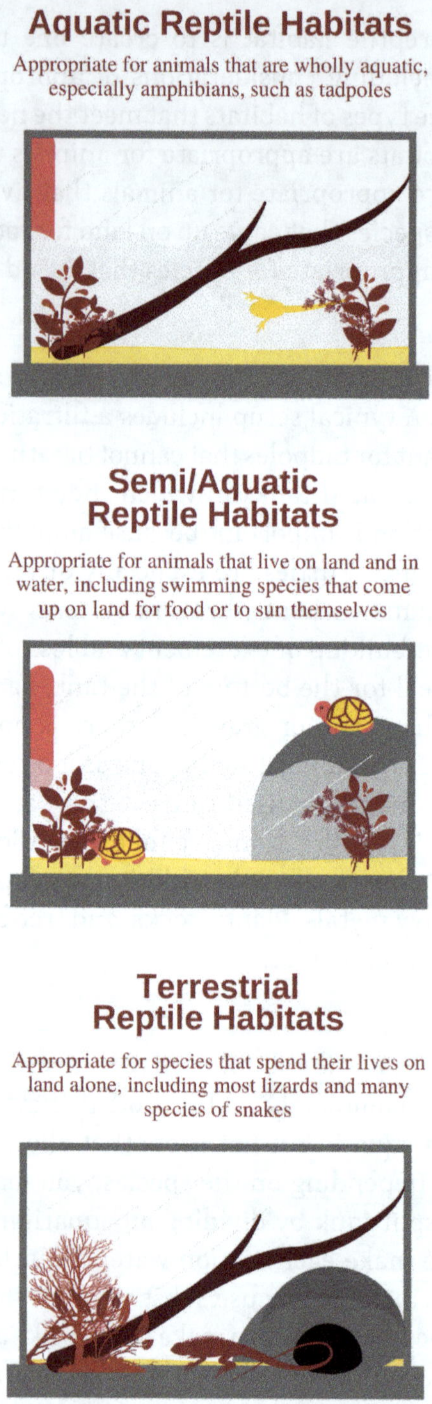
Aquatic Reptile Habitats
Appropriate for animals that are wholly aquatic, especially amphibians, such as tadpoles
Semi/Aquatic Reptile Habitats
Appropriate for animals that live on land and in water, including swimming species that come up on land for food or to sun themselves
Terrestrial Reptile Habitats
Appropriate for species that spend their lives on land alone, including most lizards and many species of snakes

Terrestrial Habitat

Many of the commonly kept reptiles require a terrestrial habitat. This entails a substrate that the animal cannot ingest, with a shelter and water bowl. Cage decorations such as fake plants and logs can be added to make the animal feel more secure. Be sure to include a bowl of water that the animal can submerge itself in if it so desires. The animal should be able to crawl into and out of the bowl freely.

Reptiles are ectothermic (cold-blooded; depending on external heat sources to regulate body temperature) and so require a heat source. When temperatures are too low, metabolism and activity decrease, leaving animals more susceptible to infections. Heating pads that lie under the tank and heat lamps are recommended. Heating pads should be connected to a thermostat to reach the desired temperature and reduce the risk of thermal burns or fire. Direct sources of heat, for example heat rocks, increase the risk for burns. Timers can be used to provide sufficient light and heat during the day with a decrease in temperature towards nightfall that mimics the natural environment. Aquatic and semiaquatic tanks will also need a way to heat water. A temperature gradient within the tank is important because these animals engage in behavioral thermoregulation to avoid overheating. The heat must be provided in a manner that permits the animal to move towards or away from the heat source to find their preferred optimum temperature zone (POTZ). Humidity must also be addressed as low relative humidity increases risk for dehydration and may impair normal shedding while too high relative humidity may predispose to skin infections. A good way to address humidity is to provide a humid hide. This is a shelter filled with a moist substrate that the animal can access when required, such as before a shed. It can be as simple as a piece of Tupperware filled with damp sphagnum moss with an access hole cut into it. Species from tropical rainforests may need sprinkler or misting systems to replicate daily rainfall of their natural environments.

Fresh water should always be available. Most lizards will drink from a water bowl. Water should be changed daily because some lizards soak in or defecate in their water dishes. Some lizards do not recognize standing water as they lap dew in the wild, like chameleons. These animals should have systems that mist the vegetation in their cages in addition to water bowls. Daily misting can also be done by hand using a spray bottle.

Reptiles should only be kept on a substrate that they are not able to ingest. There are commercial sands available that contain calcium, but these become rock-hard when they have contact with water. Many reptiles suffer from impaction while being kept on substrate that they are able to fit in their mouth like sand or gravel. They are not precise hunters, and oftentimes ingest their substrate as they eat their food. A way to avoid this is by feeding the animals in a separate enclosure that has no substrate.

Vaccinations and Disease Control

There are no vaccines recommended for control of infectious disease in reptiles. Any animal that has been kept in captivity should not be released into the wild, as they can transmit foreign diseases to local populations. Only animals raised and licensed for reintroduction should be released into the wild.

Parasite Control

Mites and ticks are not uncommon in wild-caught reptiles and are less common in healthy, captive-raised reptiles. The most common ectoparasitic mite to infest snakes and lizards is the snake mite *Ophionyssus natricis*. These mites are often vectors for diseases in reptiles and can be hard to eliminate. These mites tend to accumulate in the folds or indentations of the animal and often are found around the eye and the vent. Owners may be able to feel the mites crawling on them after handling their pet, or see the mites themselves; the mites are about the size of ground pepper. Clinical signs include decreased activity and abnormal shedding. Animals often will soak in water more than usual in an attempt to drown the parasites. The dead mites may be found in water dishes.There is a permethrin anti-parasitic agent that is approved for use in reptiles and other drugs, such as ivermectin, also have been shown to be safe and effective in some species. Ticks are readily visible and can be removed by hand or treated with medications as described above. Ticks may be associated with bacterial infections or anemia, which may require treatment as well.

All types of internal parasites are found in reptiles, although some are commonly associated with a given type of reptile. For example, trematodes are most common in turtles and snakes while tapeworms and nematodes are found in all species. Clinical manifestations of disease are most common in animals housed in crowded or unsanitary conditions. Diagnosis is by fecal flotation or direct inspection and treatment varies with the type of parasite identified.

Behavior

Specifics of behavioral concerns in the many species of reptiles will not be addressed. Veterinarians are encouraged to work with owners to ensure they know the normal feeding, shedding / molting, and hibernation / estivation behaviors of their animals, so they can tell the veterinarian if something atypical is happening. It is suggested that the owner keeps a record book of when the animal is fed, what it was fed, what vitamins and minerals were provided, the weight of the animal, when the animal shed, when the animal defecated, and any abnormal behaviors noted.

Biosecurity

In order to prevent parasites like snake mites infecting other animals, it is advised to quarantine all newly acquired animals. The animal should be placed in a quarantine tank, which is the bare minimum of requirements in a simple set-up. This allows for easy observation of the animal and any treatment that it may require. This tank should be isolated away from other animals and cleaned daily after all other cages. The animal should be quarantined for a minimum of 30 days; 60-90 days is ideal.

Transmission of bacteria, most notably *Salmonella* sp. between reptiles and humans is a very real concern, possible with many species but particularly of concern with small turtles, to the extent that since 1975, sale of turtles less than □4 has been banned by the FDA. In 2020, the CDC identified an increase in human cases of *Salmonella* sp in owners of bearded dragons. If possible, the cage and accessories and tools should be cleaned with a 1:10 solution of bleach and water, outside the home if possible. Anyone handling a reptile or any part of its housing, including food and water dishes, should thoroughly wash their hands afterward, ideally not in a kitchen sink or anywhere food for humans is prepared. Children, immunocompromised individuals, and the elderly should be particularly cautious. No one should kiss or snuggle reptiles and everyone who handles or feed reptiles should immediately wash their hands.

Nutrition

There is tremendous variety in diet of reptiles and this may vary with life stage. For example, some lizards that are primarily carnivores or insectivores as juveniles need a primarily herbivorous diet as adults, for example, bearded dragons and iguanas. Failure to change the diet appropriately with age of the animal may result in disease.

All snakes are carnivorous. Since snakes eat whole prey, they often do not have nutritional issues. Their main prey item will be species specific, as some are insectivorous and other will eat such things as lizards, mice, or other snakes. Many snakes kept in captivity have been transitioned to eating such prey items as mice, rats, or rabbits. A snake should not be offered a prey item whose circumference is larger than the thickest part of the snake's body. A live prey item should never be left with the snake, as snakes do not constrict in defense. Oftentimes, they suffer bite wounds or death from fighting with the prey. Insects may be fed live but other live prey should be avoided as they can kill the snake while defending themselves. Frozen prey can be purchased for feeding. An owner should transition the snake from live prey by offering it freshly killed prey items. There are many resources online on how to transition a snake from live to frozen prey. The snake should defecate after a meal before being fed again; with this provision, young snakes generally can be fed every 2-7 days while adult snakes can be fed every 7-21 days. Some species of snakes, like a ball python, will go for weeks without eating. If the snake begins to lose weight it should be seen by a veterinarian. Snakes that are going to shed will go off feed beforehand and become dull in color. Their eyes will turn cloudy blue when they are close to shedding, which will temporarily blind them. The snake should be left alone at this time.

Each species of reptile has its own unique dietary requirements that often require vitamin and mineral supplementation. This is especially true for tortoises, turtles, and lizards. Many of these supplements are now commercially available and tailored for some species. The frequency and types of supplementation that the animals require will change depending on species, so you will have to search for reputable sources. A good supplement will list what vitamins it provides, but also the source. Some reptiles cannot use vitamins unless they come from the correct source. Most reptiles require a calcium supplement in their diet to prevent metabolic bone disease. To properly use the calcium in their diets, reptiles require vitamin D3. This can be supplemented in the diet but is best provided through natural sunlight that is not filtered through glass or plastic as that eliminates the UVB rays they require. If that is not possible, a reptile UVB bulb should be provided. This bulb will need to be changed every 6 months to make sure it is providing not just light but also the UVB rays that reptiles require to metabolize calcium.

Always research the proper diet for the specific species of animal. For example, animals that are primarily herbivorous should not be fed high-protein dog or cat food, which makes the animal feel full without providing sufficient non-digestible dietary fiber and other components of a plant-based diet. The diet for each species will vary in protein, protein sources, and plant matter. Standard captive raised insects are not nutritionally complete enough for healthy reptiles. These prey items need to be fed a nutritious diet before being fed to a pet reptile. In addition, they should be supplemented, often through dusting with appropriate calcium and vitamins. Iceberg lettuce should be avoided, as it is devoid of nutrients. Spinach should also be avoided, as it binds calcium easily, further increasing risk of metabolic bone disease.

Diet for Lizards, Turtles, and Tortoises

- Protein Sources
    - Good staple insects: Dubia roaches, crickets, locusts, mealworms, superworms, earthworms, red worms
    - Mice can be given as a treat, but they are high in fat
    - Eggs, chicken or quail

    - Grocery store smelt
    - Feeding goldfish and rosey reds can be dangerous because it blocks thiamine absorption and destroys vitamin B1 in the animal in large quantities
- Plants
    - In general dark leafy greens can be a majority of the diet. Yellow, red, and orange vegetables like bell peppers can also be included. A good diet is often composed of a mix of collard greens, beet greens, mustard greens, broccoli, turnip greens, alfalfa hay or chow, bok choy, kale, parsley, Swiss chard, watercress, clover, red or green cabbage, savory, cilantro, kohlrabi, bell peppers, green beans, escarole, and dandelion. Fruit should be given sparingly as a treat, as it is a poor source of minerals.

AMPHIBIANS

Unique Anatomy and Classification

There are three orders of amphibians. The order Caudata is made up of newts and salamanders. The order Anura includes frogs and toads. The larval form is called a pollywog or tadpole. Tadpoles have tails and internal gills. Metamorphosis is a sudden transition from this larval stage to the adult stage. Frogs have smooth skin and long hind legs adapted for swimming. Toads do not have smooth skin and have stubby bodies and short back legs. Frogs and toads are tailless amphibians. The order Gymnophiona consists of caecilians, burrowing amphibians that resemble earthworms or snakes.

Amphibians spend their larval phase in water and the adult phase partially or completely on land. Their skin is thin and moist. Amphibians can absorb oxygen through their skin by diffusion. Amphibians do not have a diaphragm or ribs but do have sac-like lungs. Air can be drawn into the lungs through contraction of the floor of the mouth.

Amphibians are ectothermic (cold-blooded; depending on external heat sources to regulate body temperature). They have a three-chambered heart with a single ventricle.

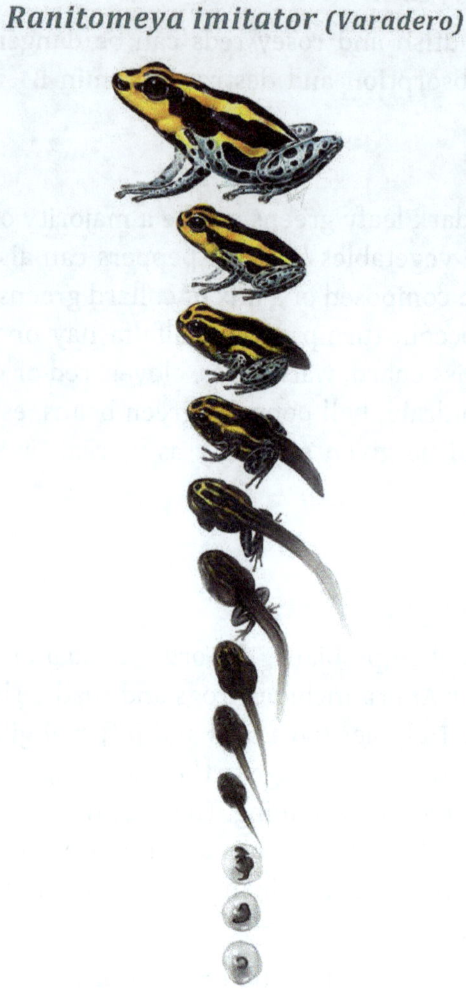

– "Digital illustration showing thumbnail dartfrog Ranitomeya imitator (Varadero) and its development in life stages", http://blog.illustraciencia.cat/2015/04/ranitomeya-imitator-varadero-mattias.html

Amphibians do not have scales. They can absorb water through their skin and lose water from the skin through evaporation. Amphibians that live in drier areas have thicker skin that helps them conserve moisture. The skin of most amphibians is covered with fluid-secreting glands that produce a slimy mucus. The mucus helps conserve moisture, prevents too much water from being absorbed into the body, and helps the animal escape predators. Some amphibians also have toxin-producing glands in their skin. The toxins produced can be deadly to predators, including humans.

Tongues of different kinds of amphibians vary considerably. Some have alterations of the hyoid apparatus that permit their long, sticky tongues to be ejected to capture prey and some do not have tongues at all. Amphibians either have no teeth or have very small teeth in the upper jaw only. They crush their prey with their jaws and swallow it whole.

Unlike birds, amphibians do have ureters and a urinary bladder and do produce liquid waste. Liquid and solid waste both are passed through the cloaca.

Amphibians generally do not have good eyesite. Their lens is fixed, decreasing ability to focus. They do not have external eyelids and instead protect the globe of the eye by pulling it back into the socket and covering it with a third eyelid, or nictitating membrane.

Specifics of anatomy and other information about amphibians can be found in the Manual of Exotic Pet Practice, pp 73-111.

Housing

Amphibian housing is similar to the housing in the above reptile section. Most should be kept individually as well to prevent stress and cannibalization of smaller cage mates. There is a wide variety of species of amphibians and an accompanying wide variety of appropriate habitats. The best guide for an amphibian habitat is to create one that closely mirrors its natural environment, including considerations of appropriate temperature and humidity. Amphibians are sensitive to chemicals, so care should be taken to thoroughly wash any décor that is placed within their enclosure. Tap water must be treated before adding it to the tank as it often contains heavy metals in addition to chlorine. Chemicals used to treat the water for fish will work for amphibians if the directions are followed. Allowing the water to sit in open containers for 48 hours to allow the chlorine to evaporate will get rid of the chlorine, but not the heavy metals.

The tank and associated equipment and tools used should occasionally be cleaned with dish soap or a dilute bleach solution. The animals must be removed from the tank and the tank must be thoroughly rinsed with water before the animals are returned. Because amphibians are directly exposed to anything in their environment through their skin, it is vital that the environment be kept scrupulously clean and that the animals not be exposed to chemicals used for cleaning.

Vaccinations and Disease Control

There are no vaccines recommended for control of infectious disease in amphibians.

No animals kept in captivity should be released into the wild. The spread of chytrid fungus, a fungus that is currently causing global amphibian extinction, has been linked to the release/escape of animals from the medical and pet trade into the wild.

Parasite Control

Amphibians can carry internal and external parasites but this is an uncommon concern in pet amphibians. Because many parasites have indirect life cycles, life cycle of the parasite cannot be completed in captive housing so the parasite population dies out. Disease is most commonly seen in stressed or immunocompromised animals, particularly those maintained outside of their POTZ.

Behavior

Specifics of behavioral concerns in the many species of amphibians will not be addressed. Veterinarians are encouraged to work with owners to ensure they know the normal feeding and hibernation behaviors of their animals, so they can tell the veterinarian if something atypical is happening.

Biosecurity

Good general hygiene should offset any concerns about passage of disease from pet amphibians to humans.

Nutrition

Amphibians are carnivores. They eat anything that will fit into their mouths, including smaller amphibians. Immediately separate if fighting occurs. Larger amphibians may consume small birds, mice, and small rodents. Tadpoles and aquatic species feed on vegetation and dead animals in the wild. In an aquarium tadpoles can be fed algae or tadpole powder available from pet stores. They can also be fed boiled lettuce, flake fish food, and fish hatchlings. As they begin to metamorphose into frogs, their diet should change to crickets, mealworms, waxworms, and other insects that are in the recommended food for reptiles. Smaller amphibians can be kept with springtails and isopods, which will clean the cage and also be a source of food. Feeding pelleted reptile food is not recommended. Amphibians are also prone to metabolic bone disease so supplementation with calcium and vitamins is required. Amphibians also are prone to hypovitaminosis A, which causes their tongue to keratinize and inhibits their ability to eat. This is also referred to as Short Tongue Syndrome. Any supplements that they receive should contain vitamin A. Some amphibians can only use vitamin A from select sources, so consult with an expert to figure out the proper supplements for the amphibian in question.

EXTRA RESOURCES

Disease control in chickens (National Poultry Improvement Program): (poultryimprovement.org).

Small and backyard poultry flocks (National Cooperative Extension service: https://poultry.extension.org

Keeping urban poultry (University of Kentucky): http://www2.ca.uky.edu/agcomm/pubs/ASC/ASC241/ASC241.pdf

Infectious and non-infectious disorders of amphibians: http://www.merckvetmanual.com/exotic-and-laboratory-animals/amphibians

Infectious and non-infectious disorders of reptiles: http://www.merckvetmanual.com/exotic-and-laboratory-animals/reptiles

Breathing in birds: https://www.whfreeman.com/BrainHoney/Resource/6716/SitebuilderUploads/Hillis2e/Student%20Resources/Animated%20Tutorials/pol2e_at_3101_Airflow_in_Birds/pol2e_at_3101_Airflow_in_Birds.html

Laryngotracheitis disease in birds: http://www.veterinaryworld.org/2008/July/Common%20Respiratory%20Diseases%20of%20Poultry.pdf

Fowl pox: https://www.hyline.com/aspx/redbook/redbook.aspx?s=5&p=35

Marek's disease in birds: https://www.merckvetmanual.com/poultry/neoplasms/marek%E2%80%99s-disease-in-poultry

CDC recommendations around salmonellosis in backyard chicken flocks: https://www.cdc.gov/features/salmonellapoultry/index.html

Specifics of anatomy and other information about various animals can be found in the Manual of Exotic Pet Practice http://www.sciencedirect.com/science/book/9781416001195

CHAPTER-15

MAMMALS

MICE

Unique Anatomy and Biology

Biology of Mice

LIFE SPAN	2 years
TEMPERATURE	98-101°F (36.5-38.0°C)
PULSE	325-780 beats/minute
RESPIRATION	40-80 breaths/minute
REPRODUCTIVE MATURITY	puberty 28-40 days, breeding initiation 50 days

House mice are 2.5-3" (6.5-7.5 cm) long and weigh 0.5-1 oz (20-40 gm). Mice sold in the pet trade are descended from house mice and have a slightly different appearance. Mice have a small head with a long, narrow snout. House mice are usually gray-brown with a light to white underbelly but pet mice can come in a variety of colors. They have large, round, black or red eyes, and large ears. Anatomy includes only 2 open-rooted (continuously growing) incisors with nerves only at the base, ability to draw the cheek folds into the diastema (space between the incisors and molars), and large masseter muscles that attach rostrally, giving them increased ability to gnaw. All rodents are obligate nose breathers.

Appearance of Mice

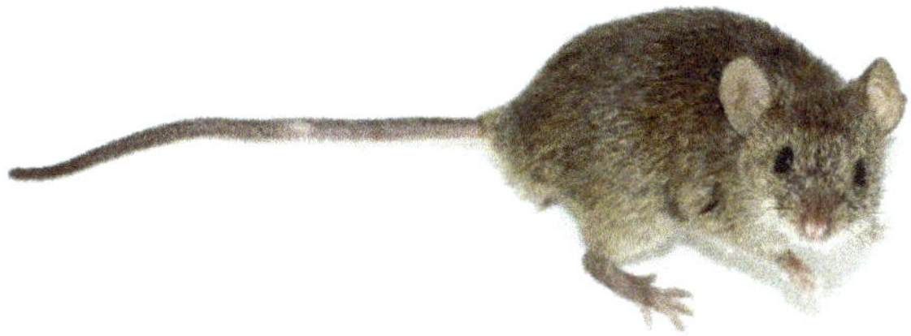

"Mouse", https://en.wikipedia.org/wiki/Mouse

Gender identification is through assessment of the anogenital distance, which is about twice as long in males as in females.

Gender Identification in Mice

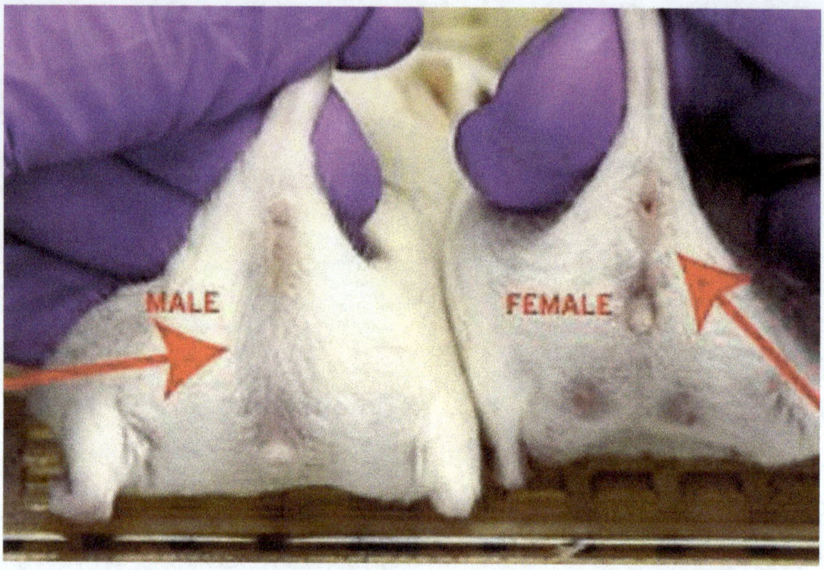

"Male vs. female mice", https://hubpages.com/animals/Why-Rats-and-Mice-Make-Better-Pets-Than-Hamsters-or-Gerbils

Specifics of anatomy and other information about mice and rats can be found in the Manual of Exotic Pet Practice, pp 326-344.

Housing

Suitable homes can be purchased or made. The bottom should be plastic or another material that will withstand gnawing and it should have closely spaced bars to prevent escape. Aquariums are excellent choices for mice. Mouse cages must have a lid or cover because mice are excellent climbers. The enclosure must be large enough for the mouse or mice, food and water, and enrichment, such as an exercise wheel. Mice also appreciate somewhere in the cage where they can hide. Appropriate bedding materials include wood shavings, ground corn cobs, pelleted sawdust, newspaper, and straw. Cedar and pine wood shavings sold as small animal bedding contain phenol that can be toxic or cause airway damage. Bedding should be replaced and the cage thoroughly cleaned 2-3 times per week. Mice don't drink a lot of water, but water should be available at all times. Open containers become contaminated with urine and feces quickly. Vacuum-type bottles with sipper tubes are ideal. Temperature, humidity, and lighting can be as that for the rest of the house.

Vaccinations and Disease Control

There are no vaccines recommended for control of infectious disease in mice.

Parasite Control

Internal parasites of mice include protozoa, pinworms, and tapeworms. These can be identified on fecal flotation or by direct inspection. Treatment varies with specific worm identified. External parasites are uncommon in captive-bred mice. Fur mites and lice can be seen, and are associated with pruritus to the point of self-mutilation and hair loss. Diagnosis is by direct inspection. Treatment is dependent on parasite identified; ivermectin is a common therapy.

Behavior

Mice are primarily nocturnal in habit but pet mice, feeling safe around humans, may come out during the day. Mice are outgoing, social creatures. They prefer the company of other mice. Male mice housed together may be territorial, and fight. Another abnormal behavior of mice housed together is barbering, the chewing away of the whiskers and the hair on the face of a submissive mouse, often by a dominant female mouse. Mice are fastidious groomers and early signs of disease often include a scruffy hair coat. Enrichment is an important component of housing to promote normal behaviors.

Dentistry

While many species of rodent require dentistry to correct or prevent overgrowth of their continually growing incisors, this is not a common problem in most mice. If malocclusion is present, the overgrown incisors easily can be identified on physical examination.

Biosecurity

Good general hygiene should offset any concerns about passage of disease from pet mice to humans; handwashing after handling rodents is essential. Many pet store mice do test positive for lymphocytic choriomeningitis virus, which can pose a risk to the unborn baby if a pregnant woman contracts the disease.

Nutrition

A commercial mouse feed that is complete and balanced with at least 14% protein is most appropriate. Treats specifically prepared for mice can be purchased. Other foods that can be offered but that should never make up any significant percentage of the animal's total food intake include leafy greens, broccoli, apples, celery, carrots, and dry bread. Mice should never be fed chocolate, peanuts, alcohol, onions, garlic, or citrus fruits.

RATS

Unique Anatomy and Biology

Biology of Rats

LIFE SPAN	2-3 years
TEMPERATURE	99-101°F (37-38°C)
PULSE	250-450 beats/minute
RESPIRATION	70-115 breaths/minute
REPRODUCTIVE MATURITY	puberty 65-110 days, breeding initiation 65-110 days

Of the 78 species of rats, only two have been domesticated as pets and for use in research, the black rat, also called the roof rat, and the brown or Norway rat. The body and head of the black rat is 5-7" (13-18 cm) long with a tail longer than its body. They weigh 4-12 oz (115-340 gm). The ears of the black rat are large and they have black or dark gray fur with a brown or gray-white underside. The brown rat is larger, with a body and head 7-10" (18-25 cm) long and a tail that is shorter than its head and body. They weigh 7-17 oz (200-400 gm). The ears of the brown rat are smaller in relationship to its head than those of the black rat. Their fur is usually dark brown to gray-brown with a lighter brown or gray underside. Pet rats descended from these two species come in a variety of colors and coat patterns.

Appearance of Rats

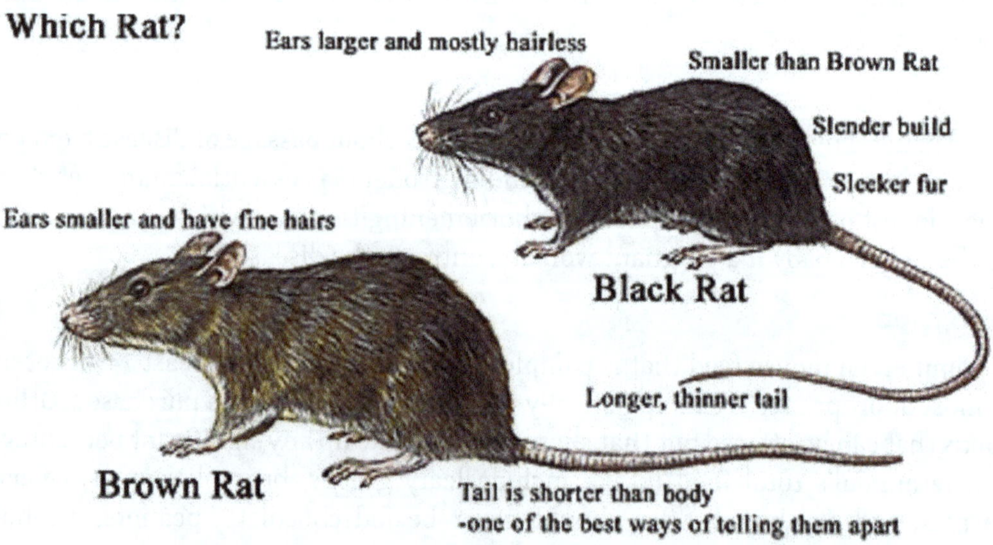
Which Rat?
Ears larger and mostly hairless
Smaller than Brown Rat
Slender build
Sleeker fur
Ears smaller and have fine hairs
Black Rat
Longer, thinner tail
Brown Rat
Tail is shorter than body
-one of the best ways of telling them apart

"Rat features", https://www.the-piedpiper.co.uk/th1.htm

Other unique anatomy is as for the mouse.

Gender identification is through assessment of anogenital distance, which is about 1.5-2 times longer in males than in females, or by direct observation of descended testes or extrusion of the penis. If the testes are not visible between the anus and genital papilla, gentle pressure on either side of the genital papilla in a male will result in extrusion of a small, red penis. Nipples are more prominent in females.

Gender Identification in Rats

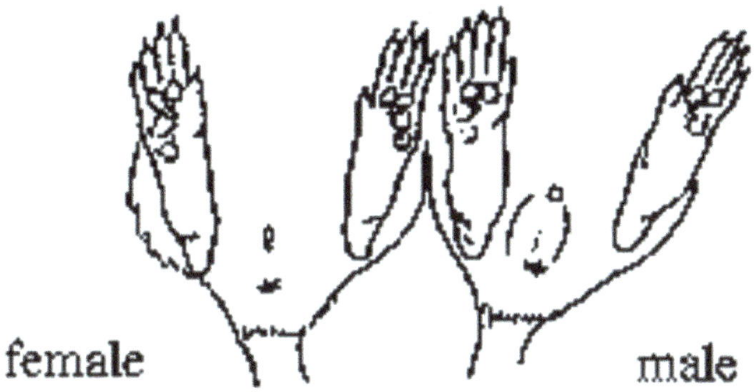

"Female vs. male rats", https://ratsinaction.weebly.com/how-to-keep-your-animals-healthy-and-happy.html

Specifics of anatomy and other information about mice and rats can be found in the Manual of Exotic Pet Practice, pp 326-344.

Housing

Wire mesh cages with solid bottoms or pull-out trays are recommended for rats. Cages can be constructed from wood and wire mesh, but materials must be thick enough to withstand gnawing. Glass aquariums work well for rats because they're easy to clean and are escape-proof with a lid. Larger cages are recommended because rats are active and benefit from environmental enrichment like ladders, ropes, and exercise wheels. Like mice, rats need a place to hide in their cage. Appropriate bedding materials include wood shavings, ground corn cobs, pelleted sawdust, newspaper and straw. Cedar and pine wood shavings sold as small animal bedding contain phenol that can be toxic or cause airway damage. Bedding should be replaced and the cage thoroughly cleaned 2-3 times per week. Rats need access to water at all times. A bottle with a sipper tube suspended from the cage is the best option. Temperature, humidity, and lighting should be as for the rest of the household.

Vaccinations and Disease Control

There are no vaccines recommended for control of infectious disease in rats.

Parasite Control

Internal parasites of rats include protozoa, pinworms, and tapeworms. These can be identified on fecal flotation or by direct inspection. Treatment varies with specific worm identified. External parasites are even more uncommon in captive-bred rats than in mice.

Behavior

Rats are primarily nocturnal, however, those kept as domestic pets are active all day and can be handled by owners. Rats are agile climbers, particularly the black rat. They use their tails for balance. They can jump up to two feet and are excellent swimmers, able to stay submerged for up to 3 minutes. They're curious and will climb a cage or stand on their hind legs to see their environment. Rats are intelligent and will learn their owner's voice and come when food or interaction is offered. Social and outgoing, rats do best when kept with other rats. Animals raised together will usually get along but, as with any animals, introducing a new rat may lead to fighting and rat fights can result in injury or death. Rat fighting should not be confused with wrestling behavior, which is affiliative play. When upset, rats can be imposing. They stiffen their bodies, arch their backs, wag their tails, and begin shaking with their hair standing on end to make them appear larger. Enrichment is an important component of housing to promote normal behaviors.

Dentistry

Because they have continuously growing incisors, if the teeth are not worn down by normal activity or if malocclusion is present, the incisors can overgrow, causing significant oral disease. This is easily identified on physical examination. Because the teeth have no nerve except at the base, they can be trimmed as needed by a veterinarian using a dental disc. Repeat trimming may be required if the underlying cause of the malocclusion cannot be resolved.

Biosecurity

Good general hygiene should offset any concerns about passage of disease from pet rats to humans.

Nutrition

Commercial pellet rations containing 20-27% protein formulated for small mammals are ideal because they are nutritionally complete and balanced. Treats specifically prepared for rats can be purchased. Other foods that can be offered but that should never make up any significant percentage of the animal's total food intake include apples, bananas, strawberries, melon, broccoli, carrots, squash, lean cooked meats, whole wheat bread, cooked beans, and yogurt. Rats should never be fed chocolate, alcohol, cabbage, high-fat or high-sugar human foods, or citrus fruits.

HAMSTERS

It is illegal in Hawaii to own a hamster. In California, it is illegal to own hamsters unless they are of the domesticated species (Syrian or dwarf hamster) and the laws are unclear regarding whether or not even those may be illegal in some municipalities.

Unique Anatomy and Biology

Biology of Hamsters

LIFE SPAN	18-24 months
TEMPERATURE	99-101°F (37-38°C)
PULSE	310-471 beats/minute
RESPIRATION	38-110 breaths/minute
REPRODUCTIVE MATURITY	puberty 42-70 days, breeding initiation 70-98 days

The most common hamster in the United States is the golden or Syrian hamster. They are 5-7" (13-18 cm) in length, with an average body weight of 4 oz (120 gm). Like mice, hamsters have 2 open-rooted (continuously growing) incisors with nerves only at the base, ability to draw the cheek folds into the diastema, and large masseter muscles that attach rostrally, giving them increased ability to gnaw. They have large cheek pouches that can be used for storage of food and bedding. They are obligate nose breathers. All hamsters have sebaceous glands on their flank, brown patches covered with fur that may appear wet and matted, especially in sexually aroused males.

Appearance of Hamsters

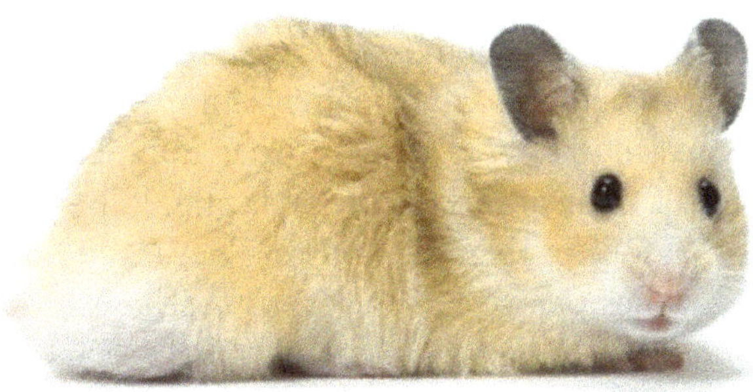

"Syrian hamster", https://hamsterpetcare.com/hamsters-care/types-of-hamsters/syrian-hamster-detailed-overview-9710.html

Gender identification is through increased anogenital distance in males, the presence of testes in males between the anus and genital papilla, and prominence of nipples in females.

Gender Identification in Hamsters

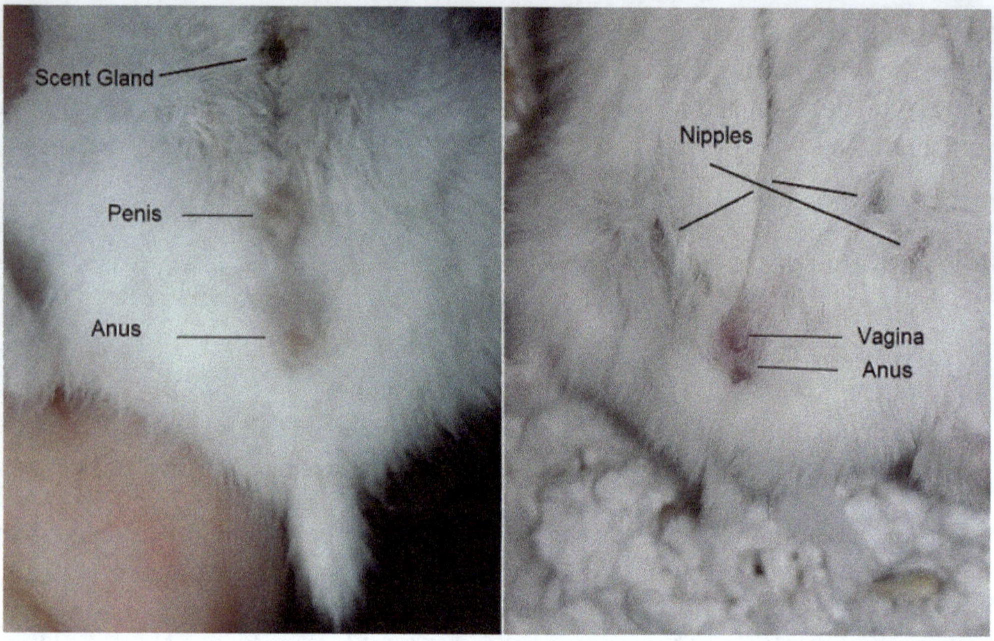

"Sexing dwarf hamsters", http://dwarfhamsterhome.com/sexing-dwarf-hamsters/

Specifics of anatomy and other information about hamsters and gerbils can be found in the Manual of Exotic Pet Practice, pp 406-432.

Housing

Hamsters are best housed alone. Hamster cages should be large enough to allow room for an exercise wheel and a place for the hamster to hide also should be provided. Simple wire cages are available in pet stores. Aquariums and custom-made hamster homes are also available; all cages should be gnaw-proof, as for other rodents. Clean fresh bedding can be paper confetti, paper strips, wood chips or shavings, ground corn cobs, hay, or straw. Corn cobs and wood shavings usually work the best because of their absorbency. Cedar should be avoided because the fumes may cause respiratory problems. Hamsters naturally hoard food; the cage should be cleaned 2-3 times per week to prevent the hamster eating old, moldy feed. Water bottles should be hung on the outside of the cage with a drinking tube extending into the cage through the side bars. This prevents the hamster from gnawing on the bottom of the water bottle and frees up space within the cage. If the water bottle is stored in the cage, it should be kept in a protective wire hanger. Hamsters prefer moderate temperatures around 70°F. If the temperature goes above 80°F, they go into a deep, sleep-like state known as estivation. This is how hamsters originally survived the hot, dry desert environment. If the temperature goes below 50°F, hamsters will hibernate. Lighting should be as for the rest of the household; a 12 hr light:dark cycle is preferred for most hamsters.

Vaccinations and Disease Control

There are no vaccines recommended for control of infectious disease in hamsters.

Parasite Control

Internal parasites of hamsters include protozoa, pinworms, and tapeworms. These can be identified on fecal flotation or by direct inspection. Treatment varies with specific worm identified. The most common external parasite of hamsters is the demodectic mange mite. Clinically normal hamsters can carry a small number of mites. Clinical disease may be seen as a secondary problem in older hamsters with other disease conditions. The signs of demodectic mange are a non-pruritic alopecia and scaling and crusting over the back and rump. Demodectic mange can be treated with ivermectin.

Behavior

Hamsters are nocturnal. Hamsters tend to be territorial and protective of food and it's not uncommon to see hoarding behavior in hamsters. They will hide food at one end of their habitat and reserve the other end for urinating and defecating. Hamsters are solitary creatures. Young can usually be kept together until they are about 5 weeks old; then they will begin to fight and need to be separated. Cannibalism may result if litters are left together for longer periods of time. Females only tolerate the male for breeding. Enrichment is an important component of housing to promote normal behaviors.

Dentistry

Because they have continuously growing incisors, if the teeth are not worn down by normal activity or if malocclusion is present, the incisors can overgrow, causing significant oral disease. This is easily identified on physical examination. Because the teeth have no nerve except at the base, they can be trimmed as needed by a veterinarian using a dental disc.

Biosecurity

Good general hygiene should offset any concerns about passage of disease from pet hamsters to humans.

Nutrition

The best way to feed a hamster is to purchase commercially prepared pellets that contain a minimum of 16% protein and 4-5% fat and are complete and balanced for hamsters. Other foods that can be offered but that should never make up any significant percentage of the animal's total food intake include most fruits and vegetables, cooked brown rice, and toast. Hamsters should never be fed chocolate, alcohol, onions, garlic, high-fat or high-sugar human foods, almonds, or citrus fruits. Uneaten soft-type foods must be removed before they spoil. Soft foods may get lodged in the cheek pouches of a hamster and become spoiled causing infection and illness.

GERBILS

Because they can damage crops and out-compete indigenous wildlife, it is illegal to have gerbils as pets in the state of California.

Unique Anatomy and Biology

Biology of Gerbils

LIFE SPAN	24-39 months
TEMPERATURE	100.4-102.2°F (38-39°C)
PULSE	260-600 beats/minute
RESPIRATION	85-160 breaths/minute
REPRODUCTIVE MATURITY	puberty 65-85 days, breeding initiation 70-85 days

The best known species is the Mongolian gerbil. On average, the Mongolian gerbil is 6-8" (15-20 cm) from tip of the nose to tip of the tail. Their bodies are 3-4" (7.5-10 cm) long and they weigh 3-4 oz (85-114 gm). Gerbils do not sweat and produce extremely concentrated urine. Gerbils have a hairless patch on their midventral abdomen that is a scent gland.

Appearance of Gerbils

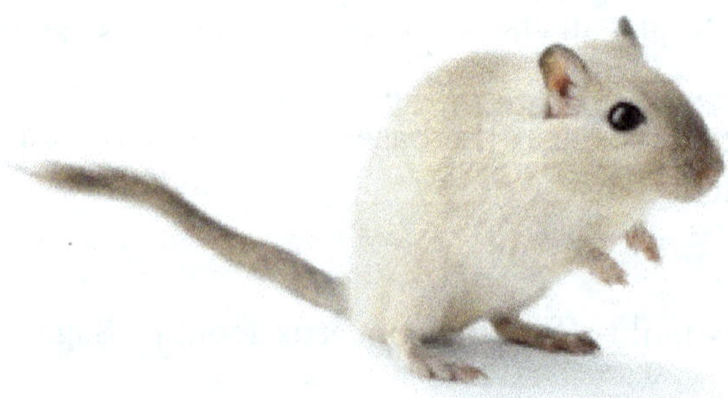

"Gerbils", https://www.omlet.co.uk/guide/gerbils/getting_a_gerbil/needs

Gender identification is by anogenital distance, which is longer in the male; by dark pigmentation of the scrotum; and by increased size of the scent gland in males and increased prominence of nipples in females.

Gender Identification in Gerbils

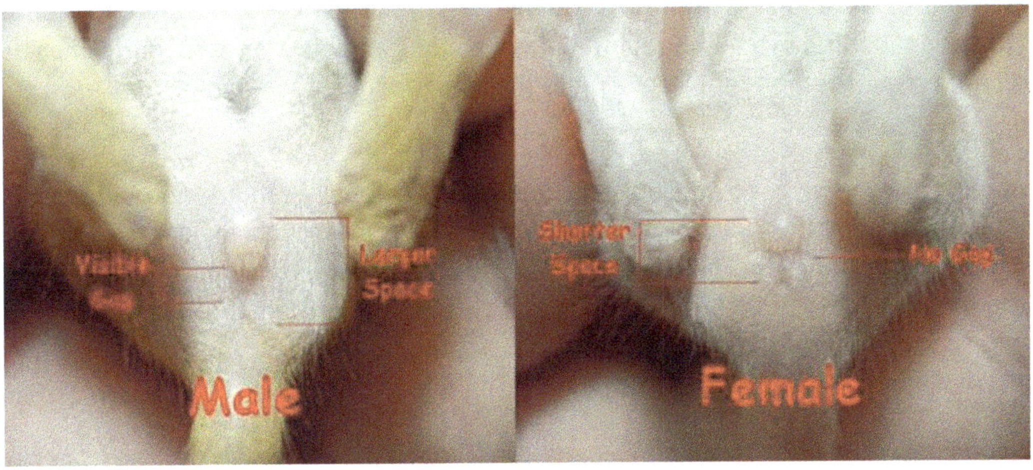

"Male vs. female gerbils", http://gerbilforum.proboards.com/thread/23303/gerbil

Specifics of anatomy and other information about hamsters and gerbils can be found in the Manual of Exotic Pet Practice, pp 406-432.

Housing

Most hamster housing is also appropriate for gerbils. Because of their highly concentrated urine, the ideal habitat for gerbils is an aquarium. It is important that the enclosure have a lid to prevent the gerbil from jumping out. Gerbils require enrichment like hamsters but caution should be used with exercise wheels, which may be associated with degloving injuries of the tail or limb fractures. Running wheels should be solid, not mesh. Gerbils also may use a sandy area in a cage for environmental enrichment. Gerbils are social animals and can be housed in pairs or family groups. If necessary, gerbils can get most of their daily water requirement from their food. Although they can survive without, free access to water is recommended. Temperature and lighting are as for hamsters. Relative humidity is best kept at less than 50%.

Vaccinations and Disease Control

There are no vaccines recommended for control of infectious disease in gerbils.

Parasite Control

There are virtually no clinically significant internal parasites routinely diagnosed in gerbils. Gerbils can suffer from demodectic mange as described for hamsters.

Behavior

Mongolian gerbils are diurnal, active during the day. Gerbils are very quiet animals. The young can be heard making squeaking noises, but the sounds diminish as they age. Gerbils communicate by drumming or pounding with their rear feet. This sound is also used as an alarm and by the male during mating. Gerbils commonly leave their scent behind by rubbing their abdomen along an object or area. Enrichment is an important component of housing to promote normal behaviors.

Dentistry

Because they have continuously growing incisors, if the teeth are not worn down by normal activity or if malocclusion is present, the incisors can overgrow, causing significant oral disease. This is easily identified on physical examination. Because the teeth have no nerve except at the base, they can be trimmed as needed by a veterinarian using a dental disc.

Biosecurity

Good general hygiene should offset any concerns about passage of disease from pet gerbils to humans.

Nutrition

The best way to feed a gerbil is to purchase commercially prepared pellets that contain a minimum of at least 20% protein and 4-5% fat and are complete and balanced for gerbils. Other foods that can be offered but that should never make up any significant percentage of the animal's total food intake include apples, pears, bananas, carrots, celery, peas, cucumbers, cooked potato, and plain popcorn. Gerbils should never be fed chocolate, alcohol, spinach, lettuce, or citrus fruits.

GUINEA PIGS

Unique Anatomy and Biology

Biology of Guinea Pigs

LIFE SPAN	5-7 years
TEMPERATURE	99-103.1°F (37.2-39.5°C)
PULSE	240-350 beats/minute
RESPIRATION	40-150 breaths/minute
REPRODUCTIVE MATURITY	puberty 6 weeks, breeding initiation 10 weeks

Adult guinea pigs reach a length of 8-10" (20-25 cm) and weigh 1-2 lb (450-900 gm). Males are larger and have larger, more rounded heads than females. The body of the guinea pig is short, stocky in build, with short legs. The nose of the guinea pig is short, blunt, and rounded. They have a small mouth with a split upper lip. There are long whiskers on the sides of the upper lip that function in the same way that cat whiskers do, allowing the animal to travel in dim light. The ears are short with little fur. Guinea pigs have very sensitive hearing and can detect frequencies beyond the range of the human ear. All of their teeth are open-rooted including the molars. Like all other rodents, they are obligate nose breathers.

Appearance of Guinea Pigs

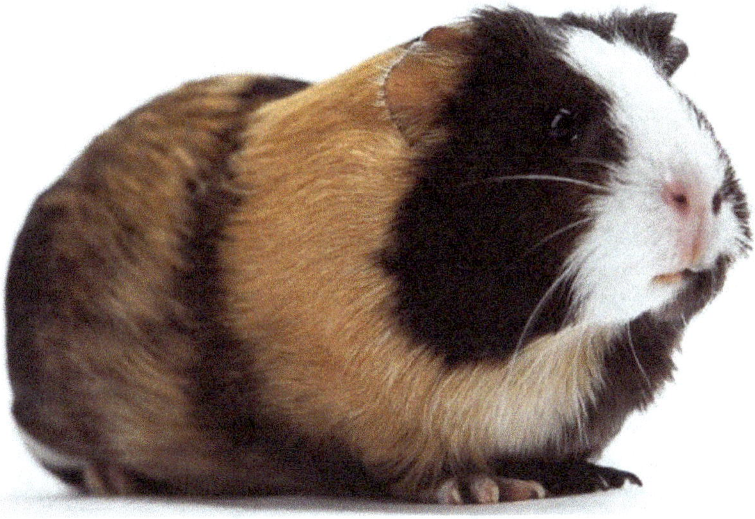

"Guinea pigs", https://www.vetcarepethospital.ca/beginners-guide-to-guinea-pig-care/

Gender identification may be done in several ways. Methods include determination of anogenital distance as in other species, examination of the genitalia itself (urethral opening a single point and area raised in males, urethral opening a slit and area flush with the surrounding skin in females), and identification of large testes to either side of the anus.

Gender Identification in Guinea Pigs

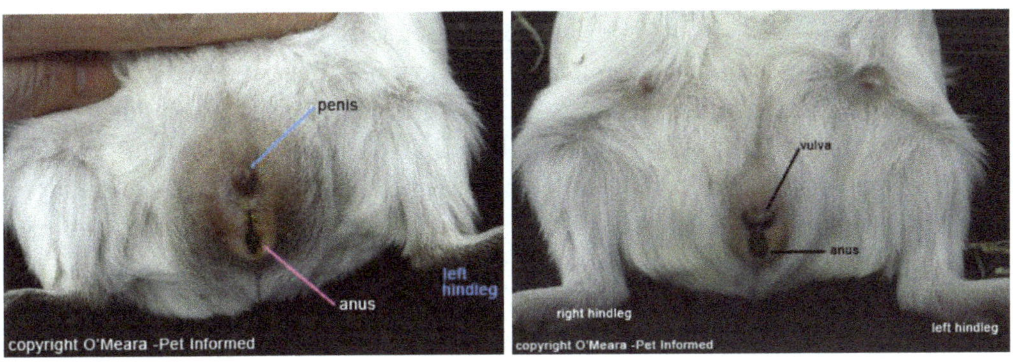

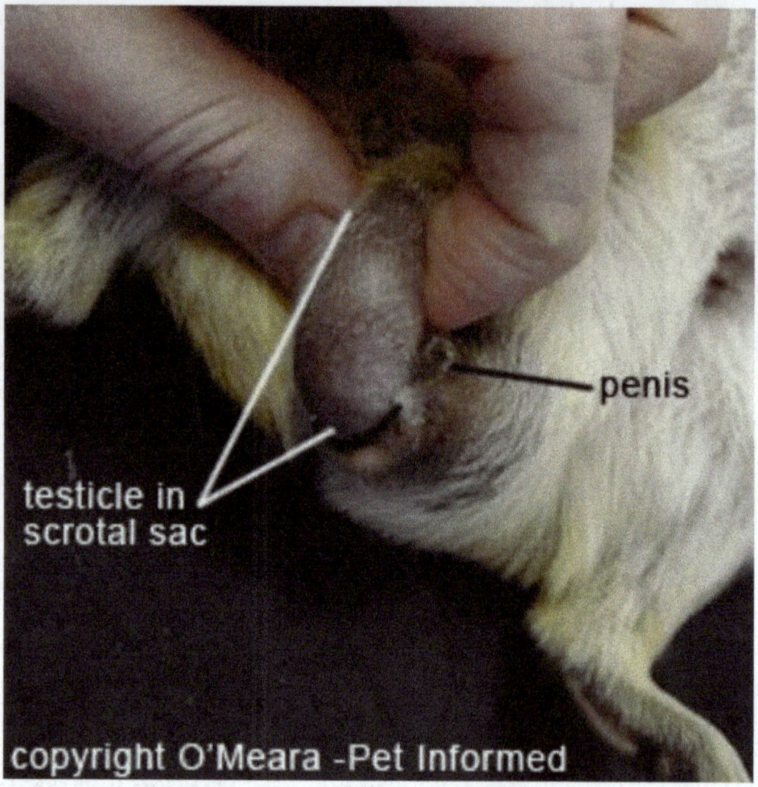

"Male vs. female guinea pigs", http://www.pet-informed-veterinary-advice-online.com/sexing-guinea-pigs.html

Specifics of anatomy and other information about guinea pigs can be found in the Manual of Exotic Pet Practice, pp 456-473.

Housing

A typical cage has a solid bottom that is 3-4" deep with vertical bars made of wire. The plastic bottom should be removable for cleaning. Deeper trays keep animals from scattering bedding or shavings out of the cage. Cages do not need covers or tops because guinea pigs don't usually climb. Appropriate bedding includes recycled newspaper products, shredded paper, and aspen shavings. Cedar and pine shavings should not be used as they may be a respiratory irritant. Cages should be cleaned 1-2 times weekly and sanitized at least once every 2 weeks. Guinea pigs will defecate into their feed and water. For this reason, an elevated feeder and vacuum-type water bottle are recommended. In the summer, guinea pigs can be kept outside once temperatures are above 50°F. Small houses, like dog houses, can be constructed to keep animals safe and protected from the elements. Outdoor housing should be portable so it can be moved when grass becomes trampled or eaten. Guinea pigs should never be housed in areas with temperature greater than 80°F or in areas of high humidity as they are susceptible to hyperthermia.

Vaccinations and Disease Control

There are no vaccines recommended for control of infectious disease in guinea pigs. However, if guinea pigs are kept in households with dogs or cats, vaccination against *Bordetella bronchiseptica* is recommended as they are susceptible and are exquisitely sensitive to contracting it.

Some husbandry that can help prevent disease in guinea pigs includes brushing and nail trimming. Guinea pigs should be brushed regularly. A guinea pig with rosettes and long hair will need to have the hair combed out in addition to brushing. Long-haired animals may also need their hair clipped around the rear to prevent matting and soiling. Guinea pigs can be bathed with a mild shampoo, for example baby shampoo. Guinea pig toenails grow constantly and need to be trimmed with regular pet toenail clippers.

Parasite Control

Internal parasites, including roundworms and coccidia, are found uncommonly in guinea pigs. External parasites, including mites, lice, and fleas, may be more commonly seen and are easily identified by inspection and treated as in other species.

Behavior

Guinea pigs are neither completely diurnal nor completely nocturnal but instead show periods of activity and sleep throughout the day. Guinea pigs may be housed in groups but two males are unlikely to live peacefully in an enclosure. In general, guinea pigs are social and respond to the activity around them with a variety of vocalizations. Enrichment is an important component of housing to promote normal behaviors.

Dentistry

Because they have continuously growing incisors and molars, if the teeth are not worn down by normal activity or if malocclusion is present, the teeth can overgrow, causing significant oral disease. Teeth can grow at a rate of up to 2 mm/week. The open-rooted molars also are predisposed to dental caries and subsequent infection. This is easily identified on physical examination but complete evaluation may require sedation and treatment requires general anesthesia. Dental radiographs may be required for complete evaluation and treatment may include trimming as in other rodents or floating to remove sharp points, as is done in horses.

Biosecurity

Good general hygiene should offset any concerns about passage of disease from pet guinea pigs to humans.

Sterilization

Elective ovariohysterectomy or ovariectomy may be performed in female guinea pigs (sows) for reproduction control. The surgery is performed as in dogs and cats, with specific care taken to avoid the large cecum on entering the abdomen, and not to tear the ovarian vessels by placing undue tension while attempting to exteriorize the ovaries. Elective orchiectomy (castration) is performed in male guinea pigs (boars) either for reproduction control or to minimize reproductive behaviors. The surgery is performed as in cats and it is required that the inguinal canal be closed on each side to prevent herniation of abdominal contents. Skin incisions are closed with suture or tissue glue.

Nutrition

High-quality hay should be available at all times. Alfalfa hay is appropriate for young guinea pigs and for pregnant sows. Timothy hay and orchard grass are appropriate for grown animals. A commercial pelleted diet formulated specifically for guinea pigs should be provided as well but should not be the primary diet as that commonly causes obesity. Fresh vegetables should make up the rest of the diet. Fruits and grains also can be provided but should never be more than 10% of the diet. Good supplementary foods for guinea pigs include bell peppers, parsley, kale, broccoli, Brussels sprouts, romaine lettuce, carrots, dandelion greens, apples, cantaloupe, and oranges. Guinea pigs cannot manufacture their own vitamin C. Vitamin C in pelleted food or offered in water breaks down quickly and provision of foods high in vitamin C or vitamin C supplements is recommended. Foods you should never give to a guinea pig include beans, rhubarb, dill, flowers, and the pits, cores or seeds of fruits.

CHINCHILLAS

Unique Anatomy and Biology

Biology of Chinchillas

LIFE SPAN	8-10 years, with some pets recorded to live up to 20 years
TEMPERATURE	100.5-102.2°F (38-39°C)
PULSE	100-200 beats per minute
RESPIRATION	40-80 breaths/minute
REPRODUCTIVE MATURITY	puberty 7-9 months, breeding initiation 7-9 months

Chinchillas resemble small rabbits with short ears and a short, bushy tail. Chinchillas range from 9-15" (23-38 cm) long with a tail of 3-10" (7.5-25 cm), and weigh from 1 to 2 lb (400-700 gm). Their thick, shiny fur is about 1" long; the most common color of chinchillas is blue-grey. The softness of the fur is due to the fewer number of guard hairs as compared with those of fur-bearing animals. Chinchillas usually shed about every 3 months. New growth starts at the neck and progresses toward the rear of the animal. The head is broad with large ears and eyes. They have very long, stiff whiskers.

Appearance of Chinchillas

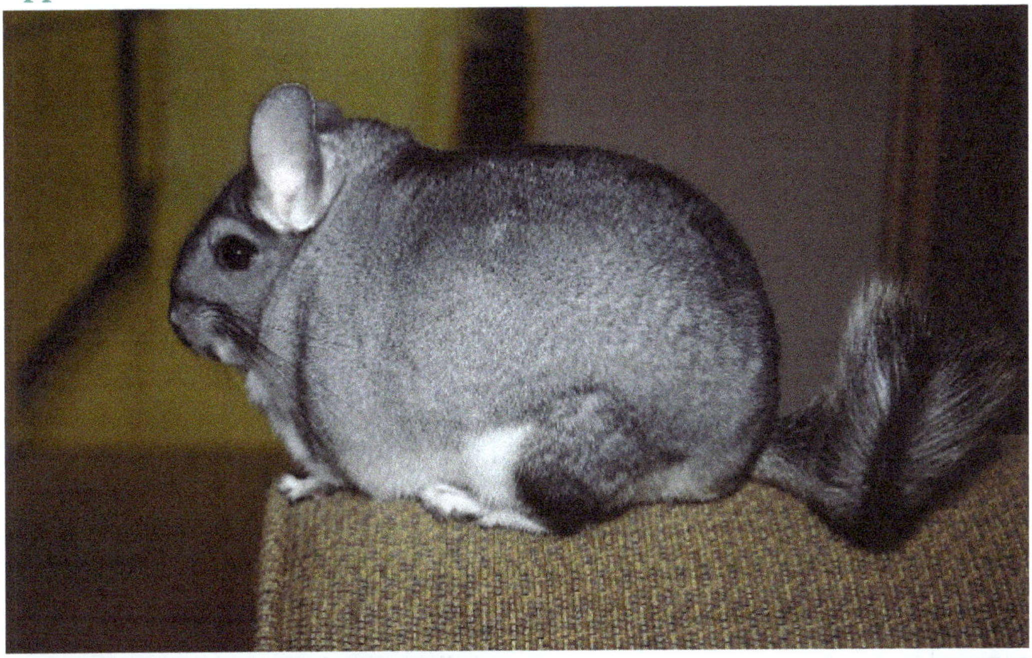

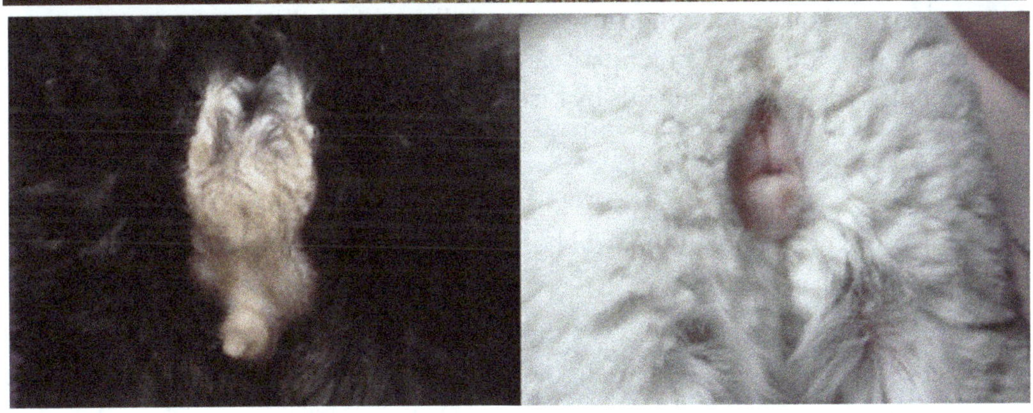

"Long-Tailed Chinchilla", https://en.wikipedia.org/wiki/Long-tailed_chinchilla

Gender identification is through anogenital distance, which is much longer in males than in females. The male below is shown on the left.

Gender Identification of Chinchillas

"Male vs. female chinchillas", http://furrytails-en.blogspot.com/2011/07/sexing-1-day-old-chinchilla-kits.html

Specifics of anatomy and other information about chinchillas can be found in the Manual of Exotic Pet Practice, pp 474-492.

Housing

Chinchillas require a relatively large enclosure with specific areas for eating, sleeping, exercising, and urinating / defecating. An area for animals to hide should be included. Chinchillas live in groups in the wild and benefit from housing with at least one other chinchilla. Dust baths should be made available as described below in the behavior section. Enclosures may have more than one level with ladders to encourage exercise. Cages should be made of metal and wire; plastic and wood will be quickly chewed through. Wire mesh is not recommended for flooring. Wood shavings and ground corn cobs are ideal bedding. Hay and straw should not be used as they may become moldy or stain fur. The enclosure should be cleaned twice weekly. Clean water should be provided in glass sipper bottles. Temperature should be kept at less than 80°F and humidity at a comfortable level for humans, as chinchillas suffer heat prostration / hyperthermia if maintained in higher environmental temperatures, especially if humidity is high.

Vaccinations and Disease Control

There are no vaccines recommended for control of infectious disease in chinchillas.

Parasite Control

Internal parasites are uncommon in pet chinchillas. Chinchillas can carry *Giardia* sp. without signs of disease. Chinchillas can be infested with fleas and mites but this is uncommon in pets. Diagnosis is by direct inspection and treatment is as in other species.

Behavior

Chinchillas are nocturnal in the wild but can adapt to a diurnal lifestyle as pets.

Chinchillas need regular baths to remove excess moisture and oil. They do not bathe in water, but in finely ground powder. In the wild, chinchillas bathe in volcanic ash of the Andes Mountains. A similar powder is available for purchase from pet stores. Chinchillas can be bathed in a small pan with 2-3" inches of powder. The pan needs to be large enough for the animal to roll around in. The powder can be used several times.

Fur chewing is a common problem of chinchillas. The animal chews the fur on the flanks leaving patches of short hair. Poor nutrition, small cages, drafty conditions, boredom, and high humidity are thought to play a role in fur chewing. Providing enough space and environmental enrichment along with a balanced diet should resolve fur chewing. Enrichment is an important component of housing to promote normal behaviors.

Dentistry

Because they have continuously growing incisors and molars, if the teeth are not worn down by normal activity or if malocclusion is present, the teeth can overgrow, causing significant oral disease. Teeth can grow at a rate of up to 2 mm/week. The open-rooted molars also are predisposed to dental caries and subsequent infection. This is easily identified on physical examination but complete evaluation requires sedation and treatment requires general anesthesia. Dental radiographs may be required for complete evaluation and treatment may include trimming as in other rodents or floating to remove sharp points, as is done in horses. The open-rooted molars also can overgrow into the jaw, causing pain and inappetance. Radiographs are used to diagnose this progressive condition, which has a very poor prognosis.

Biosecurity

Good general hygiene should offset any concerns about passage of disease from pet chinchillas to humans.

Sterilization

Elective ovariohysterectomy or ovariectomy may be performed in female chinchillas for reproduction control. The surgery is performed as in dogs and cats, with specific care taken to avoid the large cecum on entering the abdomen, and not to tear the ovarian vessels by placing undue tension while attempting to exteriorize the ovaries. Elective orchiectomy (castration) is performed in male chinchillas either for reproduction control or to minimize reproductive behaviors. The surgery is performed as in cats and it is required that the inguinal canal be closed on each side to prevent herniation of abdominal contents. Skin incisions are closed with suture or tissue glue.

Nutrition

Various pelleted foods are available today for chinchillas. These pellets consist primarily of ground alfalfa hay, corn gluten, corn tailings, wheat germ, and bran, with 16-20% protein, 2-5% fat, and 15-35% fiber. Commercially prepared foods are nutritionally complete. Chinchillas can be sensitive to dietary changes and any changes should be made gradually. Chinchillas are "hind gut" fermenters, producing cecal pellets that are reingested (coprophagy). Chinchillas also can be offered high-quality timothy or orchard grass hay and dark leafy vegetables, such as romaine lettuce and collard or mustard greens. Very occasionally, chinchillas can be offered dried or fresh apple, banana, peach, or pear, prunes, and carrot. Chinchillas should be not offered high-fat or high-sugar human treats, chocolate, corn, or acidic fruits.

EXTRA RESOURCES

Common disorders of rats and mice: http://www.merckvetmanual.com/exotic-and-laboratory-animals/rodents/mice-and-rats-as-pets

Common disorders of hamsters: http://www.merckvetmanual.com/exotic-and-laboratory-animals/rodents/hamsters

Common disorders of gerbils: http://www.merckvetmanual.com/exotic-and-laboratory-animals/rodents/gerbils

Common disorders of guinea pigs: http://www.merckvetmanual.com/exotic-and-laboratory-animals/rodents/guinea%20pigs

Common disorders of chinchillas: http://www.merckvetmanual.com/exotic-and-laboratory-animals/rodents/chinchillas

American Fancy Rat and Mouse Association: http://www.afrma.org/caresheet.htm

California Hamster Association: http://www.chahamsters.org/newsletter.html

American Gerbil Association: http://www.agsgerbils.org/

American Cavy Breeders Association: http://www.acbaonline.com/

Guinea Pigs Club: http://guineapigsclub.com/

National Chinchilla Society: http://www.natchinsoc.co.uk/

The Manual of Exotic Pet Practice: http://www.sciencedirect.com/science/book/9781416001195

CHAPTER-16

MAMMALS II / MARSUPIALS

FERRETS

California and Hawaii prohibit importation and possession of ferrets as pets. Other states may require special permits. Some local governments prohibit ownership of ferrets including New York City, Dallas/Fort Worth, and Washington, DC. Potential owners should check local and state laws before adopting or purchasing ferrets.

UNIQUE ANATOMY AND BIOLOGY

Biology of Ferrets

LIFE SPAN	5-8 years
TEMPERATURE	100.0-104.0°F (38-40°C)
PULSE	180-250 beats per minute
RESPIRATION	33-36 breaths/minute
REPRODUCTIVE MATURITY	6-12 months; virtually all pet ferrets in the United States are neutered

Ferrets are mustelids, with long, lean, slender, muscular bodies with short legs. Ferrets have oval-shaped heads and pointed snouts. Their ears are small and rounded. Ferrets have bright, clear eyes, but their sight is not well-developed. They have highly developed senses of hearing, smell, and touch. Both sexes develop a strong musky odor at maturity. Spaying or castrating, along with removal of the anal glands, can help reduce the odor; virtually all ferrets available for sale as pets in the United States are spayed / castrated. Glands in the skin also cause a musky scent.

Ferrets are unable to sweat and use changes in body posture in the environment to dissipate body heat. The fur of ferrets is dense and very soft. They change coats completely twice a year.

The heart is connected to the sternum with a ligament that often contains fat, which gives the heart a raised appearance on a lateral radiographic view. The trachea is large and the lung capacity is increased, with an increase in airway length commensurate with total body length. The intestinal tract is relatively short and the liver is relatively large. Gender identification in ferrets is as in dogs. Male ferrets (hobs) have a penis on the ventral midline of the abdomen; the penis contains a small bone, the os penis. Female ferrets (jills) have a vulva caudal and ventral to the anus. Males are usually about twice the size of females, with the average male weighing 2.2-4.4 lb (1-2 kg) and the average female weighing 1.1-2.2 lb (0.5-1 kg). Ferrets are about 18" (45 cm) in length.

Housing

An indoor cage can be provided, preferably with a solid or wire floor and wire sides, not glass. Ferrets can be housed individually but ideally are housed in pairs or groups. Ferrets need a place to hide and sleep and a place to urinate / defecate. Ferrets can be taught to use litter boxes. They prefer relieving themselves in corners. A litter box should be placed in the corner of the cage away from the food and sleep areas. Whenever left out of the cage, a litter box should be available in the room.

Ferrets are curious and can get into surprisingly small spaces. If ferrets are permitted to roam free, areas that should be blocked off include behind large appliances or immovable pieces of furniture and inside recliners.

Ferrets can be maintained outdoors but cannot tolerate temperatures below 20°F or above 90°F (< -6°C or above 32°C).

Vaccinations and Disease Control

Ferrets should be vaccinated against canine distemper virus and rabies virus. Specific vaccines approved for use in ferrets are available in the United States. Ferrets are vaccinated against distemper no earlier than 8 weeks of age, and again at about 12 and 16 weeks of age, and then annually. Ferrets are vaccinated against rabies at 12-16 weeks of age and then annually. Vaccines can be given subcutaneously; some municipalities require that rabies vaccines be given intramuscularly.

Ferrets have non-retractable claws that require regular trimming.

Parasite Control

Intestinal parasites are uncommon in pet ferrets. Ferrets presenting with diarrhea should be checked for coccidia and *Giardia* sp. and treated appropriately. Ferrets housed outside may become infested with fleas; diagnosis and treatment is as in other species. Ferrets also can pass ear mites between themselves. These are evidenced by presence of heavy brown discharge in the ears, which can be examined microscopically to identify the mites. The ears are cleaned and treated topically. Ferrets housed outdoors also may be more susceptible to heartworm, as it is carried by mosquitoes. Advantage Multi is a parasite control product recently approved by the FDA for use in ferrets that can be used as a heartworm preventative.

Behavior

Ferrets are not nocturnal but do sleep about 75% of the time. Ferrets have tough skin and while playing often bite one another. This playful bite can be painful to humans. Discipline for play biting should include a firm "no" until the ferret learns the behavior is not acceptable. As described under housing, ferrets are curious and should be carefully supervised when not enclosed. Enrichment is an important component of housing to promote normal behaviors.

Dentistry

Ferrets will develop dental tartar with subsequent gingivitis. This may be more common in ferrets fed primarily a soft diet and should be addressed with a dental cleaning by a veterinarian.

Biosecurity

Good general hygiene should offset any concerns about passage of disease from pet ferrets to humans. Ferrets are susceptible to influenza, so humans sick with the flu should avoid contact with their ferrets until they are no longer contagious. Ferrets are considered to be more susceptible to infection with COVID-19 than many other species but the CDC does not consider ferrets to pose a significant transmission threat to humans.

Nutrition

Ferrets are carnivores. Ferret food should be high in animal protein (30-40%), high in fat (18-30%), and low in fiber. Dry commercial ferret food is recommended. If a commercial ferret food is not available dry kitten chow can be used. Regular dog and cat chow, which often contains a high percentage of plant-based protein, should be avoided. Treats should be given in moderation and should be meat-based. Meat baby food, cooked meat scraps, jerky, and cracklings are appropriate. Although ferrets love raisins, dates and other sugary treats, they should not be given to ferrets because they promote tooth decay and can lead to pancreatic dysfunction. Bones should never be given as treats. Ferrets prefer to eat multiple small meals per day and will hide excess food.

Ferrets require about three times as much water as dry matter. Fresh water should be offered in more than one location and, ideally, in more than one manner. For example, water may be offered in a sipper bottle in the cage and in a crockery bowl elsewhere.

RABBITS

Unique Anatomy and Biology

Biology of Rabbits

LIFE SPAN	6-13 years
TEMPERATURE	100.0-103.0°F (38-39°C)
PULSE	130-325 beats per minute
RESPIRATION	32-60 breaths/minute
REPRODUCTIVE MATURITY	and sexual maturity 4-5 months for small breeds, 5-8 months for large breeds

There are many breeds of rabbit. Rabbits can be classified by size, by fur type, or by body type. Small breeds, those weighing less than 4-5 lb (2 kg), include the Netherland dwarf, mini-lop, and Dutch breeds. Medium breeds, those weighing 5-10 lb (2-5 kg), include the rex, English, Angora and Belgium breeds. Large to giant breeds are those weighing more than 10-11 lb (5 kg) and include New Zealand whites, English lops, British giants, and Flemish giants. Body types also can be used to classify breeds of rabbit. The commercial body type is most commonly seen in production and meat animals. These rabbits grow fast and tend to have large meaty loins. An example of this type is the New Zealand. The compact body rabbits are similar to the commercial type, only smaller. Example breeds are the American fuzzy lop and the small or dwarf breeds. There is only one representative of the cylindrical body type recognized by the American Rabbit Breeders Association, the Himalayan. The British Rabbit Council also recognizes a second breed, the Vienna. Cylindrical shaped rabbits show a straight top line with no arch. The profile shows no taper. Fully arched rabbits are built for agility and speed and resemble hares, which is where most of the bloodline comes from. The arch starts at the neck and goes right down to the tail. When viewed from the side, there's space under the belly. The semi-arch body type is common in the largest of rabbit breeds including the Flemish giant.

Rabbits have very delicate skin that can easily be torn when clipping, as for pre-operative preparation. Rabbits do not have footpads but instead have thick fur on their feet to protect them from the environment.

Rabbits' large ears are used for hearing and for thermoregulation. Rabbits have good vision but cannot see directly below their nose, relying on their stiff whiskers to identify things in the area of their mouth. Rabbits are obligate nose-breathers and have a relatively small thoracic cavity.

The skeleton of rabbits is very light and they are very muscular. This predisposes them to vertebral injury and long bone fractures. Unlike rodents, rabbits have four maxillary incisors, two large central incisors with two smaller incisors, the peg teeth, behind them. Dentistry is described below.

The large cecum of rabbits provides anaerobic fermentation of plant foods; the cecum has a capacity roughly ten times that of the stomach in rabbits. Cecal pellets are passed through the rectum and immediately re-ingested for further breakdown (coprophagy). Rabbits excrete excess calcium through the kidneys and so may have turbid urine. Color of the urine varies from yellow to red, depending on their diet.

Gender Identification in Rabbits

Gender identification is by protrusion of the penis in males. Hold the rabbit as shown below. Hold the tail with two fingers and put pressure beneath the anogenital orifice with the thumb. Pull on the tail gently but firmly and press downward on the area of the vent.

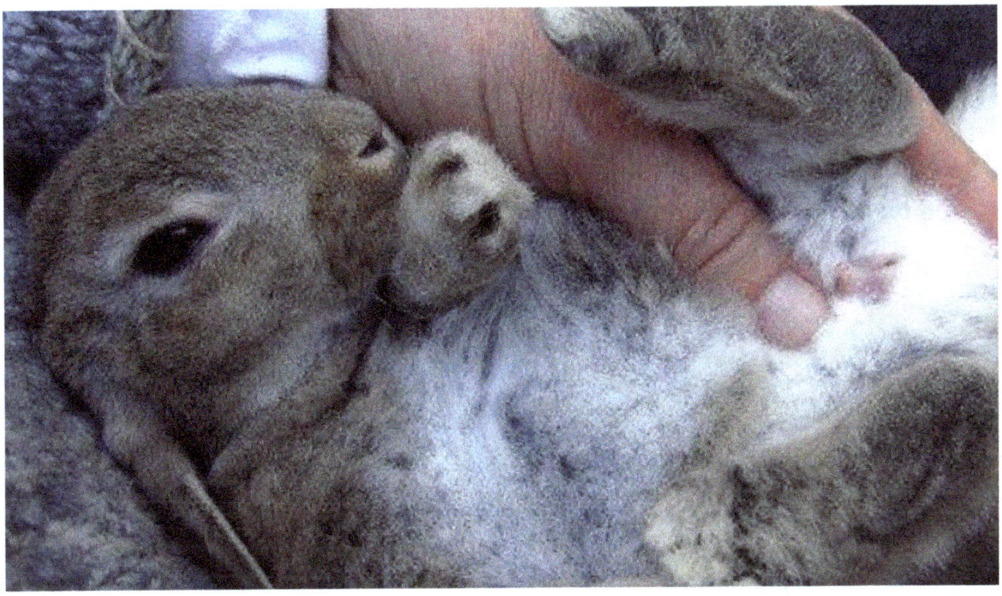

In the picture below, the tubular structure with a circular opening is the penis. In adult males, there also will be grayish areas running parallel to the long axis of the bunny on either side of the vent; these are the scrotal sacs. Inguinal canals are open throughout the male rabbit's life, so the testes can readily be drawn back into the abdomen.

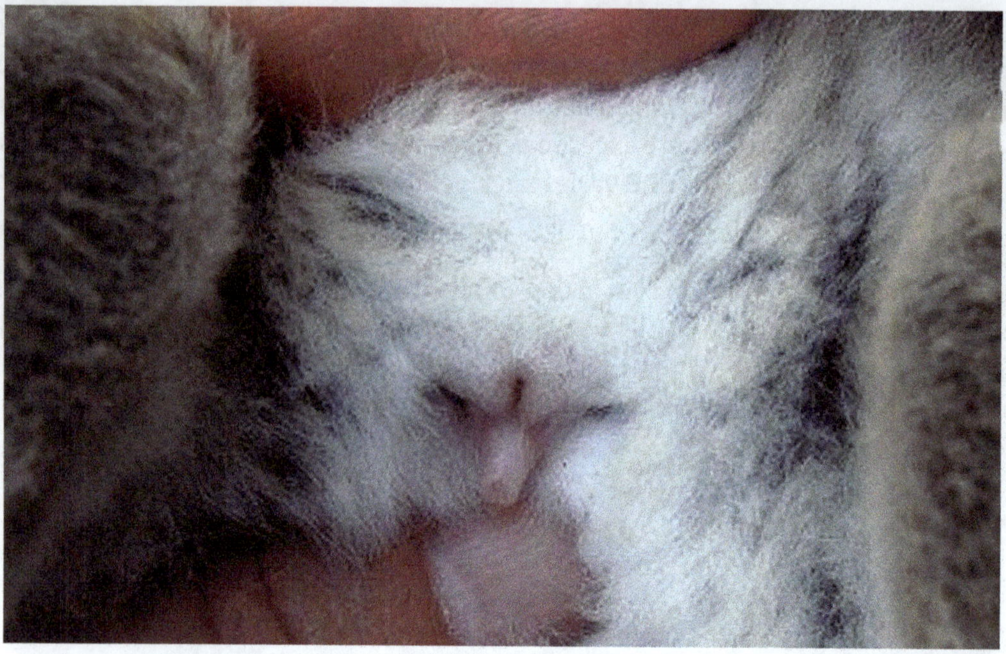

The picture below is a doe; pressure on the vent causes minimal protrusion of tissue, with a slit on it.

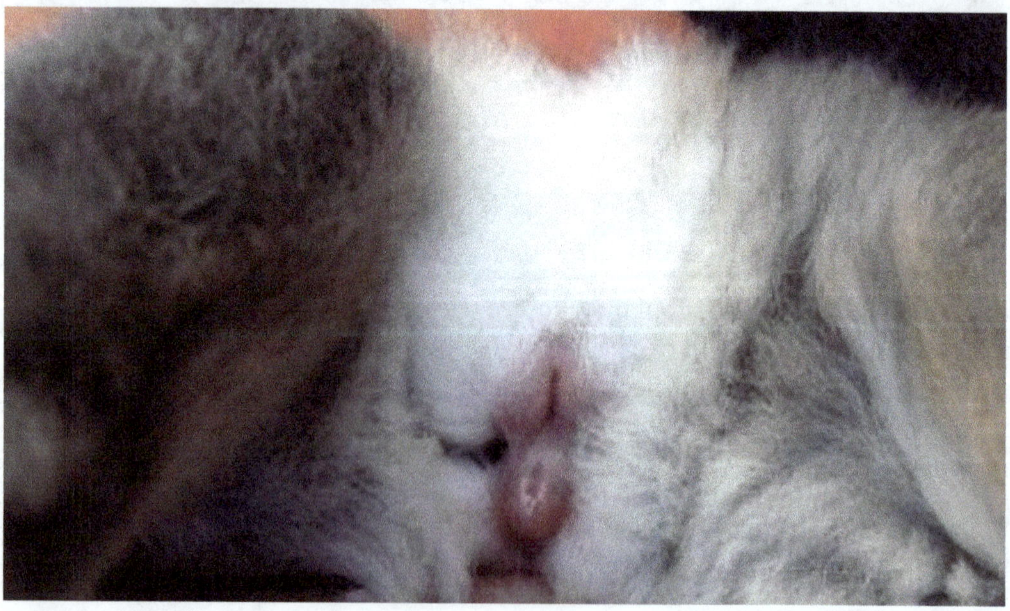

"Male vs. female rabbits", http://www.raising-rabbits.com

Specifics of anatomy and other information about rabbits can be found in the Manual of Exotic Pet Practice, pp 375-405.

Housing

The size of the hutch depends on the size of the rabbit and should include areas for sleeping, eating, and urination / defecation. Rabbits can be housed alone but ideally are housed in pairs or groups. If rabbits are to be housed in the hutch with no outdoor exercise, the hutch must also be large enough to permit the rabbit to exercise within it. The cage should be tall enough for the rabbit to sit upright without its ears hitting the top of the cage. Wire cages, including wire floors, can be used for most breeds, however, heavier rabbits should be kept on solid floors to prevent injury to the feet. Wire mesh should be an appropriate size to ensure that the rabbit's toes are not caught within mesh on the floor. All cages should include an area of solid flooring for resting. Hutches with solid floors where the rabbit will directly contact the bedding should contain timothy or grass hay, or another absorbent material. Wood shavings generally are not recommended. Urine and feces should be cleaned from the hutch daily and completely fresh bedding provided once or twice weekly. Rabbits can be trained to use a litter box. Fresh water should be available at all times in a sipper bottle or heavy crockery dish that cannot be tipped.

Rabbits are best housed at an ambient temperature from 60-75°F and humidity from 30-60%. They can tolerate colder temperatures if acclimatized and provided an enclosed shelter, however, they do not tolerate heat well.

Vaccinations and Disease Control

There are no vaccines recommended for control of infectious disease in pet rabbits.

Parasite Control

The most common internal parasite of rabbits is coccidia, of the *Eimeria* sp. These can be diagnosed on fecal examination and treated as in other species. Rabbits housed outside may become infested with fleas; diagnosis and treatment is as in other species. Ear mites also are common if the hutch is at ground level as the rabbit may have contact with wild rabbits.

Behavior

Rabbits prefer to eat in the afternoon and evening and should drink a fair amount of water every day, up to 100 ml/kg/day. Rabbits unsupervised indoors will chew and may damage furniture and woodwork or chew on electrical cords.

Male rabbits kept together may fight. Female siblings maturing together show less aggressive behavior towards one another than other rabbits. When fearful or aroused, rabbits may thump with one rear foot and may spray urine. Rabbits may pull fur from themselves or others and chew it. Fur-chewing is thought to be caused by boredom, a low fiber diet, or some unidentified nutritional deficiency. Increasing fiber seems to be effective in preventing fur chewing. Enrichment is an important component of housing to promote normal behaviors.

Dentistry

Rabbits are predisposed to dental disease by congenital malocclusion or by poor diet, without adequate wear on the continuously erupting incisors. Signs of dental disease include lack of appetite, dropping food from the mouth while chewing, and drooling. Overgrowth of incisors is easily visible on physical examination but overgrown cheek teeth require additional examination techniques. Because rabbits have a small oral cavity, complete evaluation of cheek teeth may require the use of an otoscope with a large diameter cone, sedation and passage of a speculum, and/or dental radiographs. Overgrown incisors and molars can be corrected as in other herbivore species, using a high-speed trimming dental burr or dental disc. Malocclusion is seldom "cured" by trimming and additional visits for further dental care may be needed for the life of the animal.

Biosecurity

Good general hygiene should offset any concerns about passage of disease from pet rabbits to humans.

Sterilization

Anesthesia in rabbits may be difficult due to problems with placement of endotracheal tubes for gas anesthesia. Elective ovariohysterectomy or ovariectomy may be performed in female rabbits (does) for reproduction control. Elective ovariohysterectomy should be performed in does before they reach 2 years of age to decrease incidence of uterine adenocarcinoma, a common and high morbidity tumor in many rabbit breeds. The surgery is performed as in dogs and cats, with specific care taken to avoid the large cecum on entering the abdomen, and not to tear the ovarian vessels by placing undue tension while attempting to exteriorize the ovaries. Does have a cervix at the caudal end of each uterine horn; each horn generally is ligated and transected just cranial to the cervix. Elective orchiectomy (castration) is performed in male rabbits (bucks) either for reproduction control or to minimize reproductive behaviors. The surgery can be performed either as in dogs or cats and it is required that the inguinal canal be closed on each side to prevent herniation of abdominal contents. Skin incisions are closed with buried suture or tissue glue.

Nutrition

The primary component of a rabbit's diet should be high-quality timothy or grass hay, which should be offered ad lib. Rabbits also should receive a small amount of commercially-prepared, timothy-hay rabbit pellets (less than 18% protein and 18-22% fiber) and about 1 cup of dark leafy greens daily. Types of greens includes romaine lettuce, unsprayed dandelion greens, parsley, and the tops of carrots, beets, and turnips. Rabbits do not naturally eat root vegetables and should not be given carrots, beets, or other root vegetables, which are relatively high in sugar.

HEDGEHOGS

Ownership of hedgehogs is illegal in the states of Arizona, California, Georgia, Hawaii, Maine, and Pennsylvania and in Washington DC and all five boroughs of New York City.

UNIQUE ANATOMY AND BIOLOGY

Biology of Hedgehogs

LIFE SPAN	3-8 years
TEMPERATURE	97-99°F (36-37°C)
PULSE	180-280 beats per minute
RESPIRATION	25-50 breaths/minute
REPRODUCTIVE MATURITY	puberty 6-8 months, breeding initiation 2-6 months

Gender identification is through anogenital distance, which is much longer in males than in females. The male below is shown on the left.

Gender Identification of Chinchillas

“Male vs. female chinchillas”, http://furrytails-en.blogspot.com/2011/07/sexing-1-day-old-chinchilla-kits.html

The most common hedgehog variety kept as a pet in the United States is descended from African species and is called the African pygmy hedgehog. These animals are 7-10” (18-25.5 cm) long and weigh 9-25 oz (255-708 gm). They have a long snout, four digits on each foot, and 36 teeth. They have unique musculature that permits them to roll into an almost complete ball with the spines facing outwards, for defense.

Appearance of Hedgehogs

The most notable characteristic of hedgehogs are the spines that the animal has developed as a means of defense. The spines cover the back, sides, and the crown of the head; the face, forehead, chest and underside are covered with hair. The spines are modified hairs made of keratin. Each hedgehog has from 5,000 to 7,000 spines. The outside of the spine is solid and the inside is filled with soft air pockets. Spines are soft at birth and harden within hours, with an even stiffer set of spines emerging at about 2 days of age.

Gender identification is by anogenital distance. The genitals of the female are adjacent to the anus while the penis of the male is well away from the anus, on the ventral midline, and often looks like a big belly button.

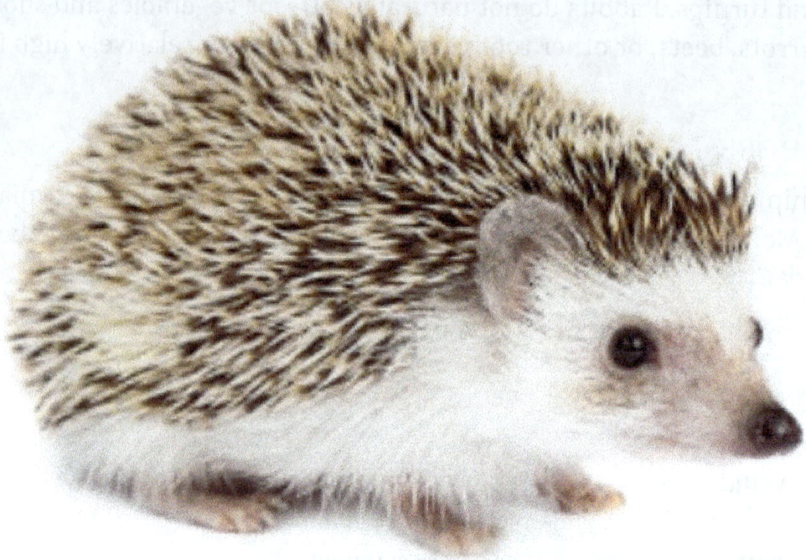

"Hedgehogs", https://www.chamblyveterinaire.com/en/uncategorized/hedgehogs/

Gender Identification of Hedgehogs

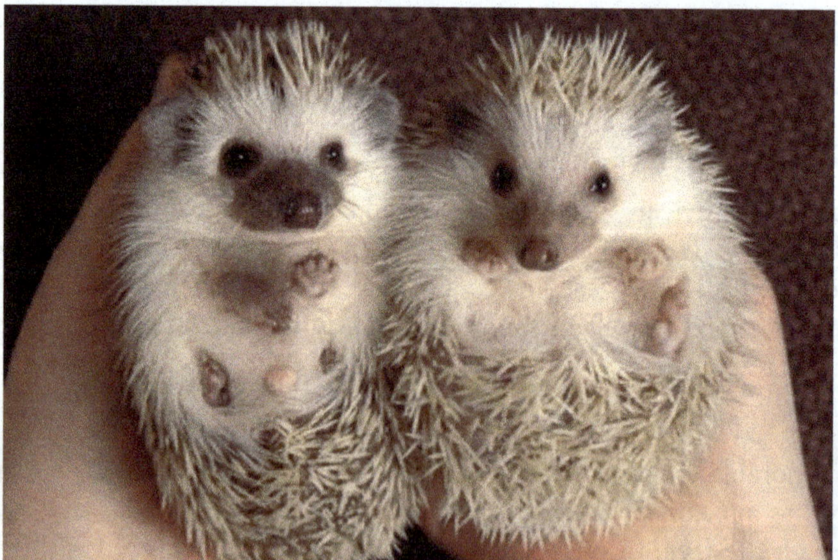

"Male vs. female african pygmy hedgehogs", https://www.factzoo.com/mammals/african-pygmy-hedgehog.html

Specifics of anatomy and other information about hedgehogs can be found in the Manual of Exotic Pet Practice, pp 433-455.

Housing

Hedgehogs are best housed individually. Aquariums, large plastic tubs, and plastic dog or cat carriers can be used as enclosures for hedgehogs. The enclosure should have smooth, high walls and a lid to prevent escape. Larger habitats are recommended to allow room for a litter pan, nest box, and exercise wheel, and to give the hedgehog room for exercise; in the wild, hedgehogs wander long distances in search of food and mates. A nest / sleeping box should be provided for the hedgehog. It should be a little longer, wider, and taller than the animal. The animal should be able to enter, turn around, and exit the box easily. Aspen or other non-aromatic shavings are recommended as a floor covering and should be changed 1-2 times weekly. Sawdust may cause respiratory problems and it can also cling to the anal and genital areas of the animal. The cage should have a solid floor. Hedgehogs can injure their legs and feet if they get caught in wire floors. Hedgehogs are clean animals and prefer to urinate and defecate in a dedicated area. A litter tray should be put in the cage. Plastic is preferred because it's easy to clean. Non-scoopable, dust-free clay cat litter can be used in the litter box. The litter tray needs to be cleaned daily and the litter should be changed weekly. Food bowls should be sturdy and non-moveable. Hedgehogs should also have a sipper water bottle. Ambient temperature should be 75-80°F. At much lower temperatures, hedgehogs will hibernate and at much higher temperatures, they estivate.

Vaccinations and Disease Control

There are no vaccines recommended for control of infectious disease in pet hedgehogs.

Parasite Control

The most common parasite of pet hedgehogs is mites. Animals may carry the mites with no signs or may show pruritus and quill loss. Diagnosis is by microscopic examination of skin scrapings and treatment is with ivermectin or permethrins.

Behavior

Pet hedgehogs generally are most active at dawn and dusk; in the wild, hedgehogs are nocturnal. Hedgehogs are solitary. They make a variety of sounds including clicking and hissing, and make and hear sounds well above the range of human hearing. One of the most peculiar and least understood behaviors of the hedgehog is the process of anointing. When the animal comes across a new smell or object, it licks at the smell or object, producing a flow of foamy saliva. The animal will then stiffen its front legs and swing its head from side to side. Using its tongue it spits and smears its spines with the saliva. The reason for the behavior is not known. Enrichment is an important component of housing to promote normal behaviors.

Biosecurity

The Center for Disease Control and Prevention reported an outbreak of salmonellosis in humans in 2019 that was traced back to hedgehogs. No single supplier of pet hedgehogs was identified as problematic. The CDC strongly encourages people to wash their hands after handling a hedgehog and any of its toys or anything in its enclosure. Never put a hedgehog near the face or kiss a hedgehog. The very young, and very old, and immunosuppressed people are at greatest risk of infection.

Nutrition

Nutritional requirements of hedgehogs have not been well defined. The base of the diet for captive hedgehogs should be a commercial insectivore diet for their species or dry, low-calorie cat or dog food. Other foods that can be provided include invertebrates such as earthworms, mealworms, waxworms; crickets; vegetables such as spinach, kale, carrots, and yams; fruits such as apples, bananas, papayas, and melon; and occasional treats of cooked egg, or meat baby food. Caution must be used to ensure hedgehogs do not become obese. Foods that should not be given to hedgehogs include grapes, raisins, onion, garlic, and dairy products.

SUGAR GLIDERS

Sugar gliders are not legal to keep as pets in Alaska and California. Special permits are required for ownership in Massachusetts and Pennsylvania.

Unique Anatomy and Biology

Biology of Sugar Gliders

LIFE SPAN	12-15 years
TEMPERATURE	96.5-98.0°F (36-37°C)
PULSE	200-300 beats per minute
RESPIRATION	16-40 breaths/minute
REPRODUCTIVE MATURITY	and puberty 3-4 months

The total body length is 10-12" (25-30 cm). The tail is usually equal to the body length. They weigh 3-5 oz (85-140 gm) with males being slightly larger than females. They have a triangular head with a short muzzle, rounded nose, and large eyes. They are soft gray in color with cream undersides. Sugar gliders have five toes on each forefoot which end with short curved claws. The inner toe on the hind foot is clawless but enlarged or bulbous which helps them grasp and hold on to branches. The second and third digits on the rear feet are fused together and have two claws.

One of the most distinguishing features of the sugar glider is the patagium, a thin, furred membrane that stretches from the wrists to the ankles. When not gliding, the membrane appears as excess skin on the side of the animal. When gliding the animal extends all four legs, which stretches the membrane out and allows the animal to glide up to 150 ft.

Appearance of a Sugar Glider

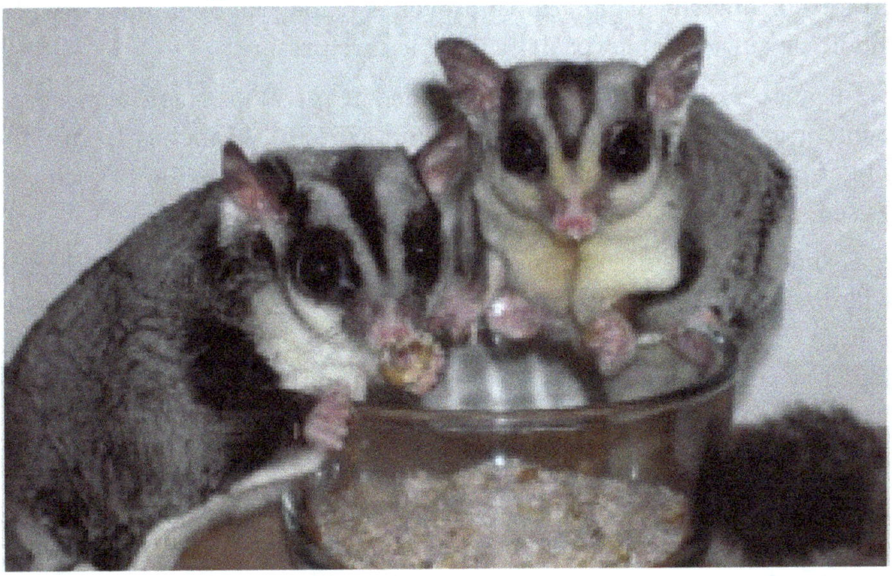

"Sugar Gliders", https://en.wikipedia.org/wiki/Sugar_glider

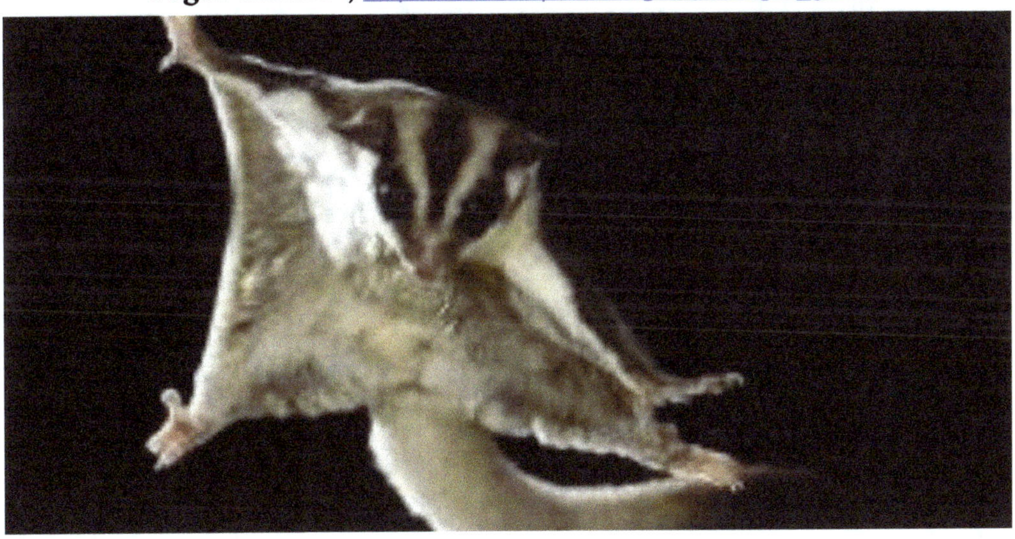

"Gliding Sugar Glider", https://mashable.com/2016/01/10/sugar-glider-instagram/

Male sugar gliders have a scrotum on their midline. The penis is bifurcated but is rarely seen extruded. Adult males have a distinctive diamond-shaped bald spot on top of their head which corresponds to a scent gland. Females have a small pouch, which appears as a ½" slit, on their abdomen.

Housing

The enclosure needs to be large enough to house more than one animal and to allow them to explore, climb, exercise, and glide. Large bird cages or aviaries may be used for housing sugar gliders. To prevent escape, the openings between wire bars should be quite small, especially if babies are present.

Tree branches or limbs should be added to give the cage a more natural environment and to encourage foraging and exercise. Branches from non-toxic woods like apple, pear, plum, or willow are recommended; conifer branches should not be used.

Cages should include a nest box and safe bedding. A cloth pouch high in the cage will be used as a place to curl up and rest. Aromatic wood shavings should not be used for bedding. Toys used for birds like swings, ladders, and bells can be enjoyed by sugar gliders. They also like pieces of PVC pipe or cardboard paper towel rolls for exploring.

Food should be placed in heavy bowls that can't be tipped over. Water can be supplied in heavy bowls or bird dishes fastened to the side of the cage. Bowls need to be cleaned daily. Food bowls should be placed high up in the cage where the gliders will feel more safe and secure. This also will prevent feces and urine from falling into them and contaminating the contents.

Ambient temperature should be 64-75°F at a minimum. At temperatures greater than 88°F, sugar gliders may suffer from hyperthermia.

Vaccinations and Disease Control

There are no vaccines recommended for control of infectious disease in pet sugar gliders.

Parasite Control

Parasitism is uncommon in pet sugar gliders.

Behavior

Sugar gliders are nocturnal and are very sociable, doing best if housed in groups of at least two. Behavior disorders such as over-grooming with subsequent fur loss, self-injury, pacing, and changes in appetite can occur in sugar gliders housed alone, with incompatible mates, or in inappropriate cages. Enrichment is an important component of housing to promote normal behaviors.

Biosecurity

Good general hygiene should offset any concerns about passage of disease from pet sugar gliders to humans.

Nutrition

Sugar gliders are omnivores. It is difficult to replicate the diet they would have in the wild. Commercial diets are available. Sweet foods are preferred by the animal and it is not advisable to have sweet food available at all times, as other foods may then not be eaten as necessary. For protein, sugar gliders can be provided with about 1 tablespoon of insects or cooked lean meat daily. Up to ½ teaspoon of chopped fruits and vegetables can be offered for a short time late in the day; good choices include apples, bananas, grapes, kiwi fruit, oranges, melon, papayas, sweet potatoes, tomatoes, corn, carrots, squash, and broccoli. Sugar gliders should not be fed insects or worms collected and brought in from outside, which may be contaminated with pesticides, apple seeds or fruit pits, and anything high in fat or sugar, such as chocolate.

EXTRA RESOURCES

Common disorders of ferrets: http://www.merckvetmanual.com/exotic-and-laboratory-animals/ferrets

Common disorders of rabbits: http://www.merckvetmanual.com/exotic-and-laboratory-animals/rabbits

Common disorders of hedgehogs: http://www.merckvetmanual.com/exotic-and-laboratory-animals/hedgehogs/diseases-of-hedgehogs

Common disorders of sugar gliders: http://www.merckvetmanual.com/exotic-and-laboratory-animals/sugar-gliders/diseases-and-syndromes-of-sugar-gliders

The American Ferret Association – colors and patterns of ferrets: http://www.ferret.org/pdfs/Ferret_Colors_and_Patterns.pdf

The American Ferret Association – ferret health and disease: http://www.ferret.org/readmenu.html

American Rabbit Breeders Association: https://www.arba.net/breeds.htm

House Rabbit Society: http://rabbit.org/

International Hedgehog Association (IHA): http://hedgehogclub.com/

Association of Sugar Glider Veterinarians – owner education materials: http://www.asgv.org/pet_owners/

The Manual of Exotic Pet Practice: http://www.sciencedirect.com/science/book/9781416001195

CHAPTER-17

MANAGEMENT OF DRUGS

This information will be repeated in pharmacology and clinical courses. Information provided in this course is intended to be an overview of veterinary drugs to help you understand what you're seeing in practices and research laboratories and to provide a frameworkfor you as you see this material again in different contexts. I here are many state and federal drug regulations practicing veterinarians are expected to know and follow. Laws change all of the time so it's good to be aware of which agencies legislate which products and to search for current information as needed on their websites or through the American Veterinary Medical Association.

- United States Food and Drug Administration (FDA)
- United States Drug Enforcement Administration (DEA)
- Minnesota Board of Pharmacy

Consumers and veterinarians are encouraged to report adverse drug experiences. This includes lack of effect of a drug, untoward or unexpected side-effects, and defects of products including poor packaging. Drug concerns are reported to the manufacturer and to the FDA. As noted earlier in the course, vaccine concerns are reported to the USDA. Flea and tick products are pesticides; some are approved by the FDA and others are under the authority of the Environmental Protection Agency (EPA). Designation for FDA or EPA approval is on the label.

DRUG APPROVAL PROCESS

The FDA defines "drugs" as "articles in the United States Pharmacopoeia, official Homeopathic Pharmacopoeia of the United States, or official National Formulary; articles intended for use in the diagnosis, cure, mitigation, treatment, or prevention of disease in man or other animals; and articles other than food intended to affect the structure or any function of the body of man other animals." For a drug to be approved, it must be demonstrated to be safe and effective in the species of interest. Safety includes safety to the animal and any food products derived from that animal, to those people handling the drug, and to the animal's environment.

A drug is defined as effective if it can be demonstrated to consistently do what the labeling claims it will do. For a drug to be approved for a given species, the drug sponsor (usually the manufacturer or holder of the patent) must provide evidence including the drug's chemistry, composition, manufacturing methods, labeling, effectiveness, adverse effects, and an environmental assessment. If the drug is intended for use in food-producing animals, methods of residue analysis must be described and safe levels for human consumption determined. The FDA rigorously evaluates this evidence and produces a summary document that includes all concerns about the drug. All warnings and precautions from the FDA must be printed on the drug label and consumers are legally required to follow the label.

Drugs may be labeled as prescription-only, over-the-counter, or VFD (see below). The FDA makes this determination based on whether a layperson can use the drug safely and effectively without guidance from a health professional. Veterinary prescription drugs can only be dispensed on the written or verbal order of a licensed veterinarian.

PRESCRIBING AND DISPENSING PRESCRIPTION DRUGS

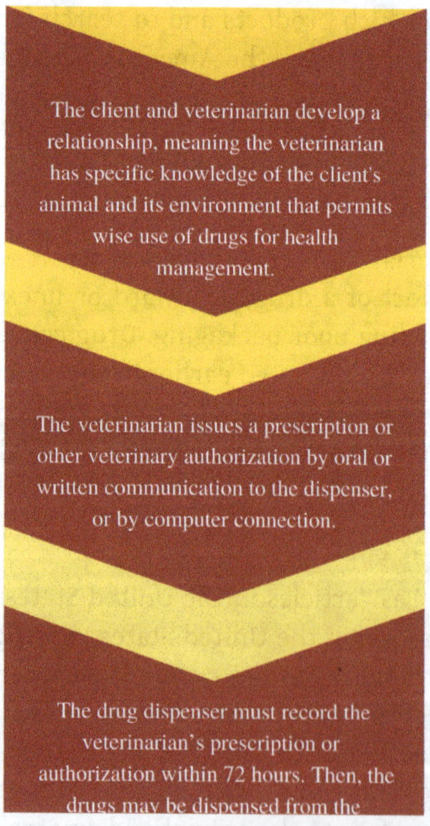

For a veterinarian to prescribe a drug for a specific animal, a valid veterinarian-client-patient relationship must exist. This relationship is defined in each state's veterinary practice act and generally refers to the veterinarian having specific knowledge of the animal and its environment that permits wise use of drugs for health management. For example, if the veterinarian has not examined the animal for a long period of time or since significant health changes have occurred, a valid relationship cannot exist. The Code of Federal Regulations defines a valid veterinarian-client-patient relationship as follows:

"A valid veterinarian-client-patient relationship is one in which: (1) A veterinarian has assumed the responsibility for making medical judgments regarding the health of (an) animal(s) and the need for medical treatment, and the client (the owner of the animal or animals or other caretaker) has agreed to follow the instructions of the veterinarian; (2) There is sufficient knowledge of the animal(s) by the veterinarian to initiate at least a general or preliminary diagnosis of the medical condition of the animal(s); and (3) The practicing veterinarian is readily available for followup in case of adverse reactions or failure of the regimen of therapy. Such a relationship can exist only when the veterinarian has recently seen and is personally acquainted with the keeping and care of the animal(s) by virtue of examination of the animal(s), and/or by medically appropriate and timely visits to the premises where the animal(s) are kept."

According to Minnesota Statute, a veterinarian may issue a prescription or other veterinary authorization by oral or written communication to the dispenser, or by computer connection. If the communication is oral, the veterinarian must enter it into the patient's record. The dispenser must record the veterinarian's prescription or other veterinary authorization within 72 hours.

A prescription or other veterinary authorization must include:

- Name, address, and, if written, the signature of the prescriber;
- Name and address of the client;
- Identification of the species for which the drug is prescribed or ordered;
- Name, strength, and quantity of the drug;
- Date of issue;
- Directions for use;
- Withdrawal time;
- Expiration date of prescription; and
- Number of authorized refills.

Prescription drugs may be dispensed from the veterinarian's facility or from a pharmacy. The label on the package of prescription-only products must state on the label the following: "Caution: Federal law restricts this drug to use by or on the order of a licensed veterinarian." Other things that must be on the package label include the recommended dosage, route of administration, quantity or proportion of each active ingredient, names of inactive ingredients, and a lot or control number to permit the drug to be tracked regarding date and site of manufacture. Veterinarians should dispense drugs in appropriate receptacles that maintain the activity of the drug and prevent inappropriate use. For example, some liquids break down when exposed to light and should be dispensed in brown bottles. The label on the drug as dispensed by the veterinarian must include the name and address of the person or facility dispensing the drug, the serial number and date of the order as filled, and name and address of the veterinarian who prescribed the drug, strength of the drug, orders for its use (dosage, route and frequency of administration), and any warnings including withdrawal times.

USE OF UNAPPROVED DRUGS

According to the Animal Health Institute, development and approval of a new drug takes about 7-10 years and costs up to $100 million. Few veterinary drugs will earn the manufacturer back enough money to offset this expense. For this reason, many drugs used in veterinary medicine are not FDA-approved for all relevant species. The FDA maintains information about all drugs approved for animals that is updated monthly. The Animal Medicinal Drug Use Clarification Act of 1994 (AMDUCA) permits the use of unapproved (also called extra label) drugs by veterinarians within a valid veterinarian-client-patient relationship when no approved drug is available for that species, the extra label drug has been shown to be safe and effective, and when the health of the animal or suffering or death may result from failure to treat. Veterinarians are only legally permitted to use drugs that are FDA-approved for use in humans or animals. The client should be informed that the drug that is being used has not been approved by the FDA specifically for use in this species and why it is being used. The FDA can declare some drugs as illegal for extra label use if they deem that drug to pose a threat to public health or if there is no acceptable method for analyzing residues of that drug in food-producing animals. Some drugs are prohibited because of concerns about creating resistant strains of zoonotic pathogens that could be transferred to humans after slaughter of food-producing animals. Drugs cannot be used extra label solely to increase production.

CONTROLLED DRUGS

Controlled substances are chemicals whose manufacture, distribution, use, and disposal require government oversight. In the United States, drugs are classified by the DEA by abuse potential, medical uses, and safety. A list of controlled drugs can be found here.

Management of controlled drugs requires the following:

- Registration
  - A designated individual is the registrant. They hold a DEA license permitting them to purchase and dispense controlled drugs. In a hospital setting, there often is one unit registrant who is responsible for the controlled drugs for a number of other people. The DEA requires different licenses for different streams of activity – for example, an individual may need one license for drugs used clinically and another license from the DEA for drugs used for research.
- Buying controlled drugs
  - Controlled drugs must be purchased by the registrant or by their designee using specific DEA paperwork. Receipt of controlled drugs includes prompt inventory to compare drugs and amounts purchased with those received and placement of controlled drugs into a safe specific to this purpose. This safe must have controlled access to authorized personnel and must be fixed in place so it cannot be removed from the room, building, or vehicle in which it is being kept, even if only temporarily.
- Storage of controlled drugs
  - All drugs must be kept in a safe that is bolted or otherwise secured to an immovable object. Drugs must be kept in the safe at all times they are not being used. Drugs can be carried in a vehicle but must be transferred in a safe that cannot be removed from that vehicle.
- Record-keeping
  - Keeping of meticulous records is vital. Specifics of record-keeping vary by state. All states require that at the time of receipt of drugs, a specific page be created in a drug log showing the following for that specific drug: the name, the strength or concentration, the form (liquid versus tablets, for example), the amount in the container, the number of containers, the date it was received, and from whom the substance was received. As the drug is used, a written record must be kept that verifies disposition of all of that chemical, including date of use, amount used, amount disposed of (if any), amount transferred (if any), and initials of user. Anyone with appropriate training can complete the log but the unit registrant is the party responsible for ongoing inventory of controlled drugs at the facility. All records must be kept for a minimum of 3 years. The DEA and appropriate state authorities may ask for records or conduct an inspection at any time.

DRUG DISPOSAL

The FDA strongly encourages laypeople to dispose of drugs as soon as they are done with them. Keeping prescription drugs in the home creates a risk for accidental or purposeful misuse.

Drugs may be collected by a variety of agencies. The DEA holds "National Prescription Drug Take Back Days" in April and October. Examples of sites that collect prescription medications near the veterinary college are the area police departments. Sites do not need to be near a veterinary college or in a large, metropolitan area; the DEA also may authorize local law enforcement agencies and pharmacies to take in drugs for disposal at any time. Some municipalities also offer mail-back programs or drop-boxes. Veterinary clinics are not required to take back drugs for disposal. It is always best to recommend to clients that they take drugs to the local law enforcement (police department or sheriff's department) or to a local chain pharmacy to dispose of drugs. This is much preferred to disposing of them in the trash. The Minnesota Pollution Control Agency provides information about disposal of unwanted medications as well. The American Veterinary Medical Association provides information for veterinarians and clients about drug disposal.

Drugs may expire in veterinary facilities or clinics may need to dispose of controlled substances. For the latter, you may wish to contact the DEA for specifics in your state. Generally the registrant is authorized to dispose of controlled drugs appropriately; any such disposal must be recorded as described above.

VETERINARY FEED DIRECTIVES IN MAJOR OR MINOR SPECIES

"A Veterinary Feed Directive (VFD) is a written (nonverbal) statement issued by a licensed veterinarian in the course of the veterinarian's professional practice that authorizes the use of a VFD drug or combination VFD drug in or on animal feed." The VFD is a component of law managed by the FDA that strives to limit antibiotic use in food-producing animals appropriately. As of January 1, 2017, the law was expanded to control use of antibiotics that are medically important for humans when provided to animals in food, even if that animal is not itself intended for food.

The law is changing over time as there are currently some contradictions. For example, only approved drugs can be used in a VFD but for some of the minor species, such as fish, there are few to no drugs available. While the rules are generally applicable to major species, veterinarians must be aware of rules and the need for antibiotics in minor species as well. Minor species, in this context, are any non-human animals other than cattle, horses, swine, chickens, turkeys, dogs, and cats. The FDA provides guidance regarding use of VFD drugs in minor species.

VETERINARY FEED DIRECTIVE REQUIREMENTS FOR VETERINARIANS – FOR VETERINARY STUDENTS

Current information available from the FDA for veterinary students is below, and is required for class and your future.

VFD Drug and Combination VFD Drug

What is a "VFD drug"?

A "VFD drug" is a drug intended for use in or on animal feed, which is limited to use under the professional supervision of a licensed veterinarian.

What is a "combination VFD drug"?

A "combination VFD drug" is an approved combination of new animal drugs intended for use in or on animal feed under the professional supervision of a licensed veterinarian, and at least one of the new animal drugs in the combination is a VFD drug.

What is a VFD?

A VFD is a written (nonverbal) statement issued by a licensed veterinarian in the course of the veterinarian's professional practice that authorizes the use of a VFD drug or combination VFD drug in or on an animal feed. This written statement authorizes the client (the owner of the animal or animals or other caretaker) to obtain and use animal feed bearing or containing a VFD drug or combination VFD drug to treat the client's animals only in accordance with the conditions for use approved, conditionally approved, or indexed by the FDA. A VFD is also referred to as a VFD order.

VFD Drugs and Prescription Drugs

What is the difference between a VFD drug and a prescription (Rx) drug?

FDA approves drugs in these two separate regulatory categories for drugs that require veterinary supervision and oversight for their use. When the drug being approved is for use in or on animal feed (a medicated feed), FDA approves these drugs as a VFD drug. When the drug being approved is not for use in or on animal feed, the drug is approved as a prescription drug.

Why VFD instead of prescription?

When the VFD drug category was created, the Federal Food, Drug and Cosmetic Act (the Act) made it clear that VFD drugs are not prescription drugs. This category was created to provide veterinary supervision without invoking state pharmacy laws for prescription drugs that were unworkable for the distribution of medicated feed.

FDA approves a drug for feed use as Over-the-Counter (OTC) or as VFD.

Veterinary Students and VFD

I don't plan to practice food animal medicine, why should I learn about VFD?

The law allows any licensed veterinarian to issue a VFD in the course of his or her practice and you may find yourself in a situation that requires one. For example, your pet owner client could ask you to issue a VFD for the flock of his/her backyard chickens.

Veterinary Students and Medicated Feed

What is really important for me to know about medicated feeds in addition to VFD?

- FDA regulates medicated feeds;
- Every use of a drug in feed has to be approved;
- There are three types of products in relation to medicated feed use:
  - Type A medicated article,
  - Type B medicated feed, and
  - Type C medicated feed;
- Type A medicated article and Type B medicated feed can be used only for further manufacture of other products. Only Type C medicated feed can be fed to animals;
- Medicated feeds are approved only as over-the-counter or VFD; they cannot be used under prescription;
- All drugs approved for use in feed are placed in two drug categories on the basis of their potential to create unsafe drug residues. Category I drugs have lower potential for unsafe drug residues than Category II drugs; and
- Finally, extra-label use of medicated feeds is prohibited by law.

How are VFD (blank) orders obtained?

VFD drug sponsors may make the VFD order for their drugs available, or, as a veterinarian, you will be able to create your own VFD.

How do I send a VFD to the feed distributor?

You must send a copy of the VFD to the distributor via hardcopy, facsimile (fax), or other electronic means. If in hardcopy, you are required to send the copy of the VFD to the distributor either directly or through the client. You must keep the original VFD in its original form (electronic or hard copy) and must send a copy to the distributor and client.

Extralabel use (ELU) of VFD feed is not permitted.

Veterinarians' Responsibilities

- must be licensed to practice veterinary medicine;
- must be operating in the course of the veterinarian's professional practice and in compliance with all applicable veterinary licensing and practice requirements;
- must write VFD orders in the context of a valid client-patient relationship (VCPR);
- must issue a VFD that is in compliance with the conditions for use approved, conditionally approved, or indexed for the VFD drug or combination VFD drug;
- must prepare and sign a written VFD providing all required information;
- may enter additional discretionary information to more specifically identify the animals to be treated/fed the VFD feed;
- must include required information when a VFD drug is authorized for use in a drug combination that includes more than one VFD drug;
- must restrict or allow the use of the VFD drug in combination with one or more OTC drug(s);
- must provide the feed distributor with a copy of the VFD;
- must provide the client with a copy of the VFD order;
- must retain the original VFD for 2 years, and
- must provide VFD orders for inspection and copying by FDA upon request.

Major and Minor Animal Species

What are "major and minor animal species"?

FDA regulations define cattle, horses, swine, chickens, turkeys, dogs, and cats, as major species. All animal species, other than humans, that are not major species are minor species.

When is a VFD needed for a minor species?

The VFD requirements apply to all VFD drugs for use in major or minor species. One VFD drug is already approved for use in minor species (e.g., florfenicol in aquaculture). Other medicated feed drugs for minor species are expected to convert from their present over-the-counter (OTC) status to VFD (e.g., oxytetracycline in honey bees) and at that time a VFD will be required for their use.

VFD and VCPR, Client

What is required for veterinarian supervision?

The veterinarian-client-patient relationship (VCPR) is the basis of professional supervision. A VFD must be issued by a licensed veterinarian operating in the course of his/her professional practice and in compliance with all applicable veterinary licensing and practice requirements, including issuing the VFD in the context of a veterinarian-client-patient relationship (VCPR).

What VCPR standard applies?

FDA provides a list of states whose VCPR includes the key elements of the federally-defined VCPR and requires a VCPR for the issuance of a VFD. If your state appears on this list you must follow your state VCPR, if your state does not you must follow the federal VCPR as defined in 21 CFR 530.3(i).

Who is the "client" on the VFD?

"Client" is typically the client in the VCPR; the person responsible for the care and feeding of the animals receiving the VFD feed.

What is an "extralabel use" of a VFD drug and is it allowed?

"Extralabel use" (ELU) is defined in FDA's regulations as actual or intended use of a drug in an animal in a manner that is not in accordance with the approved labeling. For example, feeding the animals a VFD for a duration of time that is different from the duration specified on the label, feeding a VFD formulated with a drug level that is different from what is specified on the label, or feeding a VFD to an animal species different than what is specified on the label would all be considered extralabel uses. Extralabel use of medicated feed, including medicated feed containing a VFD drug or a combination VFD drug, is not permitted.

Reorders (Refills)

When can I authorize a reorder (refill)?

If the drug approval, conditional approval, or index listing expressly allows a reorder (refill) you can authorize up to the permitted number of reorders. If a drug is silent on reorders (refills), then you may not authorize a reorder (refill).

Use of medicated feed is authorized by a VFD not Rx.

A Lawful VFD Has to Be Complete

What do I have to include in a VFD?

You must include the following information on the VFD for it to be lawful:

- veterinarian's name, address, and telephone number;
- client's name, business or home address, and telephone number;
- premises at which the animals specified in the VFD are located;
- date of VFD issuance;
- expiration date of the VFD;
- name of the VFD drug(s);
- species and production class of animals to be fed the VFD feed;
- approximate number of animals to be fed the VFD feed by the expiration date of the VFD;
- indication for which the VFD is issued;
- level of VFD drug in the feed and duration of use;
- withdrawal time, special instructions, and cautionary statements necessary for use of the drug in conformance with the approval;
- number of reorders (refills) authorized, if permitted by the drug approval, conditional approval, or index listing;
- statement: "Use of feed containing this veterinary feed directive (VFD) drug in a manner other than as directed on the labeling (extralabel use), is not permitted";
- an affirmation of intent for combination VFD drugs as described in 21 CFR 558.6(b)(6); and
- veterinarian's electronic or written signature.

You may also include the following optional information on the VFD:

- a more specific description of the location of the animals (for example, by site, pen, barn, stall, tank, or other descriptor the veterinarian deems appropriate);
- the approximate age range of the animals;
- the approximate weight range of the animals; and
- any other information the veterinarian deems appropriate to identify the animals at issue.

The veterinarian must keep the original VFD for two years.

SUBSTANCE ABUSE

There is a great deal of concern about substance abuse, both direct use of veterinary drugs by veterinary professionals and use by animal owners of drugs dispensed for animals. This concern is greatest for controlled drugs, which often have that designation because of their addictive qualities and subsequent abuse potential.

In Minnesota, the Health Professionals Services Program protects the public by providing services for all health care professionals (both human and veterinary medicine) to ensure that drug use does not impair ability of a health provider to provide safe care, and provides confidential counseling and resources for health professionals. Information about this program regularly is provided to veterinarians in Minnesota as they renew their license. A similar program is the Minnesota Veterinary Medical Association (MVMA) Wellness and Peer Assistance Committee. Their mission is the following: "Provides resource information to MVMA members on issues of suicide awareness, chemical dependence, mental health, professional burn-out and compassion fatigue. The members regard it as their responsibility to identify and/or provide assistance to MVMA members in need and to help them resume a well-balanced and healthy life."

To try to counteract the risks of owners using medications dispensed for animals, the MVMA also has created VetPMP (Veterinary Prescription Monitoring Program), as a way of ensuring that drugs dispensed for a given animal are tracked between clinics, so clients cannot "shop" for controlled substances by going from one clinic to another. This is one of many developing programs to work against the opioid abuse problem in Minnesota and throughout the US.

EXTRA RESOURCES

American Veterinary Medical Association: http://www.avma.org

United States Food and Drug Administration (FDA): www.fda.gov

United States Drug Enforcement Administration (DEA): www.dea.gov

Minnesota Board of Pharmacy: https://mn.gov/boards/pharmacy/

Reporting of adverse drug experiences: https://www.myvetcandy.com/clinicalupdblog/2019/4/3/fda-takes-new-steps-to-increase-access-to-adverse-event-report-data

The Code of Federal Regulations regarding veterinarian-client-patient relationships: https://www.gpo.gov/fdsys/pkg/CFR-2017-title21-vol6/pdf/CFR-2017-title21-vol6-sec530-3.pdf

The Minnesota Statute regarding veterinary prescriptions: https://www.revisor.mn.gov/statutes/?id=156.18

FDA Green Book – information about drugs approved for use in animals: https://www.fda.gov/animal-veterinary/products/approved-animal-drug-products-green-book

List of controlled drugs: https://www.drugs.com/csa-schedule.html

Drug disposal information:

Drop-off sites through local law enforcement offices, or local chain pharmacies: https://www.ci.inver-grove-heights.mn.us/677/Prescription-Drug-Drop-Off

The Minnesota Pollution Control Agency: https://www.pca.state.mn.us/living-green/managing-unwanted-medications

The American Veterinary Medical Association: https://www.avma.org/KB/Policies/Pages/Best-Management-Practices-for-Pharmaceutical-Disposal.aspx

FDA guidance regarding use of VFD drugs in minor species: https://www.fda.gov/animal-veterinary/development-approval-process/minor-useminor-species

FDA guidance regarding veterinary feed directive requirements for veterinary students: https://www.fda.gov/AnimalVeterinary/DevelopmentApprovalProcess/ucm455417.htm

How the Veterinary Feed Directive Will Affect Chicken and Poultry Owners: https://countrysidenetwork.com/daily/poultry/feed-health/how-the-veterinary-feed-directive-will-affect-chicken-poultry-owners/

Honeybees 101 for Veterinarians: https://www.avma.org/KB/Resources/Pages/Honey-Bees-101-Veterinarians.aspx

Use of Veterinary Feed Directive drugs in aquaculture: https://caaquaculture.org/2017/01/06/use-of-veterinary-feed-directive-drugs-in-aquaculture/

APPENDIX

OVERVIEW AND COMMON DISORDERS OF NON-TRADITIONAL PET SPECIES

Non-traditional pets are those species that are not within the standard grouping of domesticated animal companion species. For the purposes of this course, this includes backyard poultry, caged birds, fish in tanks, small mammals (mice, rats, hamsters, gerbils), larger mammals (guinea pigs, chinchillas, rabbits, ferrets), hedgehogs, sugar gliders, reptiles, and amphibians. There is great variety in this group of species. For each, information will be provided about biology, housing, nutrition, behavior, biosecurity, parasite control, reproduction control, vaccinations, and common disorders.

Many of these species are prey animals and can be quite ill before showing any signs of disease. It is good to recommend to clients that they regularly perform a brief physical examination on their pet, check the animal's housing, and note any changes in behavior. Ideally this will done on a very regular basis, for example weekly, and all results will be documented and shared with the veterinarian as appropriate.

Maintaining these animals in captivity while ensuring their physical and mental health can be challenging. Specifics of housing and nutrition will be addressed in each section. Enrichment is a term commonly used to describe the provision of physical and mental challenges for animals, to permit them to show as many of their normal behaviors as they can. This stimulation helps prevent negative behaviors such as overgrooming, pacing, and aggression. Examples of kinds of enrichment include:

- Physical enrichment – Stimulating natural behaviors such as gnawing, digging, hiding, climbing, and perching on high spots to permit them to see predators
- Mental enrichment – Incorporating problem-solving activities that permit the animal to change their environment such as tunnels or other challenges to get to all parts of the enclosure

- Social enrichment – Ensuring social species are housed with appropriate groupings that encourage normal social behaviors, such as grooming, while permitting appropriate spaces for hiding and minimizing chance of fighting
- Sensory enrichment – Changing environmental stimuli to mimic natural changes such as changes in room temperature, light, or humidity that may mimic the seasons, changing the arrangement of objects within the enclosure, and appropriately providing supervised time out of the cage or outdoors
- Nutritional enrichment – Seeking food, or foraging, is a huge part of the day for most animals in the wild. Ways to increase foraging behaviors for captive animals include scattering food, hiding food within the habitat or using puzzle toys that distribute food slowly, offering food in unique ways (frozen, hanging by a string), and decreasing predictability by offering food at differing times of day

The rest of this appendix is a brief description of the most common disorders in non-traditional pets. This is not intended to be a comprehensive listing. Species are listed in order of popularity and more information is included for the more popular species. Information is presented at the level of training of 1st year veterinary students who have had limited coursework in pathology and agents of disease and no medicine / surgery courses. Many of the concerns for which non-traditional pets present are due to improper husbandry. See the introductory modules for information about housing and diet. More information about disorders, anesthesia and surgery, and appropriate use of antibiotics and other drugs in these unique species will be available for all students in the Avian Core course and for those students who choose to take electives in 3rd and 4th year, and can be found in the following references:

Mitchell MA, Tully TN. Manual of exotic pet practice. Saunders Elsevier, St. Louis MO, 2009 (PRK will add link to electronic version available through the University library system for students).

Lafeber Vet – Students must register on this site to gain access to instructional materials; registration is free. This site has differential lists by species based on presenting complaint to aid in working through case presentations.

University of Rochester Medical Center – Body condition scoring in exotic species

CAGED BIRDS

FEATHER PICKING

Feather picking is an abnormal expression of the normal behavior of grooming or preening in birds. Causes include genetic predisposition (most common in African grey parrots, lovebirds, Eclectus parrots, cockatoos, conures, parrotlets, monk parakeets, and macaws), infectious skin diseases, allergies, liver or pancreatic disease, and trauma. This may also be a purely behavioral disorder, often due to inappropriate environment or stress. It can range from mild breaking or pulling of feathers in one area to extensive self-mutilation. Diagnosis requires a complete work-up with bloodwork and testing for specific diseases, such as psittacine beak and feather disease and polyomavirus. For treatment, underlying disorders must be addressed. Mechanical prevention of feather picking with use of an Elizabethan collar or use of noxious agents like bitter apple are not recommended. Attempts should be made to identify and remove any stressors. Owners should strive to find an alternative to persistent caging of the bird, provide enrichment for the bird, and create a stable social environment. Medical therapies for behavioral causes of feather picking have been described but should not be used as a sole form of treatment.

EGG BINDING

Egg binding is failure of one or more eggs to be laid within the normal time limits for a given avian species. Underlying causes include hypocalcemia, obesity, environmental stressors including low temperature and humidity, abnormal egg formation, cloacal masses, and disorders of the oviduct. Species at greatest risk are cockatiels and budgerigars; incidence is also high in lovebirds, canaries, and finches. Clinical signs include extreme depression, sitting on the bottom of the cage with ruffled feathers and wings spread, anorexia, straining with or without passing droppings, paralysis of the legs, and cloacal / oviductal prolapse. Retained eggs may be palpable on gentle abdominal manipulation. Radiographs may be taken; if the bird is suffering from hypocalcemia, the egg shells may be poorly mineralized and difficult to see. Abdominal ultrasound also may be used for diagnosis. The first line of treatment is supportive care (housing the bird in an environment with increased heat and humidity, providing fluids and nutritional support) and calcium supplementation (SQ, IM, or orally). Manipulation of the egg by gentle massage must be done with the bird anesthetized; the egg should be lubricated with a water-soluble lubricant and great caution must be taken not to injure the oviduct. If necessary, consider drug therapy to cause uterine contractions (oxytocin, arginine vasotocin), ovocentesis (puncture and collapse of the egg through the cloaca or through the skin) or salpingectomy (surgical removal of the oviduct). After the bird has been treated successfully for egg binding, attention must be paid to the environment and enrichment, to try to minimize excessive egg laying in the future. Simple options include no longer housing the bird with a mate, removing anything that acts as a nest box, improving quality of the diet, and ensuring a maximum daylength of 10-12 hours daily.

BEAK DEFORMITIES

In psittacine birds, the upper beak grows continually lengthwise and outward. The most superficial surface is dead, keratinized tissue, like our fingernails, that flakes or chips off. Overgrowth of the upper beak may be due to trauma, liver disease, lack of light exposure and subsequent vitamin D deficiency, hypovitaminosis A (see below), or lack of natural grooming aids to wear away the beak (cuttlebones, lava rocks, hard perches). Diagnosis is by visual inspection. Treatment involves recreating the normal shape of the beak and removing any flaked or chipped areas. Beak trimming can be done with a cutting instrument or a rotation disk tool. It is better to trim too little than too much.

HYPOVITAMINOSIS A

Vitamin A is a group of fat-soluble vitamins with similar activity that includes support of epithelial cell growth and repair, immune function, bone growth, vision, and maintenance of feather color. All-seed diets are deficient in vitamin A. Signs associated with deficiency of vitamin A include squamous metaplasia and subsequent dysfunction of mucous epithelial cells lining the respiratory and gastrointestinal (GI) tracts, sinusitis, anorexia, poor feather condition, night blindness, neurologic signs, and decreased vocalization. Diagnosis is based on history of an all-seed diet and physical examination findings. Treatment includes a change to a high-quality pelleted diet and supplementation with vitamin A.

SINUSITIS

Sinusitis in birds may be due to environmental factors (strong fumes, household temperature extremes, poor ventilation, dry air), diet (hypovitaminosis A), bacterial infections, or a combination of the above. Affected birds present with sneezing, ocular / nasal discharge, exophthalmos (protrusion of the eye(s)), anorexia, lethargy, and weight loss. Birds will have dried discharge on the feathers around the nares, will shake their head, and yawn. Diagnosis is by imaging (radiography to rule-out pneumonia) and culture of nasal flushes or choanal swabs. Treatment is supportive, with fluids and nutritional support, and may include direct administration of ophthalmic antibiotics into the nares, nebulization, increased environmental humidity, and treatment of underlying factors.

ENTERITIS

In birds, droppings include feces, created in the GI tract, and urates and urine, created by the kidneys. Diarrhea is any increase in the liquid component of droppings and so may be due to GI or urinary tract dysfunction or to any systemic condition that causes polyuria (increased urine formation). Enteritis is inflammation of the GI tract and may be due to bacterial, viral, fungal, or parasitic infections; cloacal papillomas / warts; obstruction in the GI tract; or antibiotic use. Less common causes include GI neoplasia, toxins, stress, systemic disease, or dietary changes. Affected birds show loose droppings, sometimes without an obvious fecal component, and may show non-specific signs of illness including anorexia, ruffled feathers, and lethargy. Diagnosis is through history and physical examination findings, fecal sampling for evidence of parasitism, basic bloodwork to rule out systemic disease, radiographs to assess for obstruction, and possibly specific testing for things like toxins. Treatment involves management of identified underlying causes, rehydration with fluid therapy, feeding of a low-fat, easily digestible diet, and appropriate antibiotic or antifungal medications.

NEOPLASIA

Most common cancers in birds are those of the skin, oronasal cavity, respiratory tract, and abdominal organs. Neoplasia is more common in aged than in young birds. Lipomas (benign fatty tumors) are common in obese psittacine birds and develop most commonly on the sternum and abdomen. Lipomas are fluctuant and non-painful. Diagnosis of internal masses requires radiography. Fine-needle aspirate or biopsy can be used to differentiate benign from malignant external masses and possibly to identify tumor type. Surgical removal is the most common treatment.

FRESHWATER TROPICAL FISH

ICH

This is also called white spot disease or ick, and is caused by the protozoan parasite, *Ichthyophthirius multifilis*. Infected fish present with small raised blisters on the skin or fins. Fish may also show unusual behaviors such as flashing (rubbing or banging their sides against things in the tank), gulping air at the water's surface, or jumping out of the water. The parasite life cycle includes parasitic forms on the fish and parasitic forms in the tank. One mature parasite can produce hundreds to thousands of infective offspring in less than 24 hours at a water temperature from 72-77°F. Diagnosis is by visual inspection. Treatment on the fish itself can be difficult as the parasite may be deep enough in the tissues to avoid exposure to chemical treatments. Chemicals used include formaldehyde, malachite green, and copper sulfate. Non-chemical treatment methods include adding salt to the water, increasing water temperature, and changing the water. Prevention is preferred to treatment. Because the parasite spends time in the tank, if there are no fish to infect, it will die off. Tanks should be set up with all equipment and decorations and left to run for at least one week before fish are added. Newly purchased fish should be quarantined in a separate tank for 7-10 days and verified free of parasites by visual inspection before being added to an established group of fish. Aquatic plants also should be kept in a separate tank for 5-7 days before being added to an established tank.

AMMONIA TOXICITY

Ammonia can build up in a tank from use of chemically treated tap water to refill the tank, from inadequate cleaning and subsequent decomposition of organic matter in the tank, from overfeeding and build up of decaying food in the tank, and from the fish themselves, who naturally excrete ammonia through their gills. Elevated concentrations of ammonia may be evident in the fish as their gills become red or purple, the fish start gasping at the surface for air, and they lose their appetite and normal activity level. Later in the course of the toxicity, red streaks will appear on the fish's body and fins. Eventually the fish will hemorrhage internally and externally, and will die. Diagnosis is by testing of water quality. Ammonia should be less than 1 ppm. A change in 50% of the water and lowering of the pH should be done immediately. Feedings may be discontinued or restricted to prevent ongoing buildup of organic matter. No new fish should be added to the tank until ammonia levels are normal.

FIN ROT

Fin rot is bacterial infection secondary to stress, such as overcrowding or presence in the tank of fish that fight. The condition is most common in tanks with poor water quality and low water temperature. Early in the course of disease, the edges of the fins will appear milky and start to fray, leaving a ragged edge. Fins will gradually get shorter as areas begin to slough off. Bloody patches will appear as the disease progresses. Diagnosis is by visual inspection. Treatment includes changing the water in the tank and removing debris from uneaten food. Test the water quality and ensure the pH and temperature are correct for the species of fish in the tank. Appropriate antibiotic therapy should be instituted for individual fish.

VELVET

Velvet, also known as rust or gold dust disease, is caused by a parasite that is classified by some as a protozoan and by others as an algae, named Oodinium or Piscinoodinium. Poor water quality, changes in water temperature, and other stressors may worsen disease. Similar to ich (see above), the parasite spends time on the fish and some time in the tank. Golden spots develop on the fish and may be difficult to see with the naked eye. Other physical signs of disease include fine yellow or rust-colored film on the skin, and peeling off of the skin. Behavioral signs of infection include flashing, lethargy, anorexia, and labored breathing. Diagnosis is by visual inspection. Treatment includes raising the water temperature and dimming the tank lights for several days, and treating the aquarium with salt or copper sulfate. Prevention is as for ich.

ANCHORWORM

Anchorworms are parasites commonly found on goldfish or koi. They attach directly to the fish under the scales. Females extend their reproductive structures out from beneath the scales; this gives the appearance of a short, white worm. These parasites are visible to the naked eye. As they fall off the fish, they leave behind an area of hemorrhage or fibrosis. Diagnosis is by visual inspection. Treatment requires removal under sedation so the entire parasite can be removed. The tank must be treated for juvenile forms of the parasite; over-the-counter anchorworm treatments usually are effective against juvenile forms. Alternatively, substrate and décor can be removed and the water in the tank run through a UV light. Prevention is as for ich.

DROPSY

This is an old term for edema or ascites, swelling of soft tissues due to an accumulation of water or other fluids. This is due to a bacterial infection; many fish will carry bacteria and be asymptomatic. Stress is an underlying cause of the disease and may be due to poor water quality, spikes in ammonia or nitrites, a large drop in water temperature, improper nutrition, or aggressive tank mates. Affected fish will have severely swollen bellies and their scales will stick out, giving the fish a pinecone-like appearance. The eyes may bulge and the anus may become red and swollen. Other signs include anorexia, ulcers on the lateral line, curving of the spine, redness of the fins, and swimming near the surface. Eventually the fish will undergo organ failure and death. Affected fish should be removed to a hospital tank. Water in the hospital tank should have added salt and the fish should be treated with antibiotics either in the food or in the water. Dropsy is prevented by maintaining a clean tank with good water quality, not overcrowding the tank, and not overfeeding the fish.

GILL FLUKES

Flukes are trematode parasites that live and reproduce in the gills of tropical fish. Flukes attach to the gills with hooks that may damage the gills, decreasing their ability to take in oxygen, and permitting secondary bacterial infection. Infected fish will flash and later in disease, become lethargic and spend time in a corner of the tank with the fins clamped to the body. Fish may also gasp for air and have swollen gills. Definitive diagnosis is by a skin scrape or gill biopsy. The flukes lay eggs which fall into the tank and hatch out in 2-4 days. If the newly hatched fluke does not find a host, it dies. Treatment of the tank may kill newly hatched flukes but will not affect the eggs so multiple treatments are required. A specific anti-parasitic drug should be used. Prevention is as for ich.

SWIM BLADDER DISEASE

Swim bladder disorders are most common in goldfish and bettas. Possible causes include distension of the stomach from eating too much food, eating food that expands (for example, freeze-dried foods) or gulping air; low water temperature; disorders causing enlargement of abdominal organs; parasites or bacterial infections; and trauma to the swim bladder. Abnormal function of the swim bladder interferes with the fish's buoyancy so they are unable to float or sink as they wish. Some will be perpetually at the top or bottom of the tank while others will float upside down or on their sides and will be unable to achieve normal position in the water. Initial treatment includes not feeding the fish for several days and increasing water temperature to 78-80°F. After the initial fast, consider feeding the fish cooked and skinned peas (microwave or boil a frozen pea for a few seconds, remove the skin and feed one pea per day for a few days). Other treatments include adding salt to the water, reducing flow of water if there is a strong current in the tank, and hand feeding the fish. If there is no response in a reasonable period of time, the fish should be euthanized. Prevention includes keeping the tank clean, not overfeeding the fish, feeding food that sinks, rehydrating dried foods before feeding, thawing frozen food before feeding, and not overcrowding the tank.

RABBITS

GASTROINTESTINAL (GI) STASIS

GI stasis is also called ileus, and is slow emptying of the stomach and movement of ingesta through the GI tract. Roughage in the diet is important to ensure proper digestion and ongoing function of the GI tract. When GI motility slows, hair from grooming and ingesta accumulate in the stomach. Because rabbits cannot vomit, the material in the stomach dehydrates and becomes even more difficult to pass. This condition can be caused by improper amount of roughage in the diet or by anything that causes a rabbit to stop eating. Clinical signs include anorexia, decreased production of feces, signs of pain such as bruxism (teeth grinding) and a hunched posture, and reluctance to move. Diagnosis is by history and physical examination findings; a doughy or distended and firm stomach and cecum, and gas-filled intestinal loops will be palpable. Radiographs may be used to demonstrate gastric distension with food, fluid, or gas. Treatment includes supportive care including fluid therapy; encouraging exercise; feeding fresh, moistened greens and good-quality long-stemmed grass hay as well as an appropriate pelleted diet; encouraging drinking; use of a feeding tube for animals that will not directly eat food and water; and using appropriate pain medications and gastric prokinetic agents. Some animals may require surgery to relieve obstruction. Prognosis is good if the condition is recognized quickly.

DENTAL MALOCCLUSION

Rabbits are predisposed to dental disease by congenital malocclusion or by poor diet, without adequate wear on the continuously erupting incisors. Signs of dental disease include lack of appetite, dropping food from the mouth while chewing, and drooling. Overgrowth of incisors is easily visible on physical examination but overgrown cheek teeth require additional examination techniques. Because rabbits have a small oral cavity, complete evaluation of cheek teeth may require the use of an otoscope with a large diameter cone, sedation and passage of a speculum, and/or dental radiographs. Overgrown incisors and molars can be corrected as in other herbivore species, using a high-speed trimming dental burr or dental disc. Malocclusion is seldom cured long-term by trimming and additional visits for further dental care may be needed for the life of the animal.

ABSCESSES

Abscesses can form anywhere on the body and usually develop after some sort of skin injury and colonization of normal skin flora at the site. The predominant clinical sign is a lump with localized hair loss above it. If rupture has occurred, discharge may be seen although rabbits often develop a caseous discharge that does not readily drain from the cavity. Diagnosis is by visual inspection. Because rabbit abscesses usually contain a firmer, more caseous pus than that in other species, lancing is not effective for diagnosis or treatment. Surgical excision and appropriate antibiotic treatment are recommended.

PASTEURELLOSIS

Infection with the bacterium *Pasteurella multocida* is most commonly associated with upper respiratory tract infection, or snuffles, in rabbits. This organism is common in the environment and is readily passed between rabbits. Most rabbits carry it as normal flora in the respiratory tract without signs of illness. Risk factors include stress, concurrent disease, use of immunosuppressive steroid medications, and poor husbandry. Infection usually begins with excessive colonization of the bacterium in the nose, spreading to the sinuses and bones of the face, then to the ears, eyes, and lower respiratory tract and, in extreme cases, throughout the body. Clinical signs include sneezing, clear to bloody nasal discharge, staining of the front paws, epiphora (excessive tearing), conjunctivitis, neurologic signs (head tilt or loss of balance) with infections of the inner ear, dyspnea (difficulty breathing) and non-specific signs such as anorexia and depression. Diagnosis is by history and physical examination. *Pasteurella* can be cultured from nasal discharge. Rabbits are obligate nasal breathers so treatment must include clearing of the nasal passages. Physical cleaning of the nostrils and humidification of the environment to help mobilize nasal discharge, and nebulization may be used. Address husbandry issues such as removing dusty hay or bedding, and ensuring the cage is clean with minimum ammonia concentrations. Long-term antibiotic therapy is indicated.

OTOASCARIASIS (EAR MITES)

Ear mites are transmitted between rabbits. The mites lay eggs in the wax and debris of the ear canal. Antigenic material in their feces and saliva is extremely irritating to the external ear canal, causing severe scratching (pruritus) in rabbits. The rabbit will scratch their ears and shake their head and may not want their head touched by the owner. Dark discharge will encrust the ear canal. Diagnosis is by identification of the mite in the ear discharge using a microscope. Treatment involves use of an appropriate anti-parasitic drug topically, possible use of an anti-inflammatory drug, soaking of crusts with mineral oil to help them to fall away naturally, and trimming of the nails on the hind feet to minimize trauma induced by scratching. The enclosure should be decontaminated to decrease risk of re-infestation.

ANTIBIOTIC DYSBIOSIS

In the rabbit, the intestinal microflora are very sensitive to orally administered antibiotics. Alteration in the microflora is associated with fluctuations in intestinal pH and proliferation of bacterial species that release endotoxins. Endotoxemia may lead to sudden death. When using antibiotics in rabbits, concurrent use of probiotics may minimize risk of dysbiosis and caution must be taken not to induce GI stasis.

ENCEPHALITOZOON CUNICULI

E. cuniculi is an organism that has been characterized as a microsporidian (fungal) parasite. Animals shed spores in urine that are ingested, spread to gut-associated lymphoid tissue, and then to the bloodstream and to major organs, with a predilection for the kidney and the brain. Animals may carry the organism for years with no clinical signs. Clinical signs include neurologic signs (torticollis (muscle spasm of the neck with turning of the head to one side), nystagmus (shaking of the eyeballs), ataxia, rear limb stiffness or paralysis), and urinary incontinence. Diagnosis in living animals is difficult because antibody testing demonstrates only exposure, not necessarily disease. Paired titers showing a rise in antibody concentrations supports an active infection. Treatment includes use of an anti-parasitic drug, anti-inflammatory drugs, and possibly a drug to control neurologic signs, such as meclizine (Dramamine™).

UTERINE ADENOCARCINOMA

Uterine adenocarcinoma is the most common cancer in female domestic rabbits, reported to be as high as 80% in unspayed does over 3-4 years of age. This is a slowly progressive tumor that invades locally and spreads to distant tissues late in the disease course. Clinical signs include hematuria (bloody urine), bloody vulvar discharge, and, late in disease, anorexia, lethargy, dyspnea, and anemia. Cystic mammary glands also may be seen. Diagnosis is by physical examination, bloodwork, and radiographs or ultrasound. Ovariohysterectomy (spay) is curative if the tumor has not invaded tissue outside of the uterus. Spaying does when young is preventative.

RABBIT HEMORRHAGIC DISEASE

Rabbit hemorrhagic disease is caused by a calicivirus. It is highly contagious and of high morbidity and mortality. A new variant is spreading through wild rabbit populations in the United States as of 2019 and domestic rabbits also are at risk. Updated information about this emerging concern in rabbits is available through the Minnesota Board of Animal Health.

HAMSTERS

NEOPLASIA

Benign tumors are more common than are malignant tumors in hamsters. Common tumors include adrenal tumors, and lymphoma associated with the lymph nodes, thymus, spleen, and liver. Signs may be non-specific and include anorexia, depression, abdominal pain, and diarrhea. Lymphoma may be associated with dermatitis and alopecia (hair loss). Anemia may be present. Diagnosis is by visual inspection or imaging (radiography or ultrasound). Fine-needle aspirate or biopsy may be used to differentiate benign from malignant tumors. Surgical removal is the treatment of choice.

WET TAIL

Wet tail is the common name for a variety of inflammatory conditions of the GI tract. Bacterial and parasitic agents have been implicated in the disease, which also is associated with stress, high temperature or humidity, overcrowding, malnutrition, and dietary changes. Clinical signs include diarrhea, anorexia, weight loss, dehydration, and scruffy hair coat. Diagnosis is by visual inspection. Treatment is with appropriate antibiotics and supportive care, including fluids. Mortality rate is high in young hamsters (3-10 weeks old). Use of antibiotics in cage mates to prevent disease spread generally is unrewarding.

ABSCESSES

Abscesses can form anywhere on the body and usually develop after some sort of skin injury and colonization of normal skin flora at the site. The predominant clinical sign is a lump with localized hair loss above it. Diagnosis is by visual inspection.

For treatment, abscesses can be lanced, the defect rinsed with antiseptic, and appropriate antibiotic therapy instituted.

DEMODECTIC MANGE

Hamsters may carry mange mites with no signs of skin disease. Overt disease often is secondary to an underlying problem that diminishes immune function, such as neoplasia, hyperadrenocorticism, kidney disease, malnutrition, or stress. Demodectic mange also is more common in aged hamsters than in young hamsters. Clinical signs include patchy alopecia, scaling, and crusting beginning on the neck and dorsum and gradually moving over the rest of the body. Diagnosis is made by skin scraping or tape prep to identify the mite using the light microscope. Treatment is with an appropriate anti-parasitic agent administered systemically or topically.

DENTAL MALOCCLUSION

Because they have continuously growing incisors, if the teeth are not worn down by normal activity or if malocclusion is present, the incisors can overgrow, causing significant oral disease. This is easily identified on physical examination. Because the teeth have no nerve except at the base, they can be trimmed as needed by a veterinarian using a dental disc. Hamsters should be provided with a high roughage diet and things on which they can gnaw, such as pesticide-free wood and cardboard.

LIZARDS

NUTRITIONAL SECONDARY HYPERPARATHYROIDISM

Metabolic bone disease, nutritional osteodystrophy, and rubber jaw are other names for this disorder. Calcium supports cardiac and skeletal muscle contraction, blood clotting, transmission of nervous impulses, and bones and teeth. Phosphorus also supports bones and teeth. Calcium and phosphorus must be present in a specific ratio to ensure these processes occur. Calcium is stored in bone. Normally, when calcium concentrations rise in blood, calcitonin is released and pulls calcium from the blood, depositing it in bone. When calcium concentrations are low in blood, parathormone increases absorption of calcium from the kidney and intestine and draws calcium from bone. Vitamin D is produced with exposure to ultraviolet light (UVB) and increases absorption of calcium. Nutritional secondary hyperparathyroidism is a disorder of husbandry. Animals fed a diet with inappropriately low calcium and/or inappropriately high phosphorus will perceive themselves to be in a hypocalcemic state and will produce excessive parathormone, leading to weakening of the bones and teeth, and abnormal cardiac and nervous functions. Lack of adequate exposure to UVB light and subsequent low vitamin D concentrations inhibits absorption of calcium from the diet. Affected lizards may have swollen hind legs; spinal deviations; a kinked tail; problems lifting the body and tail off the ground; jerky movements of the limbs and head; may hold their mouth abnormally with a swollen or rubbery jaw and droopy lips, and drooling; and, in chameleons, may show inability to control the tongue. Diagnosis by radiography is definitive; bones will have reduced cortical density and fractures may be evident. Treatment includes increasing calcium in the diet. Animals should be handled carefully, placed on strict cage rest, and housed with no cage mates until bone strength returns. UVB lighting should be available to increase vitamin D production. Pain medications can be used if fractures are present.

MOUTH ROT

This is stomatitis, inflammation of the mouth and gums. This is caused by infection with Gram negative bacteria. Primary pathologies are stress, improper temperature and humidity, poor diet, overcrowding, oral trauma, and hypovitaminosis A. Clinical signs include asymmetry or inability to close the mouth, red and swollen gingiva, mucus or discharge from the mouth, and open-mouth breathing. Non-specific signs are anorexia and lethargy. Diagnosis is by visual inspection. Culture of a deep pocket of infection can be used to guide antibiotic therapy. Treatment includes debridement and irrigation of inflamed tissues with antiseptic and topical or systemic treatment with anti-bacterial drugs. Husbandry issues should be addressed and underlying disease or vitamin A deficiency should be treated.

SKIN DISEASE

A very common infectious cause of skin diseases in lizards is mites. Affected lizards may be asymptomatic or may show scratching, secondary bacterial infection, and anemia. The mites are visible to the naked eye as small red dots. Topical anti-parasitic drugs can be used for treatment. Non-infectious causes of skin disorders in lizards include trauma and burns. These usually are due to housing with incompatible cage mates or to improper setup of the habitat. A final skin disorder in lizards is dysecdysis or improper shedding. Treatment includes (i) warm water soaks (77-85°F for 15-60 minutes followed by gentle pulling of old scales with a piece of gauze, (ii) correction of underlying husbandry issues, and (iii) treatment for underlying skin diseases.

EGG BINDING

Egg binding is common with a reported incidence of 10%. In non-breeding lizards, the biggest concern is egg retention or post-ovulatory egg binding, where a lizard forms one or more eggs but does not lay the eggs in a timely fashion. Underlying husbandry causes include low dietary calcium concentrations, inadequate temperature or humidity, and inadequate nesting sites. Underlying pathologies include obesity, dehydration, mechanical obstruction, reproductive tract infections, oversized or misshapen eggs, urolithiasis, fecal impaction, or oviductal stricture. Non-specific clinical signs include anorexia, lethargy, dyspnea (difficulty breathing), edema of the extremities, cloacal discharge or bleeding, straining, oviductal or cloacal prolapse, and difficulty walking. Radiography is definitive for diagnosis. Treatment by manipulation of the egg can be difficult as it may be associated with oviductal rupture or prolapse. Medical treatment involves use of a compound that can cause coordinated contractions, either oxytocin or arginine vasotocin. Treatment with calcium may be beneficial. Non-medical treatments include ovocentesis (puncture and collapse of the egg through the cloaca or through the skin) and salpingectomy (surgical removal of the oviduct). Introduction of egg yolk into the coelom is associated with egg yolk peritonitis, manifested by anorexia, lethargy, diarrhea, decreased fecal output, and many changes on bloodwork. Egg yolk peritonitis can be identified on ultrasound by presence of coelomic fluid. Treatment of egg yolk peritonitis involves fluids and exploratory celiotomy and lavage of the coelem.

TURTLES

AURAL ABSCESSES

These are ear abscesses and are common in turtles and tortoises. These are most likely to occur if the animal is immunosuppressed, as during hibernation; after trauma; if the animal is malnourished; or if it is housed in a very wet or very dry environment. The infection begins in the mouth and moves up through the internal ear canal. Because there is no external ear canal, this localizes as a pocket of pus which becomes dense and firm and will not drain back into the mouth. Clinical signs include swellings on the side of the head or, if rupture occurs, a hole in the head. They head may become asymmetrical. Diagnosis is by history and physical examination. Pus may be visible protruding from the eustachian tube into the mouth on oral examination. Surgical removal of the caseous pus and flushing of the defect is the treatment of choice. The wound is left open to heal on its own; antibiotic therapy may be required, especially if the abscess redevelops.

PNEUMONIA

Pneumonia in turtles may be bacterial or fungal. Infection develops more readily if the turtle is malnourished, is carrying parasites, is housed in unsanitary conditions, or has hypovitaminosis A. Acute disease is associated with gasping and open-mouth breathing, and sudden death. Chronic disease is associated with chronic nasal discharge and respiratory distress. If septicemia (body-wide infection) develops, the turtle may struggle to breathe, appear lethargic or uncoordinated, or convulse. Definitive diagnosis is by radiography; pneumonia is associated with fluid in the lungs. Treatment includes antibiotic therapy, housing at the mid to upper end of the optimal temperature range, nebulization, and treatment of underlying disease.

GUINEA PIGS

DENTAL DISEASE

Both the incisors and the cheek teeth are open-rooted and continuously growing. Possible causes of dental disease include lack of a fibrous diet or other things to chew on to grind down the teeth, and malocclusion. This disorder is most common in middle-aged to older guinea pigs. Clinical signs include anorexia, dysphagia (difficulty eating), decreased fecal output, weight loss, hypersalivation, and, in those with tooth root abscesses, swelling of the jaw and ocular / nasal discharge. Diagnosis is by visual inspection. Obvious malocclusion or tooth overgrowth, formation of sharp enamel points on the cheek teeth +/- oral ulceration, food impaction, and abnormal spacing between teeth may be evident on superficial oral examination. Because of the small size of the oral cavity and likelihood of significant dental disease that is not grossly evident, sedation for a full oral examination and radiographs of the skull are recommended. Trimming with a rotating dental burr in the sedated animal is the treatment of choice. Clipping instruments should not be used as they may crush or fracture the teeth. Increase roughage in the animal's diet to increase tooth wear.

PNEUMONIA

Pneumonia is common in guinea pigs and usually is due to bacterial infection from common organisms that most guinea pigs harbor without signs of disease. Stresses including overcrowding, pregnancy, and illness, increase the chance that pneumonia will develop. Clinical signs include anorexia, ocular / nasal discharge, sneezing, and dyspnea. Diagnosis is by visual inspection and radiography. Culture of the ocular or nasal discharge can be used to direct appropriate antibiotic therapy. If the animal is severely affected, oxygen supplementation, nebulization, and coupage may be required.

SCURVY

Scurvy is vitamin C deficiency. Guinea pigs and primates are two species that cannot synthesize their own vitamin C and so must have a dietary source. Pelleted guinea pig diets invariably contain vitamin C but it is a relatively unstable compound so food that is beyond 90 days from manufacture may have decreased vitamin C concentration. Similarly, vitamin C breaks down in water so supplementation in the drinking water is not effective. Guinea pigs affected with scurvy may show a rough hair coat, anorexia, diarrhea, reluctance to walk, swollen feet or joints, and ulcers on the gums or skin. Diagnosis is by visual inspection. Treatment is replacement of vitamin C.

LYMPHADENITIS

Cervical lymphadenitis is bacterial infection of the lymph nodes on the ventral surface of the neck. Abrasions in the oral cavity allow normal oral flora to colonize the area and eventually cause abscessation of the lymph nodes. Diagnosis is by visual inspection. Guinea pig abscesses usually contain a firmer, more caseous pus than that in other species, so lancing is not effective for diagnosis or treatment. Surgical excision and appropriate antibiotic treatment are recommended.

PODODERMATITIS

This condition also is called bumblefoot. Sores develop on the bottom of a guinea pig's feet, usually secondary to obesity and housing in cages with wire-bottoms or poorly cleaned floors. Abrasions on the feet permit introduction of bacteria and development of chronic, deep infections. This is a painful condition so clinical signs include lack of willingness to move, lameness, and other non-specific signs of discomfort. Diagnosis is by visual inspection. Treatment includes debridement of non-viable tissue, bandaging, and appropriate antibiotic therapy, and can be challenging.

GASTROINTESTINAL (GI) STASIS

GI stasis is also called ileus, and is slow emptying of the stomach and movement of ingesta through the GI tract. Roughage is important in the diet of guinea pigs to ensure proper digestion and ongoing function of the GI tract. When GI motility slows, hair from grooming and ingesta accumulate in the stomach. Because guinea pigs cannot vomit, the material in the stomach dehydrates and becomes even more difficult to pass. This condition can be caused by improper amount of roughage in the diet or by anything that causes a guinea pig to stop eating. Clinical signs include anorexia, decreased production of feces, signs of pain such as bruxism and a hunched posture, and reluctance to move. Diagnosis is by history and physical examination findings; a doughy or distended and firm stomach and cecum, and gas-filled intestinal loops will be palpable. Radiographs may be used to demonstrate gastric distension with food, fluid, or gas. Treatment includes supportive care including fluid therapy; encouraging exercise; feeding fresh, moistened greens and good-quality long-stemmed grass hay as well as an appropriate pelleted diet; encouraging drinking; use of a feeding tube for animals that will not directly eat food and water; and using appropriate pain medications and gastric prokinetic agents. Some animals may require surgery to relieve obstruction. Prognosis is poor if the guinea pig has stopped eating and passing feces for greater than 24-48 hours.

UROLITHIASIS (URINARY TRACT STONES)

The cause of urolithiasis in guinea pigs is not defined but likely is associated with the high mineral content of guinea pig urine due to excretion of calcium through the urine in this species. Diets that contribute to formation of uroliths are those that are lower in fiber and higher in protein and calcium, for example, pelleted diets with little feeding of grass hay, greens, vegetables, and fruits. Obesity and decreased activity may predispose animals to formation of uroliths. Clinical signs vary depending on site of the stone in the urinary tract and may include weight loss, anorexia, hematuria (blood in the urine), and straining during urination. Some affected guinea pigs will vocalize or show erratic movements while urinating, ostensibly due to pain. Diagnosis is based on clinical signs, urinalysis, and radiography; most urinary tract stones are radio-opaque. Treatment involves urethral flushing and surgery. Prevention is through dietary change with a decrease in pellets, increase in grass hay, availability of fresh water, and increased offering of greens with some vegetables and fruits. Female guinea pigs can also get concretions lodged near the urethral orifice; these are easily identified on physical examination and are easily removed.

FERRETS

ADRENAL DISEASE

Adrenal disease is more common in ferrets in the United States, where all commercially sold ferrets are spayed or castrated when very young, than in other countries where they are left intact. Cause-and-effect has not been defined. The hypothesis is that lack of feedback from the gonads leads to overproduction of hypothalamic gonadotropin releasing hormone (GnRH) and pituitary luteinizing hormone (LH), which along with exposure to long periods of daylight leads to continuing stimulation and subsequent adrenal hyperplasia, adrenal adenoma or adenocarcinoma. The adrenal produces a variety of hormones; hyperadrenocorticism in ferrets usually is associated with hypersecretion of sex steroids (estradiol, androstenedione, and 17 alpha hydroxyprogesterone). Adrenal disease is most commonly seen in ferrets 3 years of age or older. Clinical signs include progressive alopecia of the tail, tail base and trunk; vulvar enlargement in females; stranguria (difficulty urinating) and urethral obstruction secondary to prostatomegaly (increase in prostate size) in males; and pruritus (scratching). Diagnosis can be made by demonstration of increased concentrations of sex steroids and ultrasonography demonstrating unilateral or bilateral adrenal gland enlargement. Surgical removal of abnormal adrenal tissue is recommended for animals that can tolerate anesthesia. Medical therapy can be used for palliative care; leuprolide acetate, a GnRH analog, suppresses adrenal function.

INSULINOMA

This is a tumor of the pancreatic beta cells that is seen in middle-aged to older ferrets. Excessive production of insulin is associated with profound hypoglycemia and clinical signs of a dazed appearance, hindlimb weakness or paralysis, nausea (drooling, pawing at the mouth, retching), and in the end, collapse and convulsions. Diagnosis is by demonstration of consistent hypoglycemia; a fasting blood glucose concentration less than 90 mg/dL is suspicious while one less than 70 mg/dL is strongly suggestive. Mild to moderate hypoglycemia may be manageable through a high-quality, high-protein diet. Surgical debulking of the tumor is recommended. Severe episodes of hypoglycemia are emergencies and are treated with very slow normalization of blood glucose by administration of IV dextrose. Other therapies include use of glucocorticoids, which block uptake of glucose by cells and increase hepatic gluconeogenesis, raising blood glucose concentrations, and diazoxide, which antagonizes the effect of insulin.

LYMPHOMA

Lymphoma is leukemia or solid tumors of the lymphoid tissue. It is seen in young ferrets (6 -12 months of age) and ferrets 3-5 years of age. Any lymphoid tissue may be affected including peripheral and visceral lymph nodes, spleen, liver, intestines, and bone marrow. Younger animals generally show acute onset and rapid progression of disease. Older animals have a slower onset and longer survival times. Signs are non-specific and include anorexia, lethargy, weight loss, dyspnea, and coughing. If the mediastinal lymph nodes are enlarged, regurgitation may be seen; vomiting, diarrhea, and rectal tenesmus (straining to defecate) may be seen with GI disease. On bloodwork, anemia and variations in lymphocyte number may be evident. Fine-needle aspirate or biopsy of enlarged lymphoid tissues is definitive for diagnosis. Surgical removal plus appropriate chemotherapy may induce remission for as short as 3 months to as long as 5 years. Regular monitoring (blood work, complete physical examination) every 1-3 months is recommended.

RATS

NEOPLASIA

The most common tumor type in rats is mammary adenocarcinoma, with an incidence of 30-90% in aged females and 16% in aged males. Mammary tumors occur in middle-aged to older animals. Incidence can be decreased by spaying female rats early in life. The mammary tissue extends well beyond the ventrum and tumors may be seen on the ventrum, over the shoulders and neck, in the flanks, or at the tail base. Mammary tumors will be egg- or disc-shaped masses that are well demarcated and generally have only one large vessel. The mass will be well tolerated by the rat until it impedes movement, at which point it may be traumatized and become infected. Diagnosis is by visual inspection; an excisional biopsy can be submitted at the time of surgical removal, which is the treatment of choice. Recurrence is common. In intact female rats, concurrent ovariohysterectomy may or may not increase survival time and decrease incidence of recurrence. Another common tumor in rats is pituitary adenoma or prolactinoma. This tumor secretes prolactin and may promote development of mammary tumors. There is no definitive therapy for prolactinoma.

PNEUMONIA / MYCOPLASMOSIS

Respiratory disease is multifactorial, with environmental factors permitting infection. Mycoplasma is the most significant infectious agent causing respiratory disease in rats. It is highly contagious and rats that survive the disease may become lifelong carriers that are a source of infection to other rats. Poor husbandry can cause irritation of the respiratory tract. Specific problems include poor ventilation, use of dusty or aromatic bedding, and inadequate cage cleaning and subsequent increase in ammonia. Clinical signs include nasal discharge, noisy breathing (snuffling), labored breathing, red-brown tears, squinting, and a rough hair coat. Radiography is definitive for pneumonia and culture of nasal discharge defines specific organism and guides antibiotic therapy. If the animal is severely affected, oxygen supplementation, nebulization, and coupage may be required.

HEDGEHOGS

NEOPLASIA

Tumors are very common in aged hedgehogs; in one study, 30% of hedgehogs submitted for necropsy had tumors and 10% had multiple tumor types. Types most commonly seen are skin tumors, hemolymphatic tumors, GI tumors, and endocrine tumors. Surgical removal is the preferred treatment but may not be possible with all tumors, depending on extent and metastasis, and ability of the aged hedgehog to withstand anesthesia.

DERMATOPHYTOSIS

Ringworm is a fungal infection of the skin. Incidence is increased in hedgehogs housed in warm, humid environments, and in those with external parasites. Hedgehogs may harbor ringworm fungi with no clinical signs. Overtly infected hedgehogs show quill loss, and crusting and scratching at the face and pinnae. Identification of the fungus by skin scrape or tape prep, and fungal culture are diagnostic. Treatment requires use of anti-fungal drugs, either topically (localized disease) or systemically (generalized disease). Dermatophytosis is zoonotic.

SUGAR GLIDERS

NEOPLASIA

Tumors are most common in aged sugar gliders. Those most commonly described are hepatic tumors, lymphoid tumors, and mammary gland adenocarcinoma.

Diagnosis is by visual inspection. Surgical therapy (hepatic and mammary tumors) and chemotherapy (lymphoid tumors) may be attempted, with variable success.

NUTRITIONAL SECONDARY HYPERPARATHYROIDISM

Metabolic bone disease and nutritional osteodystrophy are other names for this disorder. Calcium supports cardiac and skeletal muscle contraction, blood clotting, transmission of nervous impulses, and bones and teeth. Phosphorus also supports bones and teeth. Calcium and phosphorus must be present in a specific ratio to ensure these processes occur. Calcium is stored in bone. Normally, when calcium concentrations rise in blood, calcitonin is released and pulls calcium from the blood, depositing it in bone. When calcium concentrations are low in blood, parathormone increases absorption of calcium from the kidney and intestine and draws calcium from bone. Vitamin D is produced with exposure to ultraviolet light (UVB) and increases absorption of calcium. Nutritional secondary hyperparathyroidism is a disorder of husbandry. Animals fed a diet with inappropriately low calcium and/or inappropriately high phosphorus will perceive themselves to be in a hypocalcemic state and will produce excessive parathormone, leading to weakening of the bones and teeth, and abnormal cardiac and nervous functions. In sugar gliders, this condition most often is seen in those animals on a primarily fruit diet with occasional insects or other protein sources. Clinical signs include hindlimb paralysis, muscle tremors, pathologic bone fractures, and occasional seizures. Radiography is definitive; findings include osteoporosis of the vertebral column, pelvis, and long bones. Low serum calcium concentrations will be seen on bloodwork. Treatment includes administration of calcium and vitamin D, correction of the diet, and strict cage rest.

AMPHIBIANS

RED-LEG SYNDROME

This disorder is also called pink belly disease and its official name is bacterial dermatosepticemia. This occurs most commonly in frogs and toads. This condition is due to infection with Gram negative bacteria and is associated with poor maintenance of substrate, poor water quality, and inadequate filtration in amphibian habitats, and also with overfeeding, skin trauma, and low dietary vitamin A. Clinical signs include pale pink or red lesions on the pale areas of the body including the hind legs and ventrum, ocular lesions including abnormal placement of the globe of the eye within the eye socket and corneal edema, anorexia, lethargy, prolapse of the stomach or cloaca, hemoptysis (vomiting or regurgitating blood), twitching, convulsions, and sudden death. Diagnosis is by visual inspection. Treatment with antibiotics can be attempted and biosecurity to prevent spread to other animals is vital. Prognosis is poor, with reported mortality rate of 81-100%.

NUTRITIONAL SECONDARY HYPERPARATHYROIDISM

Metabolic bone disease and nutritional osteodystrophy are other names for this disorder. Calcium supports cardiac and skeletal muscle contraction, blood clotting, transmission of nervous impulses, and bones and teeth. Phosphorus also supports bones and teeth. Calcium and phosphorus must be present in a specific ratio to ensure these processes occur. Calcium is stored in bone. Normally, when calcium concentrations rise in blood, calcitonin is released and pulls calcium from the blood, depositing it in bone. When calcium concentrations are low in blood, parathormone increases absorption of calcium from the kidney and intestine and draws calcium from bone. Vitamin D is produced with exposure to ultraviolet light (UVB) and increases absorption of calcium. Nutritional secondary hyperparathyroidism is a disorder of husbandry. Animals fed a diet with inappropriately low calcium and/or inappropriately high phosphorus will perceive themselves to be in a hypocalcemic state and will produce excessive parathormone, leading to weakening of the bones and teeth, and abnormal cardiac and nervous functions. Lack of adequate exposure to UVB light and subsequent low vitamin D concentrations inhibits absorption of calcium from the diet. In amphibians, lipoproteins transport vitamin D so animals fed a diet too low in lipoproteins may show clinical signs even if dietary calcium concentrations are appropriate. Affected amphibians will be presented with obvious skeletal deformities, abnormal posture, splayed legs, fractures, bloating, and paralysis. Diagnosis by radiography is definitive; bones will have reduced cortical density and fractures may be evident. Treatment includes increasing calcium in the diet and ensuring appropriate lipoprotein concentrations. Animals should be handled carefully, placed on strict cage rest, and housed with no cage mates until bone strength returns. UVB lighting should be available to increase vitamin D production. Pain medications can be used if fractures are present.

GERBILS

NEOPLASIA

Neoplasia is very common in gerbils over 2 years of age, with reported incidence of 8-27%. Ovarian tumors are most common, followed by skin tumors. Ovarian tumors are associated with abdominal distension and in breeding animals, with infertility. The most common skin tumor is squamous cell carcinoma of the ventral abdominal scent gland. This tumor often is associated with secondary bacterial infection. The gland will appear inflamed or ulcerated. Biopsy of the gland helps differentiate benign from malignant neoplasia. Surgical removal generally is the treatment of choice for all tumors. Appropriate antibiotic therapy can be used to control secondary bacterial infections.

ABSCESSES

Abscesses can form anywhere on the body and usually develop after some sort of skin injury and colonization of normal skin flora at the site. The predominant clinical sign is a lump with localized hair loss above it. Diagnosis is by visual inspection. For treatment, abscesses can be lanced, the defect rinsed with antiseptic, and appropriate antibiotic therapy instituted.

MICE

NEOPLASIA

The most common tumor type in mice is mammary adenocarcinoma, with an incidence of 30-70% in aged females. Other common tumors include squamous cell carcinoma, adenoma, fibroma, and fibrosarcoma. Mammary tumors occur in middle-aged to older animals. Some strains of mice have a very high incidence of spontaneous neoplasia and some mammary tumors are associated with retrovirus. The mammary tissue extends well beyond the ventrum and tumors may be seen on the ventrum, over the shoulders and neck, in the flanks, or at the tail base. Tumors are soft, highly vascular, and highly infiltrative, and readily metastasize to the lungs. Diagnosis is by visual inspection. Surgery is not recommended as it rarely is curative and is associated with extensive tissue damage.

PNEUMONIA

Pneumonia in mice generally is bacterial; viral agents and mycoplasma also may be causative. Signs are variable and include dyspnea with an extra abdominal component, snuffling, and purulent discharge on the nose and on the front paws from grooming. Sudden death may be the first sign of disease. Diagnosis is by visual inspection. Gram staining of nasal discharge may help guide antibiotic treatment. Treatment includes supportive care and antibiotic therapy.

CHINCHILLAS

DENTAL DISEASE

Both the incisors and the cheek teeth are open-rooted and continuously growing. Possible causes of dental disease include lack of a fibrous diet or other things to chew on to grind down the teeth, and malocclusion. This disorder is most common in middle-aged to older chinchillas. Clinical signs include anorexia, dysphagia (difficulty eating), decreased fecal output, weight loss, hypersalivation, and, in those with tooth root abscesses, swelling of the jaw and ocular / nasal discharge. Diagnosis is by visual inspection. Obvious malocclusion or tooth overgrowth, formation of sharp enamel points on the cheek teeth +/- oral ulceration, food impaction, and abnormal spacing between teeth may be evident on superficial oral examination. Because of the small size of the oral cavity and likelihood of significant dental disease that is not grossly evident, sedation for a full oral examination and radiographs of the skull are recommended. Trimming with a rotating dental burr in the sedated animal is the treatment of choice. Clipping instruments should not be used as they may crush or fracture the teeth. Increase roughage in the animal's diet to increase tooth wear.

CONJUNCTIVITIS

The conjunctiva is the supportive soft tissue around the globe of the eye. Inflammation occurs with excessive dust bathing, inadequate ventilation in the cage, or obstruction of the nasolacrimal duct as may occur secondary to dental disease. Bacterial infection is opportunistic, as normal flora colonize the inflamed tissues. Diagnosis requires a thorough ophthalmic examination and staining of the eye with fluorescein to define any corneal defects. A conjunctival swab should be submitted for culture. Treatment involves (i) flushing the conjunctival sac with saline, (ii) use of a species-appropriate ophthalmic antibiotic, and (iii) prohibiting dust bathing until conjunctivitis is resolved (generally about 14-21 days).

SNAKES

DYSECDYSIS

Dysecdysis is improper shedding. Remember the normal process of shedding (ecdysis): Snakes have small overlapping scales on the dorsum and sides and have ladder-like short, wide scales on their ventrum, called scutes. New scales form over the entire animal under the old scales. Lymphatic fluid accumulates between the new and old scales, dulling the appearance of the skin and markings, and making the spectacles (the scales over the eyes) opaque. The skin clears about 3-4 days before shedding begins. The snake will rub to start the shed and generally will shed the whole skin in one piece. Dysecdysis occurs when scales are not shed. Improper shedding may be due to external parasites, fungal or bacterial skin disease, hypothyroidism (low concentrations of thyroid hormone in the body) or other systemic conditions, hypoproteinemia (low protein concentration in blood), or poor husbandry (cool environment, dry environment, improper nutrition, lack of materials to rub against in the cage). Retained scales are most common on the tail and the head, including the spectacles. Diagnosis is by visual inspection. Treatment includes (i) warm water soaks (77-85°F for 15-60 minutes followed by gentle pulling of old scales with a piece of gauze, exercising great caution over the spectacles; (ii) correction of underlying husbandry issues, and (iii) treatment for underlying diseases.

INDEX

E

F

G

H

I

K

L

M

www.ingramcontent.com/pod-product-compliance
Lightning Source LLC
LaVergne TN
LVHW062219200926
848484LV00006B/1430